GLOBAL LIVESTOCK HEALTH POLICY

GLOBAL LIVESTOCK HEALTH POLICY

Challenges, Opportunities, and Strategies for Effective Action

Robert F. Kahrs

Iowa State Press
A Blackwell Publishing Company

Robert F. Kahrs worked on dairy farms as a boy; studied food science, animal husbandry, and veterinary medicine at Cornell University; and received the DVM degree in 1954. He practiced veterinary medicine, specializing in dairy cattle, in rural New York State for seven years. He returned to Cornell, earned a PhD degree, and taught epidemiology and infectious diseases to veterinary students, investigated disease outbreaks, and conducted research on bovine viral infections and vaccines.

Dr. Kahrs served on the faculties of veterinary medicine at Cornell University, the University of Florida, and the University of Missouri where he was dean for 10 years. He then spent seven years developing animal health policies and negotiating international trade agreements for the U.S. Department of Agriculture (USDA).

In 1990 he chaired a National Academy of Science Committee to evaluate the USDA's Meat Inspection System for Cattle. In 2000 he served on the International Information Committee of the National Animal Health Safeguarding Review. This study, commissioned by the National Association of State Departments of Agriculture, evaluated the disease exclusion, control, eradication, and information-sharing activities of the USDA's Veterinary Services.

Over the years, he has served on the American Veterinary Medical Association's Council on Research and Council on Biological and Therapeutic Agents. He has been active in the U.S. Animal Health Association serving on its committees on Biologics, Bluetongue and Retroviruses, Foreign and Emerging Diseases, Food Safety, Import-Export, and Infectious Diseases of Cattle, Bison, and Llama. He currently serves on the committees on Cattle Diseases and International Trade of the National Institute for Animal Agriculture.

Dr. Kahrs has written over 100 professional articles and lectured widely on livestock vaccines; investigation of disease outbreaks; international trade in animals and animal products; and livestock health policies. He is the author of *Viral Diseases of Cattle, Second Edition* (Iowa State University Press, 2001) and, several monographs on livestock health.

Iowa State Press
2121 State Avenue, Ames, Iowa 50014

Orders:	1-800-862-6657	Fax:	1-515-292-3348
Office:	1-515-292-0140	Web site:	www.iowastatepress.com

First edition, 2004

Library of Congress Cataloging-in-Publication Data

Kahrs, Robert F., 1930–
Global livestock health policy : challenges, opportunities, and strategies for effective action / Robert F. Kahrs—1st ed.
p. cm.
Includes bibliographical references (p.)
ISBN 0-8138-0204-0 (alk. paper)
1. Livetock—Diseases—Prevention. 2. Animal health—Government policy. I. Title.
SF740.K35 2004
636.089'45—dc21 2003011367

The last digit is the print number: 9 8 7 6 5 4 3 2 1

Contents

Acronyms

AAVLD-American Association of Veterinary Laboratory Diagnosticians
AI-Artificial insemination
AIDS-Acquired immune deficiency syndrome
AOAC-Association of Official Analytical Chemists
APHIS-Animal and Plant Health Inspection Service of the USDA
AVIC-Area veterinarian in charge
AVMA-American Veterinary Medical Association
BL-Biosafety Level
BSE-Bovine Spongiform Encephalopathy
BST-Bovine somatotrophin, bovine somatotrophic hormone
CAST-Council for Agricultural Science and Technology
CBP-Contagious bovine pleuropneumonia
CDC-The National Centers for Disease Control and Prevention
CEAH-Center for Epidemiology and Animal Health
CFR-Code of Federal Regulations
CJD-Creutzfeldt-Jacob disease
CODEX-The Codex Alimentarius Commission
CRD-Chronic respiratory disease
CVB-Center for Veterinary Biologics
CVO-Chief veterinary officer
CWD-Chronic wasting disease
DNA-Deoxyribonucleic acid
EBL-Enzootic bovine leukosis
EEC-European Economic Community
EID-Electronic identification devices

EP-Emergency preparedness programs, the current emergency-response capability
EPA-Environmental Protection Agency
ET-Embryo transfer
EU-European Union
FAD-Foreign animal disease
FADD-Foreign animal disease diagnosticians
FADDL-Foreign Animal Disease Diagnostic Laboratory
FAO-Food and Agriculture Organization of the United Nations
FARAD-Food Animal Residue Avoidance Databank
FAS-Foreign Agricultural Service of the USDA
FBI-Federal Bureau of Investigation
FDA-Food and Drug Administration, part of the U.S. Department of Health and Human Services
FMD-Foot-and-mouth disease
FSIS-Food Safety and Inspection Service
FTAA-Free Trade Area of the Americas
GATT-General Agreement on Tariffs and Trade
GMO-Genetically modified organisms
HACCP-Hazard Analysis and Critical Control Point
HIV-Human immunodeficiency virus
HPAI-Highly pathogenic avian influenza
IBR-Infectious bovine rhinotracheitis
ID-Identification, in animal health contexts
IIC-Inspector in Charge
ILT-Infectious laryngotracheitis
IMF-International Monetary Fund
IPPC-International Plant Protection Commission
ISO-International Organization for Standardization
IT-Information technology
LHP-Livestock health policy
MCF-Malignant catarrhal fever
MDM-Mechanically deboned meat
MLV-Modified live virus
MS&R-Monitoring, surveillance, and reporting
NADC-National Animal Disease Center
NAFTA-North American Free Trade Agreement
NAHC-National animal health culture
NAHEMS-National animal health emergency management system
NAHRS-National animal health reporting system
NAPPO-North American Plant Protection Organization
NASDA-National Association of State Departments of Agriculture

NCBA-National Cattlemen's Beef Association
NGO-Non-governmental organization
NIAA-National Institute of Animal Agriculture
NIH-National Institutes of Health
NVSL-National Veterinary Services Laboratory
OIE-Office International des Epizooties
PCR-Polymerase chain reaction
PRRS-Porcine reproductive and respiratory syndrome
R&D-Research & development
READEO-Regional Emergency Animal Disease Eradication Organization
RFID-Radio frequency identification
SPS-Sanitary and phytosanitary
TBT-Technical barrier to trade
TME-Transmissable mink encephalopathy
TPA-Trade promotion authority
TQM-Total quality management
TSE-Transmissible spongiform encephalopathies
USAHA-U.S. Animal Health Association
USDA-United States Department of Agriculture
VCJD-Variant Creutzfeldt-Jacob disease
VEE-Venezuelan equine encephalomyelitis
VMO-Veterinary medical officer
VS-Veterinary services
VS-Vesicular stomatitis
VVND-Viscerotrophic velogenic Newcastle disease
WHO-World Health Organization
WMD-Weapons of mass destruction
WTO-World Trade Organization

Preface

Purpose

This book details the complex challenges, opportunities, and strategies involved in the development and implementation of scientifically sound and credible **livestock health policies (LHPs)** in global and domestic surroundings.

Livestock health programs and activities impact human welfare, support food-safety efforts, and drive international trade. They get attention from interest groups that influence legislation, regulations, and budgets. LHP-makers must deal with scientific uncertainties, cultural sensitivities, and political realities.

Understanding these complexities will enable interested individuals and groups to cooperatively institute scientifically sound livestock health programs, solidify animal health infrastructures, enhance communication among legislators, regulators, and affected parties, and expedite the movement of livestock and poultry products in global markets.

The emphasis on democratic procedures and the use of U.S. examples reflects my experience. I don't suggest that other countries emulate U.S. practices. However these policies can provide checklists for consideration.

The world deserves transparent LHPs that consider the views of divergent interests. Policy makers in dictatorships or other totalitarian societies will find this book useful because it lays out issues they will confront in feeding their people and competing in the new global economy.

The text reaches beyond descriptive narrative to offer guidance and recommendations. These may appear prescriptive and are not applicable to all countries.

Proposed Audience

This book is intended as an indispensable reference for animal-health and trade officials, agribusiness leaders, commodity groups, financial institutions, and legislators and their staffs. It may also be of interest to importers and exporters of animals and animal products, manufacturers of biologics and pharmaceuticals, veterinarians, and leaders of the regulatory, academic, and diagnostic sectors of the agricultural and veterinary communities. The book will assist public health officials in assuring safe food, preventing zoonotic diseases, and protecting against bioterrorism. It will also be useful to consumers, journalists, and others concerned about the production, processing, and distribution of the safe, affordable protein sources needed to overcome global starvation.

Organization

This book consists of a preface, ten free-standing chapters, a chapter of discussion topics, a list of acronyms, and a glossary. It leads readers progressively through the events and decisions behind U.S. and global LHPs, and describes changing livestock production and processing methods, advances in livestock health technology, the components of competitive livestock infrastructures, and standards for international trade. It lays out the challenges facing the United States and other nations, and presents strategies for achieving policies adaptable to global dynamics, which simultaneously address the multiple issues impacting animal health, animal welfare, food safety, and global trade.

The glossary contains acronyms, initializations, definitions, disease descriptions, and web sites. Items in the glossary appear in bold print the first time they appear in each chapter or discussion topic.

Strategies for Using this Book

I suggest readers examine the background information in the first six chapters before studying the recommendations in the last four chapters.

The discussion topics in chapter 11 provide background information for group discussions of hypothetical issues. Discussion leaders can use the topics to stimulate debate. Reading the topics will illustrate the complexities of LHP-making.

A Noble Goal for this Book

The disparity between the number of starving peoples and the capacity of developed nations to profitably produce and distribute animal protein has many causes. This disparity does not result from technological shortfalls, but rather is the product of anachronistic scientific, economic, political, and cultural doctrines regarding livestock production and animal health. These doctrines are changeable to the mutual advantage of consumers, producers, processors, and distributors of animal products.

Over time, partnerships of producers, academics, processors, veterinarians, and special interest groups will be able to increase the profitability of domestic animal industries, improve the wholesomeness of animal products, expand foreign markets, and deliver affordable products to less-developed societies, while assisting them in the production of commodities adaptable to their ecosystems. These activities could substantially decrease the likelihood of hostile interactions between protein-deprived nations and those blessed with food surpluses.

The new millennium offers an opportunity for the international community to rally in response to livestock health challenges and the public concerns these challenges have created. This is an ideal time for groups sharing common goals to work together to reshape a quagmire of divisive misunderstandings into a cooperative effort that profitably addresses global starvation, food safety, food security, environmental stability, profitable animal agriculture, and the safe international movement of animal products.

This book explores the challenges and opportunities of national and global livestock health programs and the changing dynamics of a public that is increasingly critical of agriculture. It proposes strategies that could revolutionize livestock agriculture and relieve global tensions. It characterizes the leaders that should be the drivers and conscience of this effort.

I hope you find this book helpful and that you enjoy it.

Acknowledgments

Few of the ideas, concepts, and strategies proposed in this book are original. Many arose from experiences in veterinary practice, but most emerged from the thoughtful comments and questions of several generations of students and colleagues at Cornell University, the University of Florida, and the University of Missouri. I am indebted to fellow government servants at the U.S. Department of Agriculture for their tutelage in the complexities of regulatory veterinary medicine and international trade negotiations.

This book is dedicated to my wife Evelyn Payne Kahrs. Without her inspiration, help, support, understanding, and love, this book would not have been possible.

GLOBAL LIVESTOCK HEALTH POLICY

Chapter 1

Livestock Health Policy: the Basics

INTRODUCTION

The definition and implications of **livestock health policies (LHPs)** are complex and subtle. Understanding LHPs requires knowledge of their origin and development, their components, and their administration. Controversies of national or international dimension can arise over issues as fundamental as the definition of livestock.

Livestock are animals reared in captivity for the commercial production of meat, milk, eggs, and by-products. Livestock include poultry, swine, cattle, sheep, and goats. Wild species, such as deer, elk, bison, llamas, alpacas, ostriches, and emu, when reared in captivity, are considered livestock and subject to LHPs.

LHPs address an array of practices that promote the health of humans and animals and the prosperity of livestock industries using laws, regulations, and standards. The broad purview of LHPs includes livestock disease control and eradication programs and a gamut of food safety, international trade, animal welfare, and environmental issues. When it is perceived that any of these interests are threatened, voices rise to promote new policies or regulations. LHP issues are impacted by science, politics, and culture. Successful LHPs consider needs, resources, infrastructure, and programs. They require public trust and as with many endeavors, communication is the key to success when dealing with LHPs.

This chapter describes the nature of LHPs and provides an introduction to their development, application, and impact on livestock and people.

What Are Global LHPs?

Global LHPs are the traditions, practices, laws, regulations, standards, and administrative procedures that guide, manage, govern, and police the production, transportation, processing, and marketing of livestock and livestock products. Any activity involving livestock is subjected directly or indirectly to these policies. Livestock diseases, vaccines, feed additives, and the conditions under which animals are reared and processed are regulated and subjected to food-safety, environmental, and labor policies. Thus LHPs impact everyone.

The characteristics and components of LHPs vary from country to country and from state to state. Generally policy makers seek common goals that enhance the health of livestock and the best interests of people. The objectives of LHPs are diverse. LHPs encounter many opponents, but while often burdensome to those affected, LHPs usually benefit the majorities.

Livestock disease-control programs involve testing and **quarantine** procedures, disease **monitoring, surveillance and reporting systems (MS&R)**, border security, and networks of diagnostic laboratories. These activities reduce the spread of domestic diseases, prevent introduction of **exotic diseases**, and reduce human infections that involve animal-borne agents. Collectively these activities comprise **livestock health infrastructures**. LHPs and animal health infrastructures address health hazards and trade issues throughout the global food chain.

Ideally LHPs are scientifically sound, easily understandable, adequately communicated (transparent), and equitably applied (non-discriminatory). If these traits are not present LHPs cause controversy and conflict.

The components of LHPs include voluntary managerial decisions and programs developed by individual livestock producers or processors, programs designed by livestock and veterinary organizations and interest groups, and laws, regulations, and standards promulgated by subnational and national governments or international policy-making bodies.

LHPs impact producers and consumers of livestock products, animal welfare, labor practices, the environment, and society at large.

How Are LHPs Developed?

Livestock policy development procedures vary from country to country. In the United States and many democratic countries there is a sequential, transparent process with public input. The policy-development procedure involves the recognition of a need, participatory decisions on addressing the need, the drafting of laws, rules, or regulations, the presentation of the regulations for discussion and revision, and finally, the development of consensus-based policies. The policies require clearly written documentation to expedite uniform interpretation, equitable enforcement, and translation into other languages. In non-democratic countries, LHPs are often developed unilaterally with minimal public input.

Driving Forces and Framers of LHPs

Policies are driven by the concerns and problems of society (Dicks 1996). In the case of LHPs the driving forces come from multiple sources and many directions. These driving forces move irregularly, sometimes in unison and sometimes at cross-purposes, to promote actions or prohibitions to address a variety of concerns and risks.

The driving forces of LHPs come from governmental and non-governmental sources. These can include the academic and diagnostic communities, state and federal officials, or consumers. Consumers frequently comprise the driving forces on food-safety issues. In participatory democratic societies the wishes and interests of consumer-based majorities usually prevail.

Those most directly affected by LHP decisions, the producing and processing industries, are the principal **stakeholders**. Stakeholders don't often initiate regulatory action but participate actively once livestock health or food-safety measures are proposed.

The framers of LHPs, those who invent and formulate them, come from varied backgrounds and represent multiple interests. They run the gamut from individual livestock workers and veterinarians through national livestock officials, chief executives of nations, and leaders of international organizations.

LHP framers include livestock owners and the groups to which they belong, veterinarians and veterinary organizations, subnational livestock health officials, national agricultural officials, and legislators and their staffs. The complex LHP decision-making chain is influenced by a variety of food-safety, animal-welfare, labor, and environmental interests. With few exceptions, all participants in the development and implementation of LHP are also consumers who seek a variety of food products at reasonable prices and want assurances of the safety and wholesomeness of these products. However, while they share concerns as consumers, the framers of LHPs have widely varying vested interests depending on their occupation, level in the decision-making hierarchy, organizational affiliation, and source of income.

Individual Livestock Owners and Processors Generate Informal Livestock Health Policies

Individual decisions by livestock owners are generally disregarded by government officials unless they present risks to humans or animals or violate existing regulations. Livestock producers initiate private policies like nutritional programming, vaccine selection, disease treatments, decisions to sell or purchase animals, and choice of transportation methods. If successful, management practices are adopted by others and become standard practice. They can become entrenched before potential problems are suspected.

In democratic societies, the rights of livestock owners and processors are cherished possessions and, if threatened, are staunchly defended by the agricultural community. In highly competitive intensive operations the specifics of local or private LHPs may be veiled in secrecy for purposes of propriety, confidentiality, or competitive advantage.

Voluntary managerial decisions in packing plants are generally not regarded as significant LHPs as long as they are conducted within the legal framework of the territory involved. Packing-plant managers can legally invoke minor procedural changes under the watchful eye of government inspectors.

Producer and Processor Organizations Guide Policies

While individual producers or processors function unilaterally within the bounds of existing regulations (of which there are many in most countries), their organizations contribute significantly to policy making. Livestock producer or processor organizations often speak with a single voice representing a consensus of their membership. They can present realistic input on policy proposals and get the attention of legislators and animal health officials. Understandably they defend the vested interests of their industries.

These organizations carefully track the policies, regulations, and laws promulgated by national and subnational governments and develop positions by consensus or vote. They make their voices heard in support of their interests through articulate spokespersons.

In the integrated poultry industry, where producers are also processors, both voices can be heard through organizations like the U.S. Poultry and Egg Export Council or the American Association of Avian Pathologists.

Other species-based industry groups, like the National Cattlemen's Beef Association, the National Pork Producers Council, and the National Dairy Association track LHP issues. They lobby Congress and the **United States Department of Agriculture (USDA)** regularly. There are numerous other groups that represent livestock producers and meat, wool, poultry, and dairy processors. These groups are significant architects of LHP and serve as the voice of individuals who gain their livelihood from livestock.

These organizations often endorse voluntary pilot activities and quality assurance programs, to check the waters so bureaucrats don't get something etched in stone before its practicality is tested. A successful group strategy is to initiate voluntary programs, test them out, determine their benefits and shortfalls, and gradually expand them until changing conditions necessitate national resources and oversight. This strategy worked with **pseudorabies** in swine and **scrapie** in sheep. Similar programs, gaining momentum with support of some state governments, are unfolding for **Johne's disease** in cattle and **chronic wasting disease** among wild ruminants.

Producer and processor organizations are effective intermediaries between their memberships and state or federal governments who actually frame regulations affecting the national and international communities.

Veterinarians and Veterinary Organizations in LHP Development

Privately employed veterinarians aid in development of LHPs of privately owned or corporate farms. They develop customized herd and flock health measures adaptable to individual operations by detailing management, feeding, vaccination, parasite control, and breeding practices.

Veterinary organizations provide expert commentaries and science-based positions on LHPs. Veterinary organizations that contribute to U.S. policies are the American Association of Avian Pathologists, the American Association of Bovine Practitioners, the American Association of Swine Veterinarians, the American Association of Small Ruminant Practitioners, the American Association of Wildlife Veterinarians, the American Association of Public Health Veterinarians, the National Association of Chief Livestock Health Officials, the National Association of Federal Veterinarians, and others. These organizations publish journals and newsletters that inform their members of pending policy issues and persons to contact with opinions and positions. There are comparable organizations operating at the international level. There are also veterinary specialty boards that require examination for admission and involve their membership in the policy-making process.

The **American Veterinary Medical Association (AVMA)**, the veterinarian-dominated **U.S. Animal Health Association (USAHA)**, and the **American Association of Veterinary Laboratory Diagnosticians (AAVLD)** develop positions on livestock health issues through councils and committees representing the practice, academic, and diagnostic communities, and state and federal livestock officials. They prepare resolutions on timely issues for presentation to the USDA.

Subnational Officials in LHP Development

State, provincial, district, or other local governments have qualified professionals that contribute vital and thoughtful input to LHP discussions. These individuals have the authority and responsibility for controlling the movement of livestock into and within their jurisdictions and for overseeing local food-safety and food-inspection programs. Their experience is invaluable. LHP resolutions presented by the USAHA are carefully framed by these subnational livestock health officials.

On some issues subnational LHPs yield to national policies. However, subnational interests exert considerable influence, and local officials play a major role in state/federal cooperative disease-control programs. National livestock officials are most successful when they involve state and local officials and producers in the development and implementation of LHPs.

National Livestock Health Officials and Legislators in LHPs

Legislators and federal livestock officials are instrumental in the development and oversight of LHPs. They pursue comprehensive national missions of protecting livestock health, excluding exotic diseases, assuring food safety, and enhancing trade.

Legislators have a dual role of protecting the general public through food-safety activities and supporting the prosperity of livestock industries. They are accosted by pressure groups seeking conflicting programs. Legislators often rely on public officials to understand the issues and equitably address controversies.

Career officials of national livestock health and food-safety agencies are faced with the challenge of addressing controversial issues that don't have clear-cut science-based answers. Sometimes they become entrapped in bureaucratic speech and evasive behaviors that can produce counterproductive outcomes. The most controversial national livestock health issues involve food inspection, food safety and human health, the environment, and animal welfare.

As outlined in chapter 6, the key to the success of national LHPs is early consultation with all concerned parties at each stage of the policy-development process.

Role of International Organizations in Global LHP

International LHPs are shaped by trading blocs such as the European Union (EU), the North American Free Trade Agreement (NAFTA), and international organizations and governing bodies that are created and sustained by member countries. Such bodies include the **World Trade Organization (WTO)**, the **Office International des Epizooties (OIE)**, and international organizations like the United Nations.

The varying interests and agendas of countries, trading blocs, and international organizations require that LHPs generated at the international level must address the concerns of developed, less-developed, and developing countries, long-established and newly independent nations, and all regions of the world. This diverse input necessitates flexibility and compromise. The use of discretion, short of compromising scientific logic, national credibility, or personal integrity, often requires national representatives to yield on issues of importance to avoid stalemates.

Sometimes issues agreed upon in international discussions are later rejected after review by higher-level officials in national governments. This can cause embarrassment for the country's representatives and diminish the effectiveness of international bodies. To overcome such difficulties, U.S. presidents seek **trade promotion authority (TPA)**, also called **fast track authority**, which grants the right to negotiate treaties without congressional amendment privileges.

The ramifications of international LHPs are detailed in chapter 5.

Special Interest Groups in LHPs

There are numerous groups concerned with food-safety, animal-welfare, labor, and environmental matters. They represent diverse interests and issues. When their interests involve livestock products, their opinions exert credible influence on LHP development. They must be heard and considered throughout the process. The roles of these constituencies and their influence on LHPs will be elaborated on in subsequent chapters.

Elements of the Global LHP Hierarchy

Livestock health laws, regulations, and standards can originate at any level in the global policy-development chain. Consumers, organizations representing producers, processors, and veterinarians, and local, subnational, and national livestock and public health officials are included in the chain.

This policy-development process varies from country to country. LHPs are subject to various governmental styles, national hierarchies, and the guidelines of international bodies. In transparent participatory democracies, policies generally evolve from recognized national needs and pressures from professional organizations, special interest groups, subnational officials, or stakeholders. Often, action depends on state and national livestock health officials and legislative bodies who frame policies in concert with public opinion. In monarchies, dictatorships, and other autocratic systems, policies evolve from the top down and are implemented by edict.

Legislation and LHP

Legislation is the process of developing laws that establish codes of behavior. It is conducted by people who have been granted lawmaking authority by their countries or subnational governments. In democratic societies this means elected officials. Legislation differs from rulings imposed by monarchs or dictators.

Most legislators are not familiar with livestock. They draft legislation in response to pressures from constituents such as livestock producers or processors, veterinarians, or environmental, food-safety, and animal-welfare groups. Legislators usually feel that regulatory burdens must clearly benefit society in terms of food safety, livestock health, or animal welfare. They frequently act in response to requests from national livestock health officials but usually only after consulting producers, processors, or other stakeholders. They depend on others to advise them on the ramifications of livestock health matters.

Legislators usually word laws in general terms leaving the details to be codified as regulations by livestock health officials. These regulations authorize oversight of the production of livestock and inspections of meat, poultry, eggs, milk, and manufactured products of animal origin. These regulations are undertaken variously at subnational and national levels and are often overseen by multiple governmental agencies.

Subnational Laws and Regulations

State and other subnational livestock health agencies invoke livestock disease-control programs. They can exclude animal movement from adjacent areas when livestock diseases are out of control or if food-safety issues arise. In the United States, state/federal cooperative disease-control programs are common. States also develop border security measures, MS&R systems, meat- and food-inspection systems, laws for the humane treatment of animals, and standards for vaccines with limited local applications.

In many countries there is a rivalry between national and subnational governments over the authority to promulgate and enforce LHPs. Serious disagreements are usually resolved by examining legal or constitutional authorities, and in less democratic societies they are resolved by edict. In matters of territorial rights and local sovereignty, subnational interests may prevail. However, in matters with international significance, such as import regulations, national governments often have the final authority. Many countries and trading blocs deal only with representatives of national governments. Most accept correspondence or health certifications for livestock products only if they are endorsed by national officials.

Subnational officials usually, and sometimes reluctantly, acquiesce to federal officials on livestock health matters. This does not exclude them from the policy-making process or minimize the value of their input. When appropriate, national officials often yield authority to accommodate the needs of subnational territories.

National Regulations

Regulations detail procedures and practices necessary to carry out the intent of laws. LHPs usually attempt to enhance animal and human health, protect domestic livestock from exotic diseases, and preserve and enhance foreign markets for livestock products. These policies include details for conducting disease-specific control and eradication programs; testing, disease reporting, quarantine, seizure, and slaughter of infected animals; control of vaccine manufacture and use; and establishment of **sanitary measures** designed to reduce the risk of introduction of exotic diseases. These programs are expensive, and their benefits must be weighed against costs.

The oversight of national regulations requires a partnership of subnational and national livestock officials. This partnership includes technicians, scientists, and veterinarians who conduct a variety of inspection, surveillance, testing, and quarantine activities at border crossings, air and seaports, livestock and poultry markets, packing plants, and diagnostic laboratories. National regulations also authorize specific government agencies to represent the nation on matters involving international livestock health issues and trade measures.

Disease-Specific National Control Programs

Disease-specific control programs arise in countries for different reasons. Many are instituted in response to emergencies such as introduction of infectious exotic diseases. Domestic livestock populations are highly susceptible to exotic diseases, because they have never been exposed to or vaccinated against these diseases.

Some programs are implemented solely because the target diseases cause significant economic losses. Other diseases, like bovine **brucellosis** and **tuberculosis**, present additional threats by being transmissible from animals to people **(zoonotic diseases)**. Livestock farmers and ranchers often initially resist compulsory disease-control programs unless governments agree on **indemnities** to reimburse them for losses incurred through removal of infected animals. The decision to commit long-term resources to national livestock disease control or eradication programs requires careful analysis. Each country should have carefully considered criteria for disease-control decisions. These criteria are detailed in chapter 6.

The regulations and LHPs suitable for one country or region may be inappropriate for other areas for ecological, geographic, economic, political, or cultural reasons.

Exotic Disease Exclusion

The exclusion of **exotic diseases** is one function of LHPs. Many developed countries have invested in eradicating or controlling diseases that have economic or human-health impacts. Once a country is free of an infectious disease, the livestock population has negligible immunity to that disease due to lack of exposure or to vaccination that has been restricted to avoid diagnostic confusion. They are therefore highly susceptible to that disease. Some international markets demand disease-free status for exporting countries.

Retention and Expansion of International Markets

Traditionally LHPs have been directed at protecting livestock health. In recent decades, the **globalization** and free-trade movements have emphasized sanitary (health) considerations for international movement of animal products. Governments have added market access to the mission of livestock health agencies. These two goals can be compatible, because foreign markets often base import decisions on the quality of livestock health infrastructures in exporting countries. However, programs supporting livestock health can conflict with international marketing activities, because free trade is a two-way street. Disease-free nations with stringent requirements that exclude imports have few bargaining chips in their quest for foreign markets. Also the imposition of international standards creates guidelines that appear too lenient for some countries and too stringent for others.

International LHPs

LHPs promulgated at the international level are usually called standards, or guidelines, rather than laws. This avoids infringement on the sovereignty of individual nations or trading blocs. Some global tribunals, however, have the power of international law, with retributional, but usually not prosecuting, authority. This authority covers the **Sanitary and Phytosanitary (SPS)** Principles of the WTO. The details of international livestock health standards are elaborated in chapter 5.

Administration of LHPs

In democratic societies LHPs are influenced by producer, processor, and veterinary groups and by a variety of special interests. They are administered by local, state, and federal governments. National governments are usually the principal operatives and administrators of LHPs. In a global context, international bodies have widespread influence but usually recognize the sovereignty of individual nations.

Communication of LHPs

Communication is probably the most important determinant of success in the development and implementation of LHPs. This requires constant effort to openly discuss proposed or changing policies in an atmosphere of trust at all levels. Even the most logical policies can be rendered ineffective unless they are transparent to stakeholders, interest groups, and organizations.

Livestock producer and processor organizations play key roles in alerting their membership to the need for compliance and participation in disease-control efforts. The effectiveness of national and subnational livestock health agencies is largely determined by the communication skills of their employees. Communication can be enhanced by positive media relationships.

Broad-Based Constituencies and Complex Issues Create Challenges

Livestock health decisions are complicated by the multitude of people they directly affect and the numbers of interest groups with legitimate stakes in their details. The broad base of financial stakeholders in the livestock industries compounds this complexity.

Such diversity often results in conflicting and contradictory feedback from the agricultural community. LHPs are sometimes overlooked, because their stakeholders are busy with other farm policy matters such as price stability, supply and demand issues, human and animal nutrition, research funding, production and marketing controls, and dozens of other pressing economic and international issues.

Livestock is only one component of agricultural policy. Books on U.S. agricultural policy (Dicks 1996) and global agricultural policies (Bradford 1999) cover other aspects and help place LHPs in a broader perspective.

In addition to the agricultural community, the drivers and framers of LHPs must consider environmental and other consumer concerns as they strive to address livestock and food-safety issues.

Complex Interactions Among Science, Politics, and Culture

In developing and implementing LHPs, local, subnational, and national leaders must consider market forces, scientific considerations, political pressures, and cultural mindsets. These factors surface in direct, subtle, and even insidious ways.

Science, politics, and culture all come to bear in the development of local, subnational, and national priorities, policies, laws, and regulations. These factors can surface unexpectedly as consumer concerns about food prices, food safety, animal welfare, or the environment, and they inevitably come up in trade negotiations.

Animal health policy makers must be prepared to recognize and address these sensitive and frequently controversial dimensions at local, national, or international levels.

Science, Politics, and Culture in National Priorities and Regulations

Domestic livestock health policies, particularly in countries with participatory governments, are highly influenced by science, politics, and culture.

Theoretically, domestic policies, priorities, and regulations should be based on scientific facts. Science, however, is shrouded in multiple uncertainties and disagreements among experts. A common tack taken by scientists and academicians is to conclude that their findings are preliminary and that further research is needed before conclusions can be drawn. There is also a tendency to criticize colleagues who advance specific recommendations just because trivial details in their findings are lacking. This tendency can sometimes be overcome by assembling panels of experts to answer precise questions and propose specific actions.

The reluctance of the academic and research communities is offset by a sense of urgency on the part of commercial interests to get livestock health products licensed so they can be sold. This urgency can be modulated by regulatory standards for product approval and licensing.

In countries with participatory governments, political, and to a lesser extent cultural, considerations are sometimes permitted to override scientific considerations as policy makers listen to the thoughtful statements about proposed funding and regulations. Because it is difficult to reverse these decisions, policy makers must be fully informed on opposing views before moving ahead.

Impact of Science, Politics, and Culture on International Trade

The livestock industries of most countries must have foreign markets to be competitive in a global economy that is controlled by complex market forces. International prices are based on supply-and-demand factors, currency values, weather conditions, crop yields, and multiple other economic determinants.

In addition to economic considerations, the movement of livestock products in the global marketplace is ultimately governed by animal health-related import requirements called sanitary measures. Until implementation of the WTO SPS agreement in 1995, the use of sanitary measures to protect livestock industries from foreign competition was widely accepted.

The principles of the WTO SPS Agreement and the international standards of the OIE imposed a new world order that gives exporting countries clear criteria for contesting sanitary measures imposed by importing nations.

Requirements imposed on imported animals and animal products are usually spelled out in unilateral (country-to-country) or multilateral trade agreements negotiated by trading blocs representing several countries. These agreements identify diseases of concern to the importing country and specify mutually agreeable conditions for trade. These conditions, guaranteed by officials of the exporting nation, include statements of disease-freedom and details of surveillance, border security, and tests to support that status. If a disease of concern is present in exporting regions, the agreement will indicate test, or quarantine, procedures required of live animals and processing procedures required for products.

Health certificates accompanying shipments verify compliance with trade agreements, including the satisfactory completion of inspections, tests, or quarantines required by recipient countries. The certificates are endorsed by officials of exporting countries.

Agreements, and sometimes disagreements, concerning international movement of animals and animal products are subjected to complex pressures. Disagreements may arise from rapidly changing technology, global political disarray, and firmly entrenched culture-based positions.

Policy makers and trade negotiators must be able to identify the scientific, political, and cultural basis of arguments put forward by trading partners and place their validity and motivations in perspective. They must diplomatically discuss trade issues from a scientific viewpoint while understanding their political and cultural bases. If necessary they must modify their positions to accommodate unspoken political or cultural issues.

The roles of science, politics, and culture are intricately commingled with trade. These roles are discussed separately in the following sections to emphasize their individual qualities.

Science in International Trade

Science plays a significant role in the international trade of livestock and associated products. Articles 2.2, 3.3, and 5.2 of the WTO SPS agreement indicate that import measures must be based on sound science or science-based risk assessments.

Scientific data are subject to multiple interpretations and can be distorted by economic objectives. Political pressures, cultural biases, and uncertainty and disagreements within scientific communities complicate the concept of sound science. Pronouncements of scientific fact are often countered by queries about whose science is being discussed, in which journal was it published, who supported the studies, and what was the hidden agenda of the author. The role of science in international trade is confounded by subtle complications.

The scientific basis of livestock health is constantly changed by advancing diagnostic technology that permits increasing levels of differentiation among types, subtypes, and strains of animal-borne organisms. Diagnostic advances are compounded by improved monitoring and surveillance strategies and advanced **epidemiological** techniques that clarify cause-and-effect relationships and permit pinpointing of common-source epidemics.

The emergence of the **transmissible spongiform encephalopathies (TSEs)** as animal pathogens with **zoonotic** potential has added another dimension to livestock health planning and policy-making.

The scientific basis of sanitary measures is made more challenging by questions concerning how willing the importing countries are to take risks. This risk tolerance is sometimes expressed as a country's appropriate level of protection and manifested in their use of the controversial art of risk analysis.

The WTO SPS agreement grants countries the right to achieve an appropriate level of protection when importing livestock products. The international community has been unable to define an appropriate level of protection. It implies countries may define an acceptable risk level for each livestock disease and impose procedures to achieve that status.

Appropriate levels of protection have been held up as essential to free trade. They are regarded by some as an open-ended license to sidestep prohibitions on tariffs and quotas in order to protect non-competitive domestic industries.

Before science-based risk assessments are done, an acceptable risk level should be established and then used to systematically determine if a proposed import exceeds that level. Some experts, however, use risk assessments to determine acceptable risk levels, a practice that introduces circular reasoning into the legitimacy of import measures.

Risk analyses offer estimates of the dangers (risks) that an imported product can introduce diseases into recipient countries. Risk-analysis techniques are subject to controversy regarding their underlying assumptions, techniques, and biases. Some countries are criticized for establishing acceptable risk levels that are unattainably low, even approaching zero.

Scientific input into import requirements is further complicated by advancing marketing and transportation technologies that permit rapid distribution of potentially infected perishable products to areas where table scraps are fed to backyard livestock or where wildlife and birds have access to uneaten foodstuffs.

Integrated production systems and **confinement livestock operations** have produced livestock concentrations that encourage transmission of stress-related diseases. This has permitted scientists to recognize new and emerging **pathogens** with advanced diagnostic technology.

Concerns for animal welfare and emphasis on molecular biology have inhibited the use of time-tested scientific transmission studies using live animals. These studies were formerly relied upon for evaluating the risks of disease transmission by specific commodities and for determining the susceptibilities of various species to diseases of emerging importance.

Countries have differing levels of scientific capabilities. Developed countries signatory to the WTO SPS Agreement have pledged to assist less-developed countries. This adds additional dimensions to the issue of science-based sanitary measures. Trade negotiators must be willing and authorized to offer technical support to potential trading partners in lieu of criticizing disease-free claims based on insufficient information. These realities require countries to be represented by skilled and diplomatic individuals who are familiar with the scientific intricacies of animal health technology.

For all the above reasons, requirements for science-based import measures present over-simplifications that can lead to endless and heated discussions. These disagreements can be resolved only with trust and goodwill.

In some nations, scientific facts and risk assessments can be distorted by political considerations.

Politics in International Trade

Politics play a significant role in international livestock trade. Politics is variously described as the noble art of governing and decision making, or as scheming and maneuvering for personal or national gain. In livestock trade both definitions apply. Ideally, science-based recommendations should result in science-based decisions, policies, and regulations. But political considerations are inevitable.

Animal health authorities and other government officials with decision-making responsibility cannot operate in a vacuum or be shielded from the pressures of concerned constituencies upon whom they depend for political survival. They must function in a realistic domain. This requires recognizing that internationally decreed reductions of tariffs and quotas leave sanitary measures as the sole protectionist devices in the agricultural sector. Some countries may not be able to fulfill every commitment to international trade agreements due to insufficient resources or political pressures.

The first sign of politicization often appears when veterinary officials negotiating sanitary measures are told that their foreign counterparts cannot agree to mutually satisfactory arrangements without approval from higher authorities. These suspicions are often confirmed when an apparent agreement is overturned. Political overrides occur when negotiating teams lack decision-making authority, or when industry groups fear competitive pressures, object to pending agreements, and vocalize their objections to their political leaders. Countries belonging to multi-national trading blocs are further pressured to negotiate positions favored by these alliances even if they lack scientific basis and conflict with their own national interests.

The global movement toward partnering between industries and livestock health regulators, and the increasing involvement of industry groups in governmental processes, has focused increased political attention on LHPs. Political interventions can follow lengthy science-based discussions of import requirements between animal health officials. They can damage established international relationships between veterinary authorities unless intervening officials have the integrity to accept personal responsibility and admit the political basis of their decisions. Otherwise, the international credibility of the nation's veterinary officials can be undermined.

In bulky bureaucratic systems livestock health officials tire of political challenges to their professional integrity. They can fall into a counter-productive non-communicative mode of operation and work semi-secretly with their counterparts from other countries. Behind-the-scene dealings are inevitable when politically accountable officials refuse to accept responsibility for non-scientific decisions and leave underlings to accept the wrath of their professional counterparts from other nations. These arrangements frequently result in mutually satisfactory trade in livestock products, and unless challenged through political channels, such arrangements rarely come to the attention of higher authorities, who are uninterested in routine operational matters unless there are complaints from constituents or trading partners.

LHP-makers must be aware of these complications and decide if short-term trade advantage of violating requirements for science-based sanitary measures justifies long-term loss in international credibility.

The level of political influence on livestock health authorities varies from country to country. Officials in trade discussions often want to know the extent of their authority and that of their foreign colleagues. Representatives of national governments are sometimes reluctant to admit to foreign counterparts that they have heavy responsibilities but limited authority. These admissions are essential to trust-based negotiations and it is best if they emerge early, preferably over dinner rather than during formal negotiating sessions within earshot of political appointees.

There has been a global movement toward privatization of regulatory functions that in many countries were once the sole domain of full-time government employees. This trend has accompanied the evolution of voluntary disease-control and quality-assurance programs. While highly effective, these programs tend to weaken the disease control and reporting authority of national and subnational governmental units. Many countries are skeptical about dealing with governments that have relinquished any livestock health authority. Policy makers must balance transparent policies, developed with the participation of multiple interest groups, with authority to overcome illegal activities and credibly represent regulatory programs to the international community.

Importing countries are increasingly considering public concerns an SPS issue. This creates a need for clear separation of science-based regulatory policies and political-based decisions. When political interventions require livestock health officials to predetermine the outcome of literature searches, research projects, and risk assessments, the distorted status of the system soon becomes evident to the international community.

The worldwide emergence of politically influential activist groups has forced livestock health regulators and decision-makers to think beyond the interests of traditional stakeholders (livestock producers and processors). Policy makers must now consider thoughtful input from environmentalists seeking to preserve global ecological stability; from animal-welfare groups seeking humane husbandry, transport, and slaughter of animals; from human-rights interests opposing child and slave labor; and from consumer interests who want a food supply that is safe and affordable. They must also listen thoughtfully to labor groups seeking to protect the jobs and safety standards of workers and to traditional agricultural interests seeking the survival of classic agricultural practices and family and collective farms.

Many interest groups are opposing the movement to integrated corporate agriculture, mechanized feeding practices, concentrated housing of livestock, and automated slaughter and processing operations.

In the United States, this trend is balanced by national animal health coalitions such as the USAHA, the **Animal Agriculture Coalition**, and the **National Institute for Animal Agriculture (NIAA)**. These, and other groups representing agricultural interests, are seeking ever-increasing involvement in regulatory processes and are urging government officials to be more transparent and scientifically conscious in rule- and decision-making.

While political activity represents the best of democracy in action, its increasing diversity and urgency present ever-increasing challenges to LHP-makers who in good conscience seek to develop policies that address the best interests of all the people.

Culture in International Trade

Culture significantly impacts international trade in animals, poultry, and associated products. While science is rapidly advancing and political convictions can be ephemeral, cultures are slow to change.

Cultural traits become evident as the values, ideals, attitudes, beliefs, and behavioral patterns under which people live, work, and think. These traits are a product of the environment in which individuals grow up, are educated, and work. Cultural traditions are firmly embedded in societies. Most have a degree of religious underpinning and are often dearer to the hearts of people than scientific information or political affiliation.

Regulatory cultures are behavioral patterns that impact disease control and international movement of livestock products. Just as national or ethnic cultural patterns are ensconced in societies, regulatory cultures are institutionalized within government agencies. They tend to be self-protective and reluctant to change. Regulatory cultures adapt slowly to scientific advances and political or social change. They greatly influence the development and implementation of livestock disease-control programs and import requirements.

When applied to trade issues, regulatory cultures become negotiating cultures and can clash with political and scientific principles. Negotiating cultures reflect a country's regulatory culture but are dominated by personal styles and interpersonal and listening skills. In individual negotiators these attitudes and behaviors are influenced by family values, religion, and ethnic traits. These behavioral patterns are firmly embedded among those negotiating on behalf of a country, are slow to change, and are passed on to new members of the team.

Collectively, regulatory cultures and negotiating cultures can be called national animal health cultures (NAHC). They profoundly impact local policies and trade practices. They influence the effectiveness of a country's animal health programs and their success in achieving market objectives. NAHCs differ markedly between countries.

Some NAHCs, like those of the United States, are freedom-based, dollar-oriented, and impatient with the rhetoric that characterizes many trading partners. They are sometimes competitive to the extent they are considered by trading partners to be aggressive, assertive, arrogant, interrupting, condescending, bullying, and possessed of a superior attitude. The NAHCs of some other countries are more relaxed and protective. All are slow to change.

In many countries most veterinarians are in the employ of national governments and serve in regulatory capacities. In contrast, U.S. federal regulatory veterinarians constitute a minority of the veterinary profession. They play a minor role in its national leadership, which is dominated by private practitioners, academicians, and subnational officials. This trend is exemplified by practitioner domination of the AVMA and State Veterinarian domination of the USAHA, the advisory body of national livestock health policy. Compared to most countries, U.S. veterinary colleges devote a small portion of the curriculum to food hygiene, public health, exotic disease exclusion, and regulatory practice. Thus, in some parts of the world the qualifications of U.S. regulatory veterinarians are considered inferior.

The NAHC of the United States portrays attitudes characteristic of a new nation with multicultural diversity. On the other hand, the NAHCs of most trading-partners represent established social, cultural, and ethnic systems. The U.S. NAHC clashes with cultures that are based on polite step-by-step discussions undertaken after prolonged getting-acquainted rituals. The U.S. NAHC also clashes with cultures of proud, newly independent nations who crave respect and dignity and resent the superior attitudes of some U.S. spokespersons.

The NAHCs of nations moving from controlled to free-market economies retain previous ideals and only respect certificates signed by full-time employees of national governments. They consider certifications put forth by private veterinarians or corporate laboratories to be in conflict with impartial, independent, and credible regulatory practice.

Major differences on livestock health issues between U.S. and EU veterinary officials are based on cultural sensitivities regarding the use of hormones in livestock production and European concerns about integrated agriculture and confinement rearing of livestock.

Cultural differences are manifested in variations in livestock health infrastructures that make it challenging to evaluate exporting countries with respect to disease-control programs, monitoring and surveillance systems, the validity of disease reports, diagnostic capacity, and credibility of export certifications. These challenges are compounded by the preference of most livestock health officials in negotiating only with government officials of comparable rank and status. In larger countries comparably ranked officials have little knowledge of animal heath issues and little time to negotiate animal health agreements.

There is also a tendency among importing countries to mimic the SPS measures of other countries so that agreements negotiated with a single nation can have worldwide significance.

There is an increasing tendency to develop SPS issues based on public concerns, **precautionary principles**, and consumer preferences rather than science. These culturally oriented decisions indicate that all nations will not get their way in trade discussions and that power politics is rarely the best long-term strategy in international matters. Accommodating the cultural characteristics of trading partners is essential if countries are to achieve their competitive potential. Policy makers cannot ignore culture in LHP-making.

Some International Trade Realities

Multiple scientific, cultural, and political challenges will determine the future success of the international livestock trade. Most significant among these is the tendency of importing countries to use health concerns as a justification for excluding animal and poultry products as they attempt to protect domestic industries from competition.

The overwhelming competitive advantage of integrated broiler and pork industries must be carefully considered. They have the capacity, given a totally level playing field, to cause the collapse of domestic industries in countries with less-aggressive, smaller farming systems. This competitiveness must be balanced with foreign aid programs that work to support free-market economies in developing countries and in nations transitioning to democracy. The obligations of these countries to abide by the WTO SPS Agreement should help establish economic stability. The loose wording of that agreement permits member countries to apply interpretations favorable to their best interests. The vagueness of the livestock disease standards promulgated by the OIE and outlined in the International Animal Health Code also provides flexibility to countries undergoing transition in their livestock economies and political structure.

The real-world application of non-discriminatory sanitary measures to a free-market economy requires that developed countries and their stakeholders address several major realities. First, the eyes of the world are on developed nations to see if they live the rules or just talk them. Each nation's international credibility, their most cherished and fragile possession, is under close scrutiny. Their disease monitoring, surveillance, and reporting systems must be squeaky clean to establish professionalism and engender the trust of their trading partners. Privatization of regulatory oversight and volunteer programs will be attacked, when deemed advantageous, as lacking the independence and impartiality necessary to protect consumers in the importing countries.

Secondly, the trade goals of countries like the United States, with advanced **livestock health infrastructures** and integrated agricultural systems, are twofold. They strive to expand export markets and protect the health of domestic livestock. Protection of domestic livestock populations necessitates exclusion of exotic diseases, a goal that can only be achieved with stringent import measures. Because the United States does not import many livestock products, there is usually little to offer in give-and-take trade discussions.

Thirdly, while the WTO SPS Agreement grants importing countries the sovereign right to establish their own appropriate levels of protection and to impose risk-mitigating measures necessary (but not more than necessary) to achieve that level, the definition and application of appropriate levels of protection, or acceptable risk, are unresolved by the international community. Many countries are passing up a unique opportunity for global leadership by refusing to address this issue.

A major question requiring mutually satisfactory resolution in upcoming decades is how to live by the WTO SPS principles and how, short of the lengthy WTO dispute resolution process, to persuade trading partners to do so as well.

The privatization of regulatory functions, voluntary control programs, and partnering with regulated industries require careful checks-and-balances to assure that national regulators maintain the independence, impartiality, and credibility essential to sustain international trade.

International movement of livestock products encompasses the viewpoints, goals, and agendas of livestock producers and processors, veterinarians, regulators, bureaucrats, politicians, and scientists. Spokespersons for these interests represent several generations, many nations, and various political systems and cultural patterns, and speak different languages.

These complexities are compounded by the emergence of newly independent nations, the global movement toward democracy and free-market economies, the formation of multinational trading blocs, the establishment of international trade agreements, the development of international SPS principles, and the promulgation of international standards for safe trade.

Despite seemingly insurmountable odds, the world is moving slowly toward scientifically based, non-discriminatory agricultural trade practices that can eventually provide all the people of the world with safe, affordable food supplies that are produced, processed, and transported under conditions profitable to all. Achievement of this idealistic goal requires social, economic, and technological adjustments and major cultural accommodations. These adjustments will be strongly resisted but will eventually prevail.

The developed countries with participatory governments must seize the opportunity for global leadership in international trade in livestock products. Livestock health policy makers must lead the way by recognizing and compromising with the scientific, political, and cultural influences that are brought to bear on domestic policies, food safety, and international trade.

Livestock Health Information Sources

Livestock health and disease information is transmitted through producer and processor organizations at meetings and in publications. Books for non-technical audiences include *Keeping Livestock Healthy* (Haynes 2001); *The Veterinary Book for Sheep Farmers* (Henderson 1990); *The Health of Pigs* (Hill and Sainsbury 1995); and others. These books describe the characteristics and treatment of most diseases of livestock. Non-veterinarians involved in LHPs are urged to capitalize on these resources.

For veterinarians, and others willing to grapple with the vocabulary, there are many sources of information on the description, diagnosis, and treatment of livestock diseases. *The Merck Veterinary Manual* (Aeillo 1998) is a recognized encyclopedia of livestock and companion-animal medicine. There are also books on diseases of cattle (Rebuhn 1995 and Kahrs 2001); goats (Linkhalter and Smith 1993 and Mathews 1999); poultry (Saif 2003 and Charlton 2000); sheep (Martin and Aitken 2000); and swine (Straw 1999). Herd-health practices for all species of livestock are described by Radostits (2001).

The OIE publishes *The OIE International Animal Health Code* (OIE 2001) and *The OIE Manual of Diagnostic Tests and Vaccines* (OIE 2000). They are standard references for international trade. The global distribution of livestock diseases is summarized in the *Animal Health Yearbook* (FAO-OIE-WHO 2000). Those involved with LHP issues are advised to consult these and other sources to assist in developing accurate positions.

The Crucial Role of Communication in LHPs

Successful LHPs must be based on legitimate needs. They require adequate resources, solid infrastructures, and scientifically sound and equitably administered programs. Broad-based public support is essential to achieving these objectives.

Communication is the key to achieving trust, public support, and balanced media coverage. As with many activities, the amount, quality, and frankness of communication is the key to success in these endeavors. For this reason the essential channels of communication will be emphasized throughout this book.

Bibliography

Aiello, S. E., ed. 1998. *The Merck Veterinary Manual*. Whitehouse Station, NJ: Merck and Co. Inc.

Bradford, E. ed. 1999. *Animal Agriculture and the Global Food Supply*. Task Force Report Number 135. Ames, IA: Council for Agricultural Science and Technology.

Charlton, B. R., ed. 2000. *Avian Disease Manual*. 5th ed. Kennett Square, PA: American Association of Avian Pathologists.

Dicks, M. R. 1996. *How Agricultural Policy Affects You*. Moline, IL: John Deere Publishing.

FAO-OIE-WHO. 2000. *Animal Health Yearbook*. Rome: Food and Agriculture Organization of the United Nations.

Haynes, N. B. 2001. *Keeping Livestock Healthy*. 4th ed. North Adams, MA: Storey Books.

Henderson, D. C. 1990. *The Veterinary Handbook for Sheep Farmers*. Ipswich, UK: The Farming Press.

Hill J. R. and W. B. Sainsbury. 1995. *The Health of Pigs*. Burnt Mill, England: Longman Scientific and Technical.

Kahrs R. F. 2001. *Viral Diseases of Cattle*. 2d ed. Ames: Iowa State University Press.

Linklatter, K. A. and M. C. Smith. 1993. *Diseases and Disorders of the Sheep and Goat*. London: Mosby-Wolfe.

Martin, W. B. and B. W. Aitkin. 2000. *Diseases of Sheep*. Ames: Iowa State University Press.

Mathews, J. G. 1999. *Diseases of the Goat*. 2d ed. Ames: Iowa State University Press.

OIE. 2001. *The OIE International Animal Health Code*. Paris: Office International des Epizooties.

OIE. 2000. *The OIE Manual of Diagnostic Tests and Vaccines*. Paris: Office International des Epizooties.

Radostits, O. M. 2001. *Herd Health: Food Animal Production Medicine*. Philadelphia: W. B. Saunders Company.

Rehbun, W. C. 1995. *Diseases of Dairy Cattle*. 2d ed. Baltimore, MD: Williams and Wilkens.

Saif, Y. M. 2003. *Diseases of Poultry*. Ames: Iowa State Press.

Straw, B. E. ed. 1999. *Diseases of Swine*. 8th ed. Ames: Iowa State University Press.

Chapter 2

Twentieth Century Progress and Change in Livestock Health

INTRODUCTION

During the twentieth century livestock health steadily improved throughout the world. This progress resulted from changing production and management systems, improvements in reproductive efficiency, control of metabolic, toxic, parasitic, and infectious diseases, and better understanding of immunology. These changes were accompanied by increased understanding of animal-derived foods; mechanization in meat, poultry, and dairy processing; improvements in refrigeration and transportation of perishables; and the emergence of international guidelines for the safe movement of livestock products.

This progress coincided with global dynamics that revolutionized **livestock health policies (LHPs)** and emphasized the importance of animal health to national economies and human health.

The future holds challenges and opportunities in livestock production and processing and for LHP-makers the world over. Recognizing these challenges and seizing these opportunities requires an understanding of twentieth century progress and its complexities. This chapter describes developments affecting livestock health and management over the last century and lays a foundation for topics that follow.

Changing Livestock Production and Management Systems

The twentieth century brought nutritional advances, farm management improvements, confinement housing, and increased numbers of animals per farm. Scientists, nutritionists, and feed manufacturers combined their efforts to determine the dietary requirements for each life-stage of every livestock species. Advances in livestock and poultry nutrition were accompanied by mechanization of equipment for planting, harvesting, transporting, storing, grinding, and feeding the plant products that comprise most livestock diets. These advances found common application in feedlots and pork, poultry, egg, and milk production units.

Establishment of nutritional standards permitted the formulation of totally mixed rations of vitamins, minerals, protein, carbohydrates, fiber, and growth promotants to permit maximum conversion of feed to meat, milk, and eggs. Computer algorithms were developed to formulate least-cost rations permitting profitable production of quality, affordable products.

The sizes of poultry, swine, beef, and dairy farms increased rapidly in the United States and other developed countries. Family farms that raised a few cattle, pigs, chickens, and sheep gave way to single-species operations of increasing size.

There was an emergence of **integrated production systems** with livestock production and processing operations under common ownership. Some integrated operations control the origin of the animals, their feed sources, their management during growth or lactation, and the processing, packaging, and merchandising of the products. Integration reduces middlemen and assures tighter control, more uniform products, improved bio-security, higher-quality health care, and uniform disease prevention strategies. In the United States, this progress has provided a wide variety of meat, milk, and poultry products to consumers at affordable prices.

Studies indicate animal-derived foods can be a vital component of constantly changing human diets. In the United States they can provide up to 70% of dietary protein and up to 40% of required calcium, magnesium, iron, thiamin, and vitamin A (Beitz et al. 1997). The down side is the health concerns surrounding the fat and cholesterol content of these foods.

Highly efficient integrated operations can also have negative effects. They often confine livestock and poultry in close quarters, which can induce stress, lower resistance to disease, generate odors, and cause waste disposal problems.

The progress in livestock production and processing has raised concerns about food safety, animal welfare, the environment, **genetically modified organisms (GMOs),** and the decline of small farms. Most of these problems deserve discussion. Sometimes however, they are founded on naive perceptions of animal agriculture or advocacy group agendas that are only distantly related to available scientific facts.

Countries with less-competitive livestock industries have used concern over the negative effects of integrated and confinement livestock-production practices on the environment and food safety to manipulate prices and block international trade. In the future, such practices may accelerate if scientific standards for international movement of foods of animal origin are extended to include animal well being and other social concerns about livestock and poultry.

Advances in Livestock Breeding and Reproductive Efficiency

Reproductive performance is a crucial determinant of livestock health and production efficiency. During the twentieth century there were advances in the diagnosis and prevention of infertility and abortion and the introduction of artificial insemination, estrous synchronization, **embryo transfer (ET)**, sex-sorting of semen, and **cloning** of livestock.

Diagnosis and Prevention of Infertility and Abortion in Livestock

At the opening of the twentieth century livestock owners experienced losses from infertility caused by **vibriosis** and **trichomoniasis** and abortion storms from brucellosis and other infections. In the United States, brucellosis abortion gradually declined to negligible levels due to education, refinement of diagnostic tests, and a State-Federal Cooperative **Brucellosis** Eradication Program. This program initially encountered resistance. It utilized vaccination and blood testing to establish cattle herds as brucellosis-free so they could meet requirements to ship milk and move cattle.

Despite progress in the brucellosis program, producers continued to report sporadic (and occasionally epidemic) abortions in livestock. Advancing diagnostic technology revealed over 50 bacterial, viral, protozoan, fungal, hormonal, and toxic causes of abortion in cattle, swine, and other species. These were addressed by the introduction of artificial insemination (AI) and vaccines for **leptospirosis**, **bovine viral diarrhea**, **infectious bovine rhinotracheitis**, **porcine reproductive respiratory syndrome (PRRS)**, and other infections. In the new millennium, nonetheless, abortions continue to occur sporadically at levels adequate to cause economic concern and diagnostic challenges. The partial control of many abortifacient agents has been followed by focus on newly emerged and identified causes of abortion, including ***listeria***, a bacterium that causes abortion in most livestock species, and ***Neospora caninum***, a **protozoa** that causes abortion in cattle and small ruminants.

However, in spite of these advances in knowledge, lack of reproductive efficiency inhibits efficient livestock production in some parts of the world.

Artificial Insemination

The development of AI in cattle and other species was a major livestock health event of the twentieth century. It permitted rapid replication of genetic traits enabling farmers and ranchers to select characteristics such as high milk production, desirable conformation, and optimum growth rates by purchasing semen from sires proven by multiple breedings to transmit these characteristics. AI resulted in reduction of sexually transmitted diseases that caused infertility and abortions and permitted the exchange of livestock genetics between regions where movement of live animals is limited by disease considerations. Disease-specific standards for international movement of livestock semen are detailed in the **International Animal Health Code** published by the **Office International des Epizooties (OIE)** (OIE 2001).

Introduced on a commercial level in the late 1930s, AI offered immediate and inexpensive distribution of valued genetic traits. AI eliminated the need for small farmers to keep a bull to breed a few cows, which was a costly and dangerous proposition often bypassed by leading cows over to a neighbor's bull. Initially, semen used in AI was collected, diluted, and distributed daily. This fresh semen required refrigeration and remained fertile for only a few days. With the development of frozen semen it became possible for semen to remain fertile for years. This permitted the use of superior genetic material even years after the death of the donor.

AI had two phenomenal impacts on the cattle industry. AI allowed the large-scale replication of genetic traits conducive to increased milk production and breeding efficiency, which, along with nutritional and disease-prevention advances, increased livestock production profitability. And, when antibiotics were added to commercial semen in the 1940s, the use of AI virtually eliminated vibriosis and trichomoniasis, two sexually transmitted diseases that cause early embryonic death, abortion, and delayed conception.

Initially, trained AI technicians or veterinarians inseminated animals with semen provided by cooperatives or commercial organizations. Eventually farmers and ranchers bred their own livestock with purchased frozen semen. Sperm-sorting technology, based on automatically measuring the **deoxyribonucleic acid (DNA)** content of sperm in flow cytometers, is undergoing evaluation. If successful, cattle breeders may be able to choose the gender of calves by using sex-sorted semen.

Estrous Synchronization

AI must be performed at a precise time in the female's reproductive cycle, called the estrous or heat. Careful estrous detection is crucial to livestock health. Hormonal induction of estrous can be accomplished by injecting hormones that stimulate ovulation. Hormone treatment of groups of animals, estrous synchronization, permits their simultaneous insemination. This enables livestock owners to predict the dates of group births, provide oversight of the birthing process, and market animals of uniform ages. Estrous synchronization has provided improved breeding efficiency, particularly in beef herds.

Embryo Transfer (ET) and In Vitro Fertilization

Commercial ET enhances the genetic potential of livestock and permits production of 50–100 offspring per year from highly productive, rapidly growing, or otherwise genetically meritorious animals. ET also offers disease control options that permit the international exchange of livestock genetics without the disease risks involved in the movement of live animals.

ET involves non-surgical harvest of fertilized ova from planned matings of superior males with females that have been super-ovulated by hormone injections. The embryos are then implanted into donor females that serve as surrogate mothers and ultimately produce highly desirable offspring.

Embryos harvested from healthy animals are unlikely to transmit diseases if they are appropriately handled and washed. This makes ET a useful vehicle for the international movement of animals in circumstances where live animal importations would be excluded because of disease risks.

In vitro fertilization, an extension of ET, has been applied to cattle, sheep, goats, and swine. It involves the harvest of unfertilized eggs, or oocytes, from valuable females that have difficulty conceiving, are already pregnant, are too young to breed, or are dying. The eggs are fertilized in the laboratory with semen from selected sires. The fertilized eggs are then implanted in recipient females. *The Manual of the International Embryo Transfer Society* (Stringfellow and Seidel 1998) details ET procedures that meet the import requirements of most countries.

Cloning of Livestock

Cloning, the production of genetically engineered multiple identical replicas of desirable animals, has potential in the replication of rare individuals and the preservation of breeds or endangered species. It also has potential in the production of cows and goats genetically engineered to produce milk proteins of medicinal value. Cloning has been successfully accomplished with varying degrees of success in sheep and other small ruminants, cattle, and horses.

In its developmental stages animal cloning is a costly and risky process. It is currently conducted in research institutions and on a limited commercial basis. When cloning is perfected and becomes readily available, it will have the potential to develop highly productive, disease-resistant herds and flocks that could make foods of animal origin available throughout the world.

Cloning of cattle has resulted in the birth of calves with variable birth weights, oversized bodies, undersized organs, and a variety of prenatal and neonatal abnormalities. In order to survive, cloned calves often require expensive veterinary support in intensive care facilities. The complications in bovine cloning procedures may be forewarnings of potential problems in other species, including humans. Cloning is controversial and raises moral, ethical, and religious issues, but cloning must be explored as future work promises to be less problematic and the potential benefits appear to be worth pursuing.

The cloning process involves harvesting unfertilized oocytes from females, removing all nuclear (genetic) materials, and replacing them, using microsurgery techniques, with the nuclear material of rapidly dividing cells from the animal chosen to be duplicated. The semen of cloned animals could command high prices because of rapid growth, high milk production, or disease-resistance characteristics of the cloned individual. In the cloning process the transplantation of the nuclear materials is done under magnification and requires meticulous attention to detail and timing. The inserted genetic materials are fused with structural elements of recipient oocytes and nurtured in the laboratory until cell division is apparent. The fertile eggs, now actually embryos, are then implanted into recipient females who, if all goes well, give birth to valuable offspring that are practically identical to the selected parent.

The application of cloning and other genetic manipulation to human reproduction raises controversial moral and ethical issues that could spill over into livestock cloning and complicate LHPs. LHP-makers face the question of whether animal cloning should be regulated. If so, how and by whom? This decision depends on whether or not cloned animals, and the foods they produce, are a hazard to food safety or the environment.

According to a 2002 U.S. Food and Drug Administration report, cloned animals probably are safe food sources, but their use could reduce genetic diversity. Further study is needed on their nutrient values and eventually some regulatory oversight on the cloning of food animals may be required. The report also indicated that cloned animals, which are exact genetic replicas of existing animals, differ from transgenic animals, in which genes from one species have been inserted into another species or genus, and that the safety of food products from transgenic animals requires further study. This uncertainty could produce consumer backlash about all GMOs (Holdredge and Talbot 2001) if the public fails to recognize the distinction between clones and transgenic animals (see chapter 3).

Advances in Diagnosis and Control of Metabolic Diseases

In addition to progress in livestock nutrition, reproduction, and management, the twentieth century produced advances in the diagnosis and control of metabolic, toxicologic, parasitic, and infectious diseases of livestock and poultry. Metabolic diseases alter the complex physical and chemical control mechanisms in the body. Metabolic processes regulate growth, development, reproductive activity, and essential bodily functions such as neurological function, circulation, respiration, digestion, and the maintenance of normal body temperature. Some metabolic disorders have a genetic basis but these are rare in livestock.

Most metabolic diseases of livestock result from imbalances of nutrient intake under the demands of the production of milk, meat, or eggs. They are often associated with dietary change or bearing and rearing of newborns. Because metabolic disorders are sporadic, non-contagious, rarely affect human health, and can be addressed locally, they rarely become subjects of LHP-making or international trade discussions.

Advances in Diagnosis and Control of Toxicologic Diseases

Toxicology deals with the properties, modes of action, effects, and diagnosis of toxic substances (toxicants) in animals and humans. The twentieth century brought the recognition and description of numerous livestock and food toxins and their diagnosis by laboratory tests. Today, many toxicological tests are automated and most veterinary diagnostic laboratories have a toxicology section.

A wide variety of toxicants can cause acute illness, sometimes death, or chronic changes in animals. Their effects are dose-dependent, and most exert detrimental effects on a broad range of species. In a given species, a toxicant in low dosage may cause undetectable effects and at certain levels some potential toxicants, such as trace elements and other micro-nutrients, meet essential nutritional requirements or may even have therapeutic effects. However, the same substance, in higher dosages, can cause sickness and in still higher dosages may be lethal.

There are hundreds of elements and compounds that are toxic to livestock and people. They are absorbed into animal bodies by varying mechanisms, have different modes of action and different target organs, and are metabolized or eliminated by multiple routes.

Many toxicants are naturally occurring substances present in soils or plants. Others, called **mycotoxins,** are produced by fungi. **Botulism** and **tetanus** toxins are produced by bacteria and require specific conditions for their formation. Many compounds synthesized by humans for agricultural use, like herbicides and insecticides, are potent toxicants if they contact the skin or are swallowed in adequate amounts.

Toxicants can accumulate in animals or animal products and may contaminate foods of animal origin. Unlike infectious agents, toxicants, unless being produced by living organism such as bacteria or fungi, don't multiply in animals or animal feeds. They can, however, accumulate in individual plants or animals, in the environment, or in ecosystems. Over time, concentrations of some toxic residues are gradually metabolized in living animals and may dissipate in animal feeds and human foods through dilution. Toxicants in foods can best be minimized by controlling their production, monitoring their addition to animal and poultry feeds, and restricting their farm and garden applications.

Advances in Diagnosis and Control of Parasitic Diseases

Parasites are organisms that live and feed in or on other organisms or animals. They usually inflict damage in the process. Technically, bacteria, viruses, and fungi are all parasites. Because of unique infectivity patterns, tissue-penetrating capabilities, and disease-producing capacities, bacteria, viruses, and fungi are called infectious agents rather than parasites. This difference in invasiveness is reflected in terminology. Bacteria, viruses, and fungi are said to infect their hosts. With some exceptions parasites are said to infest their hosts. Unless present in overwhelming numbers parasites generally inflict less profound damage than bacteria or viruses.

Parasites of livestock include internal parasites (endoparasites) that dwell within the animal's body and external parasites (ectoparasites) that infest the skin and can transmit diseases. Endoparasites occur in all livestock and cause subtle losses that reduce feed conversion and productivity. These losses are often subclinical but can cause observable damage. They are occasionally life threatening. Principal endoparasites are worms (helminths) including roundworms, tapeworms, strongyles, and flukes. Some helminths have complex life cycles involving intermediate hosts and have specific ecosystem requirements that limit their geographic distribution. Most are transmitted by fecal-borne eggs or larvae acquired from contaminated feed or pastures. After the eggs or larvae are eaten, most of them penetrate the stomach or intestinal wall, undergo developmental stages in digestive or respiratory tissues, and excrete infective immature forms in the feces. The concentration of endoparasite eggs or larvae on pastures fluctuates with the stocking density of animals, the temperature, and the ambient moisture of the pasture or feed. Intensely grazed pastures can become highly infective in tropical regions and after summer rainfalls in temperate zones. In developed agricultural settings helminths are usually controlled by timely pasture rotation and administration of various worm medications called **anthelmintics**.

There is a growing array of anthelmintics available in developed countries. Most are effective against a broad range of parasites and have wide margins of safety. They present challenges, because they can induce the emergence of drug-resistant parasites, though drug resistance can be avoided by shifting the products used in a herd. Anthelmintics can also produce residues in meat or milk, and their use must be carefully controlled by licensing procedures, drug withdrawal times, and milk-discard guidelines.

Principal ectoparasites of livestock are flies, gnats, lice, ticks, mosquitoes, and other biting insects. They cause subtle losses through blood sucking and agitation of animals. Significant losses result when their numbers become overwhelming, when they transmit infectious agents, or when their migration within the host's body causes damage. Mange mites and grubs damage hides, and ticks and some blood-sucking flies can produce anemia. **Screwworms,** the larvae of a subtropical fly called *Cochliomya hominivorax*, infest wounds, destroy flesh, and can be fatal.

Ectoparasites transmit several important protozoan diseases of livestock including **cattle tick fever,** also known as piroplasmosis or bovine babesiosis. Ectoparasites also transmit viral diseases such as **vesicular stomatitis** and **bluetongue,** endemic in parts of North and Central America. Some major insect-borne viral infections of livestock are currently confined to tropical regions including **Rift Valley fever**, **lumpy skin disease**, **ephemeral fever**, and **Akabane.** These diseases are of concern in areas currently free of them.

U.S. policy makers were startled in 1999 by the appearance in the United States of **West Nile fever**, which can be lethal to humans, horses, and many species of birds. It was probably introduced from the Middle East by the arrival of an acutely infected person. This alerted officials to the fact that temperate regions can have environments that support disease-carrying insect populations usually confined to tropical or subtropical ecosystems. The West Nile virus gradually became established **(endemic)** in the United States. Controlling this virus will require effective vaccines, mosquito control measures, and educational programs.

Control of external parasites requires integrated pest management systems that combine sanitation, application of parasiticides, reduction of breeding sites, environmental sprays, and weed and vegetation controls. Some regions have developed biological controls, such as the release of larvae-eating parasitic insects.

Parasiticides are drugs directed against internal or external parasites. Safe and effective antiparasitic compounds have been developed for use in livestock. In general, these compounds have wider margins of safety, and their residues are of less concern than hormones and **antimicrobials**. Parasiticides must be used with caution to maximize their economic efficiency, minimize the development of drug resistance, prevent residues in food, and avoid their being used as trade barriers.

Advances in Diagnosis and Control of Infectious Diseases

Infectious diseases cause most of the health problems that impact livestock production, food safety, or international trade. The twentieth century brought progress in the diagnosis of existing and emerging livestock infections. Infectious agents, such as viruses and bacteria, multiply exponentially and mutate in human and animal bodies. Bacteria can survive and multiply at temperatures conducive to their reproduction in the presence of fecal material or other nutrient substances such as meat, milk, and eggs. Viruses survive only briefly outside of living cells.

Throughout the twentieth century, there was continuous advancement in the capacity to diagnose infectious diseases and identify parasites of livestock. This progress began with techniques for finding and identifying parasites and bacteria under the microscope and by capitalizing on their ability to grow in non-living culture media. Bacteriology flourished via continual refinement of isolation and identification techniques.

The age of bacteriology led to virology, the study of smaller, but equally pathogenic, infectious viral agents that cannot be viewed with ordinary microscopes and are not treatable with **antibiotics**, the miracle antibacterial compounds. Viruses can be cultivated only in living animals or in living cells derived from animals, plants, or insects. The isolation, cultivation, and identification of viruses require technology more sophisticated than that of bacteriology. Both viruses and bacteria can mutate and sidestep the disease-control technologies that have been developed. Viruses have been more amenable to control by vaccination than bacteria.

Advances in bacteriology and virology gave rise to **serology**, the study of the clear fluid **(serum)** that exudes from blood as it clots. Serologic tests detect specific **antibodies** that appear in the serum days or weeks after an infection. Serology, while subject to errors in interpretation, is a superb diagnostic and epidemiologic tool for studying infectious diseases of livestock. It can be used to estimate the prevalence of infections in populations and to establish disease-free status of regions or countries for export purposes. A single positive serologic test indicates the tested animal has been exposed to the infection. Serological determination that a specific infection is associated with a disease episode requires two blood specimens. In order to determine that the animal developed antibodies at the time of the observed disease, an initial specimen, called the acute sample, collected early in the disease must be negative, while a second specimen, the convalescent sample, collected 2–3 weeks later should be positive.

Hyper-immune serum, generated by inoculating animals with disease-producing agents, can be used in the treatment of infections or poisonings; for passive, or temporary, immunization; for the treatment of certain tumors; and to specifically identify infectious agents or toxins. For diagnostic tests highly specific antibodies, called monoclonal antibodies, are generated by tumors of antibody-producing cells that are maintained in laboratory mice or organ cultures.

The recognition of **prions**, which cause **bovine spongiform encephalopathy (BSE)** and other **transmissible spongiform encephalopathies (TSEs)**, introduced a third level of sophistication to animal-disease diagnosis. All these levels of complexity have been upgraded by the molecular revolution that has added detail and accuracy to work on disease agents.

The application of advancing diagnostic technology heralded specialization and costly improvements in animal disease laboratories and in the technology needed for tracing diseases. These technologies permitted scientists and regulatory officials to pinpoint the causes, geographic distribution, and impact of multiple types, strains, and subtypes of disease-causing bacteria, viruses, internal and external parasites, and prions. These developments raised new expectations for rapid progress in the war on infectious agents that reduce production efficiency, threaten human health, and inhibit international trade.

Many of these advances utilized molecular and genetic technology, which presents the capability of characterizing the complete genetic sequences of animals and infectious agents. This technology multiplied the costs of diagnostic and regulatory programs and presented challenges to regulators and policy-makers who must prioritize programs and activities in the face of political pressures, scientific uncertainties, changing disease and market conditions, and the demands of individuals and groups with a variety of agendas, some of which include an anti-science component.

The **polymerase chain reaction (PCR)**, one of many useful molecular techniques, brings an increased level of sensitivity and specificity to the detection and identification of disease-causing organisms. The PCR permits amplification of nucleic acid sequences in test materials to achieve quantities of test materials that would otherwise be undetectable. This allows the identification of agents that are difficult to detect with classic microbiological procedures or that have ceased multiplying by the time samples reach laboratories. The PCR and other rapid molecular procedures can detect genetic differences among infectious agents, strains, and subtypes of organisms. These differences impact control efforts and diagnostic tests. Genetics dictate an organism's pathogenicity; its resistance to environmental influences, disinfectants or antimicrobials; and its immunologic properties that are important in diagnosis and vaccine effectiveness. Efforts are under way to improve surveillance for exotic diseases by incorporating PCR-based **foot-and-mouth disease (FMD)** detection procedures into commonly used tests for domestic infections (Hietala et al. 2002).

Emergence of Antimicrobials in Livestock Health

Along with advances in livestock health and production efficiency, the twentieth century introduced a variety of biologically active substances, called antimicrobials, that increase growth rates and feed efficiency, eliminate animal parasites and infectious agents, prevent or cure infectious diseases, and prolong animal life. These materials increase the efficiency of livestock production, but they have public health ramifications and trade implications and generate complex scientific and political issues for LHP-makers. With respect to LHP, these substances are best grouped according to their intended outcomes.

Antimicrobials inactivate, kill, or retard the growth of microorganisms. They include antibiotics and other antibacterial substances, antiviral agents, and parasiticides. These compounds are variously administered by mouth (either directly or as feed additives), by injection or implanting, or by application to the skin as sprays or pour-ons. Some can remain as residues in meat, milk, or other animal products. To reduce the risk of their presence in foods many governments have established mandatory withdrawal times, or intervals during which treated animals or their products must be withheld from market following their last use.

These therapeutic and prophylactic products generate different emotional responses in their opponents in public interest groups and in their supporters in the livestock and pharmaceutical industries. Regulators who approve, or prohibit, the use of drugs and biological products in livestock attempt to resolve these differences by instituting licensing and labeling requirements specifying approved animal species, indications and contraindications for their use, and withdrawal times.

In regulating animal health products, policy makers must assure their use is safe for the treated animals and the food-consuming public. Each country's regulations should be harmonized with international standards, fulfill the expectations of trading partners, protect the legitimate rights of livestock producers and pharmaceutical manufacturers, and protect the public. These conflicting concerns must be addressed transparently throughout decision-making processes.

One class of antimicrobials, the antibacterials, exert a detrimental effect on bacteria. They are frequently collectively referred to as antibiotics, and many antibacterials are true antibiotics. Technically, however, antibiotics are substances produced by living organisms. They are harmless to mammalian cells but kill or inhibit the growth of sensitive bacteria. Many antibacterial agents are not true antibiotics, because they are neither derived from living organisms nor synthesized replicas of naturally occurring antibiotics. The collective term antimicrobials is favored for compounds used to treat bacterial and other infections. Use of the word antimicrobial conveniently bypasses the semantic exercise over the precise meaning of antibiotic.

In the early twentieth century it was believed bacteria were not susceptible to therapy. This changed in 1935 with the discovery that prontosil, a red dye, killed streptococci. An uncolored portion of prontosil, called sulfanilamide, was the active component. A series of related compounds, the sulfa drugs, soon followed. In livestock, the sulfas were used to treat protozoan and bacterial infections of the respiratory, reproductive, and gastrointestinal tracts. They were also effective for bacterial infections, such as **footrot**, in cattle, small ruminants, and swine. Sulfa drugs are still used today but have largely been replaced by newer antimicrobials.

Penicillin, the prototype antibiotic, was discovered in 1920 by Sir Alexander Flemming who noticed that molds of the *penicillium* species secrete substances that inhibit bacterial growth. This discovery lay idle until 1939 when British scientists developed penicillin for treatment of battlefield wounds and U.S. scientists developed fermentation technology for its mass production. This process was soon used for production of numerous other antibiotics. Once their chemical structure was determined, antibiotics and other antimicrobials were synthesized.

The introduction of penicillin, which soon became readily available and reasonably priced, initiated the antibiotic era that revolutionized human and veterinary medicine. Penicillin and other antimicrobials gave those responsible for livestock health a previously unimagined therapeutic arsenal.

Antimicrobials can be bactericidal or bacteriostatic. Bactericidal compounds cause the death of bacteria, and bacteriostatic substances slow their growth. These compounds exert their effects by various mechanisms including interference with the organism's ability to develop essential components or impairment of essential functions such as synthesis of protein or DNA, the highly stable material in the nucleus of living cells that transmits genetic information and controls bodily processes. The spectrum of bacteria affected by a specific antimicrobial may be limited to a single organism, a few organisms, or a wide variety of organisms.

In the post-WWII era, penicillin was frequently injected in combination with streptomycin in non-specific treatment of infectious livestock diseases. Use of this mixture to achieve a broad spectrum of antibacterial activity was considered indiscriminate antibiotic therapy and discontinued in favor of newer antimicrobials.

From the time of their initial development antibiotics have had ever-increasing applications. In addition to being used to treat infectious diseases they are used as feed additives to increase growth rates. Another use, called metaphylaxis, involves antimicrobial disease prevention in healthy high-risk animals. Livestock subjected to metaphylaxis are usually young animals assembled from several sources, commingled, trucked long distances, and subjected to sudden changes in feed or weather.

In the last quarter of the twentieth century, antimicrobial use in animals gave rise to fears that residues in meat and milk could trigger allergic episodes in people with sensitivities to certain products, particularly the penicillins and sulfonamides. More controversy, however, surrounds the suggestion that antibiotic use in livestock may contribute to the emergence of strains of pathogenic bacteria resistant to antimicrobials used in human medicine.

The susceptibility or resistance of a bacterium to a given antimicrobial determines its therapeutic effectiveness. The susceptibility of bacteria to antimicrobials is ascertained by antibiotic sensitivity tests that determine the appropriate therapy for each infection. In these assays, discs impregnated with antimicrobials are placed on agar plates and inoculated with organisms isolated from infected patients. Zones of growth inhibition around the discs indicate susceptibility of the isolate to the drug.

Antimicrobial-resistant bacteria include some classes of organisms that have a natural or innate resistance, usually genetically determined, to a given drug even if they have never been exposed to it. Some antimicrobial resistance occurs as a result of random mutations.

Of more concern is acquired antimicrobial resistance that develops in the face of exposure to specific products. Acquired antimicrobial resistance in previously susceptible microorganisms can occur in several ways. One mechanism involves natural variations in drug susceptibilities among offspring of individual bacteria. The more resistant bacteria survive the treatment longer than their kin. If a drug is administered in marginally effective dosages, or is withdrawn prematurely, the survivors continue multiplying. This process establishes bacterial populations that are resistant to antimicrobial drugs.

Another established mechanism, called transferable drug resistance, involves exchange of resistance-controlling genes among closely related organisms and sometimes between bacteria of distinctly different species.

As antimicrobial use in humans increased, more and more resistant organisms appeared. They sometimes emerge in hospital settings and can produce serious or even fatal human infections.

The suggested association between the development of resistance to antimicrobials and their therapeutic or sub-therapeutic use in livestock remains neither proven nor disproved despite 30 or more years of study (Brown 1999). This alleged cause-and-effect relationship is complex, unpredictable, and controversial. An equally appealing, yet unproven, hypothesis is that the misuse and overuse of antimicrobials in human medicine has contributed to the development of antimicrobial resistance (Reeves 2000).

The continued appearance of bacteria that resist antimicrobial treatments is likely the result of random mutations and overuse of antimicrobials in both animals and humans. Even careful use of antimicrobials can induce the emergence of resistant organisms, but it is believed that their improper or indiscriminate use accelerates the process.

Educating physicians, pharmacists, and patients about the potential of inducing antimicrobial resistance with indiscriminate use, improper dosages, or inadequate duration of treatment hasn't resolved the issue. Some experts think antibiotic treatments of livestock diseases and their use as growth promotants amplifies the problem. It is estimated that about 70% of antibiotics produced in the United States are fed to livestock. Some countries prohibit the use of an antimicrobial in livestock if the same antimicrobial is also used in human medicine. Other countries enforce withdrawal times for treated animals. Many countries test foods of animal origin for antimicrobial residues and impose penalties on livestock owners who fail to follow recommended withdrawal times.

Antimicrobial resistance presents a dilemma that is currently unresolved by medical technology. This uncertainty underlies an ongoing turf war between a small faction in the human-health community and livestock interests. One school of thought, put forth by opponents of sub-therapeutic antimicrobial usage, supports a total ban on their use in healthy livestock. The more moderate school suggests that sub-therapeutic antimicrobial usage be phased out based on the results of science-based risk assessments. It contends that further study is needed to clarify the issue. Antibiotic-resistant organisms will probably continue to emerge. Most new drugs will eventually encounter resistant microorganisms.

This enigma requires that leaders in both sectors cooperatively address their areas of responsibility and develop scientifically sound solutions. These policies must harness the forces of free-enterprise economies, address political realities, and ultimately be based on sound science.

There are many approaches to controlling antimicrobial use in livestock and to preventing chemical and antimicrobial residues in food. Appropriate approaches will depend on the species involved, the management system under which they are maintained, and the ultimate use of the product.

National governments are likely to use approaches consistent with their regulatory styles, be they voluntary, compulsory, or cooperative. In many cases voluntary programs are of limited success and do not command the respect of trading partners. Compulsory programs, particularly when initiated unilaterally by government agencies, tend to be resisted and fail unless inordinate resources are expended in their oversight. Cooperative programs, on the other hand, particularly those initiated transparently with the input and cooperation of involved producers, practicing veterinarians, the academic communities, and subnational animal health officials, usually produce better results, but they take time and effort to develop.

Quality assurance programs accompanied by producer education and price incentives have moderate success in some countries but require continual development and attention to detail. Residue avoidance is complicated by the multiplicity of available drugs and **biologicals**, the numerous indications for their application, the variable withdrawal times, the high cost of testing for residues, and the complexities of tracing residues to the source in marketing systems without mandatory animal identification.

Antimicrobials are used extensively to treat bovine mastitis, an inflammation of milk-producing tissues, and can appear in milk for variable periods. They are also used as growth promotants in livestock operations and to treat a variety of diseases in all livestock species.

Several antiviral drugs appeared late in the twentieth century. They were far more difficult to develop than antibacterial agents and anthelmintics, because virus replication is an intracellular process directed by host cell DNA. That means antiviral drugs must enter living cells of treated animals and interfere with cell metabolism without damaging vital pathways. Testing viruses for sensitivity to potential antiviral therapeutics is more complex, more expensive, and less reflective of clinical results than testing bacteria for sensitivity to antibacterial drugs.

Although broad-spectrum antiviral agents are under development, most antiviral drugs affect a narrow range of viruses. A specific virologic diagnosis is generally needed for their effective use. Antiviral drugs are costly. They have specific applications in human medicine, limited application in pets, and less application in livestock. Their use in livestock is limited by cost, by having a narrow range of effectiveness, and by the fact that vaccines have been the traditional control mechanisms for animal viral infections.

As viral technology advances, less expensive and more effective antiviral drugs will be used in food-animal medicine. These will require new strategies on the part of national governments to guarantee the safety of treated animals and the consuming public. Caution must be observed to assure that these products do not compromise procedures for safeguarding against the entry of exotic viral infections by masking infections or obscuring laboratory test results. As antiviral drug use in livestock appears on the horizon, it will become an issue requiring thought and understanding on the part of LHP-makers.

In the United States, a successful educational program promoting reductions of residues in foods of livestock origin is the **Food Animal Residue Avoidance Databank (FARAD)**. Since 1982 this USDA-supported online data bank offers livestock producers, veterinarians, and other interested parties constantly updated information on availability, legal uses, dosages, and withdrawal times for drugs used on livestock.

In upcoming decades debates over antimicrobials for food-producing animals may increase. These debates will challenge the credibility of scientists, the integrity of livestock and pharmaceutical interests, the character of regulators, and the knowledge, skills, and wisdom of policy makers.

Advances in Immunology

The late decades of the twentieth century brought new understanding of the immune system of humans, experimental animals, and livestock. Immunity is the collective term for protective responses to foreign substances that access the body, including tumor cells, toxins, and other foreign particles. Livestock health focuses on bacterial and protozoan parasites, viruses, and other disease-producing entities called **pathogens**. To date, workers have not detected classic immunologic responses to prions, the agents associated with the TSEs.

The immune system generates, transports, and regulates a complex armamentarium of proteins, enzymes, and cells that identify, remember, debilitate, and eliminate pathogens from the body. The breakdown, neutralization, and inactivation of pathogens utilize proteins in stepwise reactions. The complex details of immunology are almost incomprehensible to average citizens.

Rapid progress in immunology offers visions of miracles to those who erroneously consider it a panacea for protection against infectious diseases. Some of these hopes may eventually materialize. However, each new detail presents fresh complications and further questions rather than simple solutions. Genetic predisposition, age, stress, nutrition, overall health status, and exposure rates also contribute to the probable outcome of an infection.

When functioning effectively and in appropriate balance, the immune system recognizes each individual's own cells, tissues, and fluids. This complex self-tolerance mechanism instructs the immune system to ignore normal bodily components. Effective immune systems recognize markers, called **antigens**, on foreign invaders and launch an immune response of cascades of proteins and cells to eliminate them.

The first time an individual's immune system sees a foreign antigen it initiates a time-consuming primary immune response that records the intruder's identity before undertaking destructive action. Subsequent invasions by the same organism invoke a more rapid and profound secondary immune response that usually aborts the infection.

When malfunctioning or defective, immune systems ignore infections or cancer cells. When unregulated, or over-functioning, the immune system produces allergies, auto-immune diseases, or cancer of the lymphoid system (lymphoma).

Twentieth century immunologic advances introduced techniques to diagnose and track disease and develop and evaluate vaccines. This set the stage for a century of sophistication in livestock health.

Improved Vaccines for Livestock Diseases

Major twentieth century advances resulted from continually improving vaccines against livestock diseases. Animal health policy makers need an understanding of the strengths, limitations, and trade impacts of livestock vaccines. Thoughtful regulatory control of vaccine production and administration is needed to protect treated animals, safeguard the food supply, and address potential trade issues.

There are many bacterial vaccines, **modified live virus (MLV)** vaccines, inactivated viral vaccines, and vaccine combinations available for livestock. Each product has advantages, disadvantages, and unique indications and contraindications (Kahrs 2001). Vaccination is just one component of disease control and must be complemented with sound management.

Vaccinations can reduce the likelihood of catastrophic losses but will not prevent all infections or all disease. Livestock vaccines are constantly changing due to the frequent appearance of new infectious agents, and the development of new immunologic information, new technologies, and improved products. Policy makers continually face legitimate disagreements regarding the safety, effectiveness, and conditions for use of individual and combination vaccines.

Vaccination programs must be tailored for geographic areas and specific production and management systems. Vaccine users must adhere to manufacturer's recommendations and national and local regulations.

The development and evaluation of vaccines requires scientific expertise, laboratory facilities, and specialized equipment (Pastoret et al. 1999). In the United States and most developed countries vaccines are developed by private industry, university scientists, or government laboratories.

Vaccine development begins with the isolation and purification of a strain of the disease-producing infectious agent. The candidate organism must be readily propagated in the laboratory and have adequate antigenic properties to induce a protective response in vaccinated animals. It must be decided if the proposed vaccine is to be a live vaccine or an inactivated product. Thereafter, technical procedures are initiated to develop a product that meets standards for purity, potency, safety, and efficacy. The process is completed when regulators examine and approve all the procedures, all testing requirements are met, and the product is licensed.

The regulation of vaccines is an essential part of LHPs. In the United States, the **Center for Veterinary Biologics (CVB)** of the **Animal and Plant Health Inspection Service (APHIS)** of the USDA is responsible for animal vaccines, diagnostic reagents, and antiserums. These are collectively designated biologics. Around the world most livestock biologics are regulated by national governments, and many countries have national programs for regulating vaccine production, distribution, and utilization.

National governments usually retain the right to exclude the production, entry, sale, or use of vaccines, antiserums, and diagnostic reagents within their boundaries.

International standards for veterinary biologics are outlined by the OIE in the *Manual of Diagnostic Tests and Vaccines* (OIE 2000).

Some state and subnational governments regulate vaccine use by only permitting the use of nationally licensed products. Some states license products with limited local applications. In the United States state-approved biologics can only be used within the licensing state and cannot be transported across state lines. The USDA requires federally licensed vaccines to be pure, potent, safe, and effective.

Vaccine purity means freedom from contamination with pathogenic or inactivating substances and is determined by bacteriological culture and viral detection techniques. Vaccine potency implies a vaccine dose adequate to induce a satisfactory immunologic response. Potency is determined by testing products for antigen concentration, measuring **antibody** responses in vaccinated animals, or by challenging vaccinated animals with strains of the organism that causes obvious disease in unvaccinated control animals. The latter is called a vaccination and challenge study.

Vaccine safety means the vaccine is free of hazard to vaccinated animals or unvaccinated herd mates. Demonstrating vaccine safety requires vaccinating animals that are in contact with carefully observed unvaccinated susceptible animals followed by testing the unvaccinated herd mates to assure the vaccine did not spread. Spread of vaccine to herd mates occasionally occurs with products containing living organisms. It can cause abortion in unimmunized pregnant animals or induce immunological responses that could exclude breeding stock from export.

Efficacy implies the vaccine does indeed protect against the disease. Efficacy is usually evaluated by inoculation of vaccinated animals with a government-approved strain of the pathogen that is capable of producing defined clinical signs in unvaccinated controls. Where no disease-producing model is available, blood tests for vaccine-induced immune responses are used to demonstrate vaccine efficacy.

The level of immunity and degree of protection induced by vaccines for any given disease varies among individual animals and products. The success of vaccinations depends on the type of product selected, its effectiveness in stimulating the animal's immune system, and the characteristics of the vaccinated animals. The animal-related variables include the animal's pre-vaccination immune status, its overall immunocompetence, its age, its general health status, and the amount of stress present at the time of vaccination.

Vaccines are intended to induce antibody production and cell-mediated immune responses without causing disease or other harm to vaccinated livestock or their herd mates and without producing food-safety hazards or injection-site blemishes. These simple sounding goals become complex when it comes to developing measures to assure their accomplishment.

Most vaccines against bacterial diseases are **bacterins,** which are preparations of killed bacteria, or **toxoids,** which are inactivated bacterial toxins.

Bacterins and toxoids usually require two initial doses and repeated boostering to maintain protection. Because they do not multiply in vaccinated animals, it is crucial that each dose contain an adequate antigenic mass. Live bacterial vaccines are relatively uncommon compared to bacterins or live virus vaccines but have been used successfully for bovine brucellosis, **anthrax**, **contagious bovine pleuropneumonia** and some ***Salmonella*** infections.

Both live and inactivated viral vaccines are used in livestock. MLV vaccines are viruses manipulated so they remain capable of infecting vaccinated animals and stimulating an immune response. When they work properly, MLV vaccine infections are mild and do not produce disease. MLV vaccines are the most commonly used and most effective of the livestock vaccines because they replicate in vaccinated animals without producing disease and engender immunological responses similar to natural infections. Their use requires consideration of the age, health, and pregnancy status of the animals to be vaccinated. Some MLV vaccines are capable of inducing abortion and should not be used on pregnant animals.

Inactivated-virus vaccines contain viruses that have been killed or otherwise rendered non-infective. In general, inactivated vaccines tend to be safer and less subject to damage during storage but live vaccines generally produce more effective and longer-lasting immunity.

It is common to combine vaccines to facilitate administration, control costs, and reduce the stress of catching and restraining animals. Vaccine users must be instructed to only use mixtures prepared by licensed manufacturers, because the diluents, **adjuvants,** antibacterial components, preservatives, and active ingredients are delicately balanced and must be compatible. Products can be inactivated and rendered ineffective when improperly mixed.

Vaccines can be administered by intramuscular, subcutaneous, nasal, or oral routes. As inspection procedures and quality control programs focused on injection site blemishes in muscle meat in the latter years of the twentieth century there was a shift from intramuscular to subcutaneous injection of vaccines.

Livestock vaccines present numerous challenges to LHP-makers. Policy makers must assure that safe and effective vaccines are available for major diseases of economically significant livestock species and that the costs of the vaccines are justified by the economic risks of the diseases. They must assure that vaccines authorized for use in this country do not compromise foreign markets by causing false positive tests. These rigorous goals require credible regulatory oversight of the manufacture and use of livestock vaccines. When countries report they are free of a disease, vaccination against that disease threatens the credibility of that status.

Progress Toward Understanding Vector-Borne Diseases

The twentieth century brought new knowledge and attention to a group of insect-transmitted livestock diseases that have unique transmission cycles and require special ecosystems for their survival.

Vectors are carriers of disease-producing organisms. Vector-borne diseases have intermediate hosts, usually insects, that transmit infectious agents from mammalian or bird reservoirs to susceptible victims.

With few exceptions, vector-borne diseases are less problematic in livestock than in horses and people. Principal human vector-borne diseases are mosquito-transmitted malaria; yellow fever; eastern, western, Japanese, St. Louis, and **Venezuelan equine encephalitis (VEE); West Nile fever**; and **Rift Valley fever**. There are also tick-borne and flea-borne diseases such as plague.

Most vector-borne diseases have complex life cycles. In their native habitat, they are usually **endemic** with regular, often sub-clinical, and non-fatal activity in natural wild reservoirs. This activity provides a source of infection for secondary human or animal hosts at levels adequate to maintain relatively immune populations.

When ecological equilibrium exists among wildlife reservoirs, mosquito populations, and humans, vector-borne diseases remain confined within distinct geographic niches. They overflow these boundaries when increased moisture or other changes produce insect population explosions that coincide with waning immunity of individuals on the periphery of infected areas.

Incursions into previously uninfected areas can result from the introduction of infected insects into supportive ecosystems or from migration of infected animals or birds into areas with existing vector populations. Permanent establishment requires an ecosystem supportive of insect reproduction and a susceptible population of mammals or birds.

Control of vector-borne diseases can be accomplished with a combination of vaccination, public education about periods of maximum insect activity, and insect-control activities. Successful insect vectors rapidly develop resistance to insecticides like DDT, which was briefly regarded as the answer to yellow fever and malaria.

In the United States, localized areas experience vector-borne infections due to bluetongue and vesicular stomatitis viruses, which can impede international trade in sheep, cattle, and swine.

Emergence of Growth Promotants

Growth stimulants, commonly called growth promotants, are substances that induce increased growth rates and feed conversion (Roche 1998). They are used in beef cattle and swine and to a lesser extent on animals raised for milking or breeding purposes. They are rarely used in poultry production, because they produce erratic results in avian species. Additionally, the short life span of most commercial poultry does not allow time for growth promotants to be metabolized and eliminated before poultry products reach market.

The use of growth promotants has raised public concern about residues in meat and created trade issues. Two main classes of growth promotants are hormones, which stimulate growth directly, and antimicrobials, which alter the microbiological makeup of the gastrointestinal tract permitting efficient utilization of nutrients and increases in growth and weight gain.

The use of growth promotants has caused the erection of trade barriers and this has erupted into a newsworthy international controversy. Objections to growth promotants come from the European Community, which refuses to import U.S. beef because of fears of the alleged dangers of hormones. These fears have been determined to be unfounded and without scientific basis by international tribunals. They are considered by U.S. officials to be protectionist measures in violation of the requirements for transparency, non-discrimination, scientifically based risk assessment, and equal national treatment of the WTO SPS Agreement to which both parties are signatory (see Discussion Topic 1).

Hormonal growth promotants are widely used in livestock production. Hormones are biologically active substances secreted directly into body fluids by endocrine glands, including the thyroid and parathyroid glands, the pituitary and adrenal glands, the pancreas, testes, ovaries, and the placenta. Hormones produced by these glands arrive at distant body locations via the blood or lymph where they exert a wide variety of highly specific stimulatory effects on the structure or function of target organs and tissues.

Most hormones are steroids. The natural steroid hormones used as growth promotants in livestock production are the sex hormones progesterone, testosterone, and estradiol. They can influence growth and bodily distribution of proteins and fat. They are usually administered as pellets implanted in the ears of cattle or small ruminants. The ear is used, because it is usually discarded at slaughter eliminating likelihood of residues or injection site blemishes. Hormonal growth promotants may increase growth rates from 5–15%.

Synthesized steroids are also administered as ear implants. Synthetic nonsteroidal hormones have similar effects on growth. One of these, diethylstilbesterol, is banned in many countries because of its capacity to cause DNA alterations (Roche 1998). The kind of hormones administered depends on the age, sex, and intended use of the treated animals. Hormonal growth promotants are usually contraindicated for animals used for breeding purposes.

Bovine growth hormone, usually called bovine somatotropin (BST), is produced by the anterior pituitary gland. It acts directly on growing tissues and stimulates the liver to produce growth factors. In 1994, an injectable, recombinant BST produced by genetically engineered bacteria was approved for use in the United States in lactating dairy cattle to increase milk production and reduce feed costs. In the early years of its use, there were concerns that consumer objections would force the labeling of the milk from treated cows, and that there would be negative health effects on treated animals. There were reports that BST-treated animals may have a higher incidence of mastitis, a chronic inflammation of milk-secreting tissue that results in the appearance of flakes and clots in the milk. A scientific basis for this claim, however, was difficult to establish, because mastitis is common among dairy cattle not treated with BST as well. Arguments were put forward that mastitis is associated with the high milk production rather than with BST per se. Early reports indicated these concerns were unfounded (Collier 1995). U.S. regulators have rejected the claims that there were health issues in the treated animals. The injectable product, which is administered every two weeks, is heavily used in lactating dairy cattle.

The use of BST is banned in the European Union, which applied precautionary measures as a justification even though their technical reviewers found BST safe for cattle and for the consumers of the milk and meat from treated animals.

After the turn of the century the use of BST to stimulate increased milk production remained the subject of some controversy (Kronfeld 2001). There were also efforts to demonstrate economical growth-promoting value for BST in swine and beef cattle, but these never achieved commercial application.

The complex technology and multiple public concerns about the use of hormones in livestock cast an ominous shadow on the future of some markets for livestock products produced using biotechnologic methodology. The BST story challenges regulators and policy makers to move thoughtfully in the face of scientific uncertainty.

Antimicrobials and probiotics are widely used in livestock production. Antimicrobial growth promotants, fed in sub-therapeutic levels, increase growth rates and feed efficiency by altering the microbial makeup of the gastrointestinal tract. In ruminants, this occurs through altering rumen energy metabolism or reducing methane production that drains energy from animals. Low-level antimicrobial feed additives inhibit microorganisms that cause mild infections and slow growth. The result of these combined effects is an increase in growth rate.

As discussed above, the use of sub-therapeutic antimicrobials is sometimes said to speed up the development of antimicrobial resistance among pathogenic bacteria. Supporters of the use of antimicrobials downplay this thesis stating that the compounds involved are rarely used in human medicine and mostly remain in the animal's intestinal tracts. Nonetheless, animal health policy makers can anticipate challenges to their use.

Probiotics are not antimicrobials. They are living organisms, principally bacteria and yeasts, that increase livestock growth rates and feed efficiency by competitively shifting the balance of microbe populations in the gastrointestinal ecosystem. Unlike antimicrobials, which inhibit bacteria, probiotics are living cultures of non-pathogenic lactobacilli, streptococci, or yeasts. They compete with potential pathogens and high-energy consuming bacteria in the animal's gut and result in accelerated growth. The results of probiotic feed additives vary. They appear most effective in young animals whose systems are not yet infected with potentially pathogenic bacteria.

Mechanized Systems for Processing Meat, Poultry, and Dairy Products

Increased speed and mechanization of slaughter, processing, packaging, and shipping of meats, poultry, and dairy products have decreased food prices; offered a variety of standardized products; and presented the potential to improve human diets. These efficiencies have forced small slaughterhouses out of business; attracted the attention of food safety, animal welfare, labor and environmental groups; and presented challenges to policy makers. The mounting volumes, increased line speeds, and low wages in food processing plants reduced production costs, increased corporate profits, and made quality products available to larger segments of the population.

These changes have created a need for updated regulations and inspections. For years traditional meat-inspection systems focused on visible evidence of disease or gross blemishes on carcasses. Such inspection procedures don't detect bacteria or residues of hormones, antibiotics, and chemicals. These hazards can now be identified and traced by improved technology. Through media coverage and pressure from interest groups, food safety has become an object of thoughtful public concern (Wasserman et al. 1985) and a focus of international trade restrictions.

In the 1990s these concerns stimulated officials of the USDA **Food Safety and Inspection Service (FSIS)** to initiate a radical and controversial inspection system, based on **hazard analysis and critical control point (HACCP)** strategies. This system was put into effect in U.S. meat plants and foreign facilities that export to the United States. Food inspectors, labor unions, and some food-safety groups resisted the HACCP system, because it decreases individual inspections and focuses on surveillance, spot checks, and intermittent testing in high-risk areas known as critical control points.

This new system addressed the disconnect between modernized animal production and processing and an antiquated meat inspection system based on outdated statutes and regulations. The HACCP system arose from the need to shift to science-based techniques. The HACCP system, initially implemented in 1998, recognizes that zero risk is unachievable. It reduces the number of inspections and focuses on points most likely to permit product contamination or to support the multiplication of pathogens, and it shifts much of the responsibility for meeting standards to meat packers. It relies on testing small random samples for chemical and biological residues and disease-producing bacteria such as ***Camplobacteria***, *Listeria*, ***E. Coli* O157:H7**, and *Salmonella*. These organisms inhabit the intestinal tracts of livestock and people and are transmitted via fecal contamination. Visible excrement has always been trimmed from carcasses, but much bacterial contamination is not visible to the naked eye. Carcass-scanning devices that can examine entire carcasses and detect invisible contamination are under development. This equipment employs fluorescent beams to detect unseen manure-borne by-products of photosensitization.

Salmonella organisms with origins in human, animal, and poultry feces are globally ubiquitous. They require sanitary measures to limit their spread at all levels of the food chain (Anonymous 1999). The **Codex Alimentarius Commission (CODEX)**, the international standard-setting organization for foods and pharmaceuticals, indicated that HACCP, no matter how imperfect, is the best available program for reducing human food poisoning caused by *Salmonella*. HAACP has produced progress in lowering levels of bacterial contamination of meats but requires constant refinements and improved technology.

Policy makers need to continually review inspection and testing procedures and strive for improvement in food safety through total quality management programs throughout the food chain. This will permit advancing technology to minimize the risks of contaminated products entering the marketplace. Risk-based systems address the major sources of product contamination and points of cross contamination within packing plants but are not a total answer to food safety. As they conduct ongoing efforts to improve the safety and quality of meat and poultry products, policy makers must focus on cost efficient inspections, surveillance, testing, and product-handling efforts in areas most amenable to detection and most vulnerable to interdiction.

Some experts suggest the meat industry should follow the lead of the milk industry, which took a giant step in food safety, despite considerable objections, by introducing sterilization by pasteurization. As technology advances, the prospects for safely irradiating high-risk meats such as hamburger and poultry products continue to improve. Irradiation, also called cold sterilization or electronic pasteurization, appears logical as an addition to ongoing efforts to protect animals, farmers, food handlers, and products from microorganisms that are ubiquitous in the environment. Electronic sterilization is a process similar to milk pasteurization. It uses ionizing energy from electronic beams, x-rays, or gamma rays to kill bacteria. It is best conducted on cut or ground, already-packaged products that will be no longer exposed to the multiple sources of contamination in processing plants. However, once the package is opened, it is still subject to recontamination from unsterilized products, utensils, or human carriers in kitchens. Electronic sterilization is, therefore, no panacea. Lukewarm public perceptions have slowed its progress. Nonetheless, sales of electronically sterilized meats are increasing and major supermarket chains are making them available. As with other innovations, public understanding and acceptance will gradually overcome objections to this technology but this will require education and an adjustment period.

Improvements in Refrigeration and Transportation of Perishable Foods

Twentieth century advances in refrigeration, transportation, processing, handling, and distribution of perishable livestock products have expedited supplying meat, milk, and eggs to all parts of the world on a year-round basis. These advances ushered livestock health into the globalization movement.

The transportation of perishables permits global marketing of livestock products by surplus-producing nations. All countries cannot feed their exploding populations. These needs can be met by external providers. In a free-market economy, this may cause collapse of some cherished rural societies that survive by subsidies, quotas, tariffs, and trade barriers.

Like other resources, transportation and refrigeration capacities are unequally distributed among nations. Attempts to capitalize on modern production and processing methodology with ancient transportation and refrigeration techniques can create health hazards. Accusations of ineffective inspection and processing can emerge when spoilage and food-borne disease is associated with foreign perishable products transported in inadequately refrigerated conveyances or left unrefrigerated at points of consumption.

Importance of Animal Health to Livestock Profitability, Human Health, and Food Safety

The events of the twentieth century brought the awareness that animal health extends beyond livestock profitability to impact human health and food safety. There are many **zoonotic** diseases shared by humans and animals. Some are mild infections in animals that are rarely evident to people. Some, like BSE, remain unrecognized for long periods during which they can spread through the food supply. Until it was realized that plants were also a source of food-borne diseases, food-safety attention focused on products of animal origin as sources of disease.

Livestock profitability requires that animals and poultry grow at maximum rates, efficiently utilize foodstuffs, produce maximum amounts of milk or eggs, and remain in good condition until they are marketed as meat. In incentive-based and profit-oriented economies, health is a key ingredient of successful livestock industries, and unprofitable farms soon go out of business or become hobbies supported by other incomes.

Healthy human populations require affordable, adequate, nutritionally balanced diets and a variety of wholesome foods. Healthy livestock populations are the basis of safe foods of animal origin and are essential to supplying safe and affordable milk, eggs, and meat.

Twentieth Century Global Dynamics' Impact on National Economies, Livestock Health, and Human Health

Twentieth century progress in livestock health coincided with world population expansion, upheavals of political systems, movements to democracy and free-market economies, and advances in communication technology. These dynamics introduced new public concerns and created challenges and dilemmas for LHP-makers in the twenty-first century.

The recent monumental political and ideological changes set the stage for a shifting role of livestock health in the global economy. The emigration from rural to urban areas resulted in the need for more food to be produced by a shrinking number of farmers.

Changing governing styles have increased public dependence on national agencies and provided citizens with the freedom to criticize. The demise of non-competitive regimes that offered little incentive for productivity was climaxed by the collapse of the Soviet Union and its division into thirteen independent nations. Each of these new nations faced, overnight, a transition to capitalism, transparent governance, and incentive-based economies.

The world rapidly evolved into a massive free market economy and the one-world concept of **globalization** fell upon unprepared societies that were unfamiliar with the complexities of such an economy.

North America languished in food surpluses. They had readily available meat, eggs, and dairy products to provide essential proteins, vitamins, minerals, and micronutrients. New concerns about the health of diets containing excessive quantities of red meat and dairy products soon surfaced, and vegetarian and **vegan** interests pioneered anti-meat movements.

Throughout the twentieth century many parts of the world faced starvation. Advancing technology offered potential solutions, but correction of the imbalance was prohibited by economic, political, and cultural differences.

Progress Produces Challenges and Presents Opportunities

The livestock-production dynamics of the twentieth century revolutionized the world's livestock industries, changed human diets, engendered food-safety and environmental concerns, and impacted international trade. The United States' contribution to this advancing technology was a result of investment and return from the **land grant system** that encouraged and supported agricultural research, education, and information transfer. This success promoted U.S. agriculture, benefited the American people, and reached out to many parts of the world.

The closing years of the twentieth century revolutionized the biological sciences and introduced a controversial biotechnological era with techniques for manipulating animal, plant, and human genes and altering the activities of pathogenic microorganisms. With these developments came new hopes for overcoming livestock diseases, human pestilence, and global starvation. The production of GMOs, cloning of animals, insertion and deletion of genes in living organisms, and the introduction of stem cell technology all raise thoughtful, though divisive, moral, ethical, and ecological questions (Holdredge and Talbot 2001). Policy makers cannot ignore these questions.

The extent to which livestock health interests have marketed their agendas to national governments varies throughout the world. LHP-makers must seek public support and educate officials about the importance of protecting the health of each nation's livestock.

The twenty-first century promises more progress. With it will come technologic, economic, political, and ethical challenges for livestock producers and processors. This progress will provoke thoughtful resistance from interest groups concerned about the environment, animal welfare, food safety, the transmission of diseases from animals to humans, and the potential dangers of the genetic manipulation of animals or their feed. There will be concerns about the safety and ethics of GMOs, embryo transfer, animal cloning, and **stem cell technology** and their possible spillover into human medical applications.

Before rendering decisions, LHP-makers must understand the scientific bases of these technologies. Successful strategies for the coming decades require that they listen thoughtfully to the supporters of these changes as well as to the strong opposition these changes generate.

Bibliography

Anonymous. 1997. *Food Safety From Farm to Table: A National Food Safety Initiative: A Report to the President.* Washington, D.C.: U.S. Environmental Protection Agency, U.S. Department of Health and Human Services, and U.S. Department of Agriculture.

Beitz, D. C., L. A. Berner, G. F. Combs et al. 1997. *Contributions of Animal Products to Heathful Diets.* Task Force Report, Number 131. Ames, IA: Council for Agricultural Science and Technology.

Brown, C. 1999. Historical Evaluations of Antimicrobial Resistance and Food-producing Animals. In *Proc US Anim Health Assoc* 103:84–86.

Collier, R. J. 1995. An Update on Bovine Somatotropin. In *Proc US Anim Health Assoc* 99:390–394.

Hietala, S., P. McCready, T. McKenna et al. 2002. Diagnostic Surveillance for Foreign Animal Diseases. In *Proceedings of the 45th Annual Conference of the American Association of Veterinary Laboratory Diagnosticians 45:4.*

Holdredge, C. and S. Talbot. 2001. Sewing Technology: The Ecologic Argument against Genetic Engineering Down on the Farm. *Sierra: Magazine of the Sierra Club*. July-August.

Kahrs, R. F. 2001. *Viral Diseases of Cattle*. Ames: Iowa State University Press.

Kronfeld, D. S. 2001. Concerned About Use of BST in Dairy Cattle. *J Am Vet Med Assoc* 219: 291-292.

OIE 2000. *The OIE Manual of Diagnostic Tests and Vaccines.* Paris: Office International des Epizooties.

OIE 2001. *The OIE International Animal Health Code.* 9th ed. Paris: Office International des Epizooties.

Pastoret, P. P., J. Blancou, P. Vannier, and C. Verschueren, eds. 1999. *Veterinary Vaccinology.* Amsterdam: Elsevier Science Publishers.

Reeves, D. E. 2000. Characterization of Antimicrobial Resistance. In *Proc US Anim Health Assoc* 104:479–486.

Roche, J. F. 1998. Growth Promotants. In Aiello, S. E. and A. Mays, eds. *The Merck Veterinary Manual.* 8th ed. Whitehouse Station, NJ: Merck and Company.

Stringfellow, D. A. and S. M. Seidel. 1998. *3rd Manual of the International Embryo Transfer Society.* Savoy, IL: International Embryo Transfer Society.

Wasserman, R. H., J. C. Bailar, F. Bryan et al. 1985. *Meat and Poultry Inspection: The Basis of the National Program*. Washington, D.C.: National Academy Press.

Chapter 3

Thirty Years That Shaped Livestock Health Policy

Introduction

Effective policy-making requires an appreciation of events that have forever changed livestock health. Recent decades saw outbreaks of **foot-and-mouth disease (FMD),** the appearance of the **transmissible spongiform encephalopathies (TSEs)**, an increasing emphasis on new and emerging diseases, new disease-control and eradication campaigns, and the emergence of captive and free-ranging wildlife as **livestock health policy (LHP)** issues. In the 1990s the globalization movement reached into LHPs, and the **Sanitary and Phytosanitary (SPS) Agreement** of the **World Trade Organization (WTO)** established guidelines for international movement of livestock products.

These events coincided with growing consumer involvement in food safety, animal welfare, and the environment; new recognition of the role of livestock in public health and international trade; and the emergence of epidemiology and risk analyses as influential livestock health disciplines. These events created needs for new understandings, changed outlooks, and decisive actions by policy makers.

Impact of Outbreaks of FMD

FMD has ravaged global livestock populations for centuries. In recent history massive outbreaks in Taiwan, Great Britain, the Netherlands, and elsewhere have caused huge economic losses. Graphic media coverage provoked public outcries over the environmental and humane implications of the slaughter and disposal of millions of FMD-infected and exposed animals.

FMD is the worst-case scenario among livestock diseases, because it spreads rapidly, is difficult to control, and infects many domestic and wild species. The FMD virus resists drying and survives on inanimate objects and in chilled and frozen meat. It can withstand many disinfectants and environmental influences. The measures needed to exclude, eradicate, or control FMD are stringent enough to control most other contagious livestock diseases.

When introduced into FMD-free regions, FMD can devastate livestock industries, raise food prices, and limit exports. FMD affects cloven-hoofed animals such as swine, cattle, sheep, goats, wild **ruminants**, and many exotic species. Sheep and goats experience mild infections and can surreptitiously spread FMD long before it is suspected.

FMD is **endemic** in parts of South America, Africa, Asia, and Europe where it reduces production efficiency and impedes trade. It is usually fatal only in newborn animals. It causes inappetence, painful lameness, and severe debility due to blister-like **vesicles** on the mouth, feet, and teats. Similar lesions are seen in **vesicular stomatitis (VS)** and other diseases.

Laboratory tests are needed for a positive diagnosis and to distinguish among seven **serotypes** of FMD virus. Spread is rapid and FMD is difficult to eliminate or control once established in an area, particularly if wild ruminants or feral swine become infected.

In regions where FMD is endemic it is partially controlled by vaccination. When it appears in FMD-free areas, it is eradicated by slaughtering affected and exposed animals to prevent spread.

Vaccination is invoked only as a last resort, because it is expensive, only partially effective, must be repeated frequently, and complicates diagnostic test results. FMD vaccines have a limited shelf-life. Immunity to FMD is of limited duration and separate vaccines are needed for each of the seven serotypes. Natural infection or vaccination affords partial, rather than absolute, protection from infection. Vaccinated or recovered animals can subsequently develop mild and undetected infections and can spread the disease. In addition, animals that recover from infection with one serotype are usually susceptible to infection with others and can develop full-blown disease.

FMD-free countries avoid vaccination and prefer the stamping-out technique, because vaccination involves an endless outlay of resources, provides herd immunity capable of masking clinical signs thus permitting widespread dissemination before infection is recognized, and limits the efficiency of surveillance activities. Also, vaccination is discouraged, because outbreaks have been traced to escape of FMD virus from vaccine production facilities. Occasionally vaccines have actually induced outbreaks.

In cattle, FMD can be confused with **bovine viral diarrhea (BVD)**, **rinderpest**, **malignant catarrhal fever (MCF)**, **bluetongue**, and **papular stomatitis**. It can be misdiagnosed as respiratory disease or **footrot,** which are common ailments of cattle. The teat lesions can be confused with poxvirus infections or **bovine herpes mammillitis**.

In swine, FMD resembles **vesicular exanthema of swine** and **swine vesicular disease**. In sheep and goats it must be differentiated from footrot and other causes of lameness and from **sheeppox**, **goatpox**, **sore mouth,** and other mouth disorders that also cause drooling.

Laboratories undertaking diagnosis of **vesicular diseases** must have high-level biosecurity ratings and batteries of specific reagents for identifying viruses. In North America, specially trained exotic-disease diagnosticians are available on short notice to collect diagnostic samples and send them to national laboratories for testing. Specimens from suspected FMD cases must be collected and packaged carefully to avoid spreading the disease.

While there have been efforts to eradicate or control FMD, there are many areas where FMD viruses are ensconced. These include parts of South America, Asia, Africa, and portions of Eastern Europe.

FMD-free areas include Australia, New Zealand, Japan, many Pacific islands, and all of North and Central America. Countries contiguous to infected areas or that regularly import livestock products from infected regions are at high risk and occasionally experience costly FMD introductions.

The contagiousness and resistance of the FMD virus multiply the risk of introducing FMD into disease-free countries. The United States Department of Agriculture (USDA) has regulations and requirements that mitigate each risk. In approximate order of gravity these risks include:

- Importation of live animals to be placed in contact with susceptible livestock
- Importation of wholesale quantities of contaminated meat, scraps of which could be fed to swine
- Entry in passenger baggage or postal packages of contaminated meat, scraps of which could be fed to swine
- Importation of semen or embryos of infected animals to be implanted directly into livestock
- Entrance of people with shoes or clothing contaminated with FMD virus who may then visit the premises where susceptible livestock are kept
- Importation of horses that have hoofs, coats, or tack contaminated with FMD virus and subsequently enter premises where susceptible livestock are kept

- Entrance in cargoes or passenger baggage of antiques, vehicles, or used farm equipment from infected regions, which end up on premises housing livestock
- Entrance of hunting trophies, including animal heads, antlers, and hides
- Entrance of vaccines, pharmaceuticals, soaps, serums, diagnostic specimens, and other biological materials
- Zoo animals imported from FMD-infected regions

Live swine, ruminants, and other cloven-hoofed animals from most of the world cannot enter the United States without elaborate quarantine and inspection procedures. Canadian or Mexican cattle designated for direct slaughter or for fattening in quarantined feedlots are an exception. By special permit, and with accompanying health certificates, zoo animals may enter for quarantine and consignment to approved zoological parks. Also by permit semen and embryos from excluded species can be imported if they are collected and processed according to standard conditions under USDA supervision in the country of origin.

Over 3,000 live horses from all parts of the world arrive at New York's JFK airport annually. Without ever touching the ground horses are moved in disinfected transporters to sealed trucks operated by private contractors and transferred directly to the quarantine station at Newburgh, NY. There they are examined, disinfected, and quarantined awaiting results of required tests performed on blood samples submitted to the **National Animal Disease Center (NADC)** in Ames, Iowa. Grooms accompanying imported horses must disinfect their shoes before leaving the airport.

Horses arriving without proper paperwork (health certificates from veterinary officials in the county of origin and a U.S.-issued import permit) are left on the aircraft for return to the sender. The majority of imported horses perform in one or more equine events and then leave the country, sometimes to continue on the international show circuit. Planes carrying horses into the United States must be disinfected under USDA supervision before departure.

Birds and poultry imported for agricultural enterprises and for consignment to inspected and approved zoological parks are transported to a USDA-supervised facility for inspection, quarantine, and testing. Hunting trophies require permits and must be transferred under seal to approved and inspected taxidermy facilities.

These procedures markedly reduce the risk of FMD introduction by legal importations but don't cover smuggled items.

In FMD-free areas, the slightest suspicion of FMD must be reported to regulatory officials. Immediately upon diagnosis, the **stamping out method** is invoked. This consists of:

- Immediate quarantine of all infected, exposed, and high-risk premises (usually involving area quarantines that restrict movement of animals, people, or vehicles)
- Depopulation of infected and exposed cloven-hoofed animals
- Disinfection of infected premises
- Investigation to determine the source of infection
- A period of 30 days or more during which no animals are permitted on the premises
- Trial re-population and eventual restocking
- Educational programs
- Strict controls on the movement of people, livestock, and vehicles
- Restrictions on commercial or private undertakings that could expedite spread of the disease

The stamping out method can become impossible to implement if widespread infections occur. If economic realities or public pressures force officials to halt eradication efforts, the affected area will be permanently infected.

The timing of the decision to abandon eradication efforts and initiate vaccination is based on many factors. Ring-vaccination around depopulated and infected areas can be used to limit spread until later efforts narrow infected areas enough to permit logistically feasible eradication approaches.

FMD has been successfully eradicated from Great Britain and parts of Western Europe, the United States, Canada, and Mexico by the stamping out method, which is feasible in newly infected areas when prompt action is taken. In 2001, FMD was reintroduced into Western Europe, probably from swine consuming scraps of meat illegally imported from an infected country.

Once FMD is ensconced in an area, eradication requires monumental efforts including slaughter of livestock populations and wildlife reservoirs. Eradication programs in areas where FMD is well established must be preceded by careful study of the logistical, environmental, and economic feasibility of the project.

If resources and infrastructure are available and domestic industry and neighboring countries are cooperative, the long-range economic benefits of FMD eradication are considerable. Greater progress results from programs based on governmental partnerships with producers and industry groups than when govern-and-command tactics are utilized by regulatory authorities.

Eradication by developing countries seems unlikely, especially in Africa where wildlife reservoirs exist. South Africa has used extensive testing, surveillance, and control efforts. They have limited wildlife movements by fencing and almost eradicated FMD from the entire country with the exception of the Kruger National Wildlife Preserve.

Animals and related products from infected regions are excluded from many world markets or subject to stringent risk-reduction measures such as special processing, quarantines, and testing. FMD-free countries have protected themselves from a variety of diseases by restricting commerce in bovine and porcine commodities from FMD-infected regions.

While FMD is an old disease, the extent of media coverage and the cost of the outbreaks at the end of the twentieth century will undoubtedly cause the test and slaughter approaches to future outbreaks to be revisited (see Discussion Topic 10).

Appearance of the TSEs

The recognition of **bovine spongiform encephalopathy (BSE)** in the mid-1980s introduced a new chapter in livestock-disease history and added new dimensions to LHP-making. BSE is not a classic contagious disease or virus infection. It belongs to a group of unconventional subviral disorders known as TSEs, or prion diseases. It is an insidious, chronically progressive, inevitably fatal, neurodegenerative disease of cattle manifested by behavioral, postural, and locomotor disorders.

BSE has caused international concern and distrust, trade barriers, uncertainty within veterinary services worldwide, dissension within the **European Economic Community (EEC),** and OIE efforts to develop new standards for movement of livestock products and new criteria for countries to be recognized as BSE-free.

BSE was first recognized in the United Kingdom in 1985–86 and called mad cow disease. Starting as just a few cases, it soon became a major **epizootic**. By 2000 it had killed over 200,000 cattle and caused the slaughter of almost four million exposed animals. By 1996, BSE was a European problem and no longer confined to the United Kingdom.

BSE probably originated from protein supplementation of cattle diets with meat and bone meal containing rendered offal from **scrapie**-affected sheep. Meat and bone meal produced from BSE-infected cattle probably amplified the epidemic. In the early 1980s the United Kingdom instituted energy-saving measures that lowered rendering temperatures in the feed production process. This new process may have permitted the survival of the scrapie agent (or a mutation thereof) in feed and its dissemination among cattle.

Like other TSEs, BSE causes spongy degeneration of neurons in the brain and spinal cord. These lesions cause progressive loss of body condition and neurologic function that result in behavioral changes, incoordination, staggering, recumbency, and death, but cattle don't develop clinical signs until two to eight years after infection.

It has been convincingly demonstrated that embryo transfer (Wrathrall et al. 2002) will not transmit BSE. This affords an opportunity for trade in bovine genetics between BSE-free and BSE-affected countries.

As of 2003, BSE had not occurred in North or South America with the exception of a single case in 1993 in Canada in a cow imported as a three-month-old calf from England in 1987. The absence of BSE in the United States as compared to the United Kingdom was presumed to be due to its smaller sheep population, fewer scrapie-infected sheep, and less feeding of ovine offal. There could be strain differences between U.K. and U.S. scrapie agents.

The TSEs are a perplexing group of slowly progressive fatal diseases that have been described in several animal species and in humans. They were originally called slow virus infections due to their long incubation periods and progressive clinical courses. They are now called TSEs, because classical viruses have not been isolated.

Some TSEs occur sporadically, widely separated in time and space, and appear unrelated. Others are geographically clustered and associated with exposure factors such as cannibalism and trans-species carnivorism. They sometimes appear to have a familial or species-related susceptibility component that is difficult to distinguish from common exposures to sources of infection, toxicosis, or deficiency. Different TSEs are caused by unique agents that can be distinguished by molecular technology and by their incubation periods and lesions in experimental mice.

The human TSEs include kuru, fatal familial insomnia, Gerstmann-Straussler-Scheinker syndrome, and **Creutzfeldt-Jacob disease (CJD)**. Until recently, human TSEs have occurred sporadically and have generally been regarded as non-transmissible biochemical defects. An exception is kuru, which was virtually eliminated when the custom of eating the brains of dead relatives ceased among affected populations in Papua New Guinea.

CJD is a chronic, fatal, degenerative neurologic disorder that occurs sporadically worldwide in approximately 1:1,000,000 people. Until 1993 it was regarded as a genetic, or metabolic, defect. Then a new variant form **Variant CJD (VCJD)** was recognized in England. VCJD differs from classic CJD by having an earlier age of onset and slightly different clinical signs and microscopic lesions. The agents of CJD and VCJD are biologically indistinguishable.

VCJD probably results from people eating BSE-contaminated meat. Its recognition caused further bans on cattle and beef from the United Kingdom, criticism of British handling of BSE, allegations that agricultural interests were neglecting consumer safety, and movement of animal health responsibilities from agricultural to consumer-oriented agencies in the European Union (EU). Milk, milk products, gelatin, and properly rendered tallow were considered safe, but cosmetics, pharmaceuticals, and products derived from glands became suspect.

The TSEs of animals include scrapie, BSE, feline spongiform encephalopathy, **chronic wasting disease (CWD)** of deer and elk, and **transmissible mink encephalopathy (TME)**.

Scrapie is the prototype TSE. It occurs in sheep and rarely in goats. It has been endemic in Great Britain for several centuries. Scrapie was first diagnosed in the United States in 1947. Presumably, it was introduced by Suffolk sheep imported from the United Kingdom. Following an incubation period of one to two years or more, affected sheep develop locomotor incoordination. They exhibit behavioral changes including rubbing against objects, staggering, tremors, and walking in circles, progressive weight loss, and ultimately death. Scrapie is seen mostly in black-faced sheep that are between two and eight years old. Scrapie received revived attention due to the relationship of BSE to VCJD.

Chronic wasting disease (CWD) of deer and elk is progressive and fatal. It has received increasing attention with growing concerns about TSEs. CWD was first identified in the United States in 1977. Its spread is probably linked to increasing population densities and environmental contamination. The geographic distribution and prevalence of CWD in free-ranging and captive **cervids** (deer, elk, and moose) appears to be expanding, partly due to increased surveillance activities. Determining the exact magnitude of the CWD problem awaits the perfection of techniques for mass testing of live animals.

CWD is characterized by weight loss and emaciation. Affected animals drink more frequently than usual and salivate and urinate excessively. They may have blank stares in both eyes, and they develop life-threatening pneumonia, which is frequently the cause of death. The differential diagnosis of CWD includes malnutrition, parasitism, chronic pneumonia, renal or enteric disease, weather stress, and inhalation pneumonia. Although they have spongiform brain lesions CWD patients rarely exhibit behavioral changes, nervousness, hyperexcitibility, hyperaesthesia, teeth grinding, or pelvic ataxia.

Preliminary studies indicate the etiologic agent of CWD is probably distinct from both scrapie and BSE. Knowledge of CWD will probably expand with further surveillance and advancing diagnostic technology. The disease has been found in an expanding number of areas in the western United States. The domesticated-cervid industry, in cooperation with state governments and the USDA, is undertaking a CWD herd-certification program based on postmortem surveillance, animal identification and trace back, depopulation, and quarantine. Its long-term goal is control and eventual eradication of CWD. The plan is to only permit interstate movement of cervids in herds participating in the program.

Transmissible mink encephalopathy (TME) is a rare, fatal, neurodegenerative disease of mink. Its clinical signs and lesions are similar to those of other TSEs. It was speculated that TME may result from feeding mink the meat from downer, or non-ambulatory, cows (Marsh 1990). This conjecture was never confirmed, but it has been used by the EU as evidence that BSE is present in the United States.

The unfolding TSE saga is one phase of the focus on **emerging diseases** that will challenge LHP-makers throughout the millennium.

Increasing Attention to Emerging Diseases

The closing years of the twentieth century brought increasing attention to new and emerging animal diseases, particularly those transmissible to people. From a policy perspective these concerns must be addressed cooperatively by multiple national and subnational regulatory authorities.

This new focus began with the emergence of **human immunodeficiency virus (HIV),** the cause of acquired immunodeficiency syndrome (AIDS). It was accelerated by BSE, the other TSEs, diseases like **Nipah** virus, West Nile Fever, and other vector-borne zoonoses, and the revival of interest in **anthrax** and human **tuberculosis**. The ecological impact of increasing population densities, advancing diagnostic technology, and potential bioterrorism will increase this attention.

Emerging disease activities are being tracked in a monthly journal (CDC 2002). The U.S. **National Center for Disease Control and Prevention (CDC)** has undertaken a program to update and revitalize the nation's capacity to protect against emerging diseases. This program involves improving disease surveillance and outbreak-response capacity, supporting research on emerging infectious diseases, improving infectious disease prevention and control programs, disseminating public health information, and upgrading the infectious disease component of the public health infrastructure (CDC 1998).

Role of Zoos in the Surveillance of Emerging and Exotic Diseases of Livestock

Zoos provide ideal sentinels for emerging exotic and vector-borne diseases by offering a unique variety of species in an environment accessible to insects. They also have staff veterinarians. Many zoos have serum banks that archive specimens permitting chronological comparisons. The American Zoo Association and the CDC have cooperated to monitor the spread of West Nile Fever in the United States. Such activities can play a vital role in public health surveillance programs and national livestock health-reporting systems.

New Disease-Control and Eradication Campaigns

Global efforts to control BSE and FMD emerged in the latter years of the twentieth century. In the United States there were also revived efforts to control scrapie and Johnes disease. During this period some EU countries developed national programs to control several livestock diseases that are globally endemic including BVD, **infectious bovine rhinotracheitis**, and **enzootic bovine leukosis**.

Growing Importance of Captive and Free-Ranging Wildlife to Livestock Health

There has also been increasing attention paid to diseases of free-ranging, wild, or exotic species. Many of these species are domesticated in commercial animal parks, state and national parks, or hunting preserves. Others are raised under semi-traditional farming conditions and ultimately slaughtered for specialty meats.

Animals considered to be captive wildlife in the United States include bison, water buffalo, the cervids, llamas and alpaca, and the flightless birds (ostriches, emu and rhea). These species often originate in regions infected with livestock diseases not present in the United States. Little is known about their capacity to carry disease or their long-term impact on local ecosystems should they escape.

Captive wildlife are examined for disease less frequently than traditionally farmed livestock. They can experience silent infections and transmit diseases to domestic herds if they commingle.

It is challenging to identify or capture free-roaming species to diagnose illnesses, test them for programmed diseases, vaccinate them, or conduct other disease-control procedures. Many captive wildlife operations have limited restraint facilities. Species differences and wording technicalities, such as the definition of **ruminants**, sometimes exempt them from regulations imposed on traditional livestock. Zoos also keep captive wildlife, but they are of less concern as they usually have veterinary supervision, carefully observe their animals, and comply with import and public health regulations.

Captive and free-ranging wildlife can carry tuberculosis, brucellosis, FMD, and many other diseases. They often contact traditional livestock and can impact disease-control programs.

Efforts to control captive and free-ranging wildlife can cause battles between conservationists and animal health authorities such as occurred over bovine brucellosis in bison and elk in Yellowstone National Park.

Resolution of conflicts can be expedited by involving wildlife or zoo veterinarians that share the interests of both sides. This helped in planning procedures for controlling tuberculosis in captive and free-roaming deer in northeastern Michigan in the late 1990s. Local stakeholders were invited to participate in the planning, and this resulted in a cooperative effort.

Issues surrounding captive and free-ranging wildlife and exotic species complicate livestock disease-control programs and present thought-provoking challenges to LHP-makers.

Role of Feral Animals in LHP

Feral animals comprise an expanding dimension of LHPs. Some dictionaries define feral as wild, or non-domesticated. In LHP jargon feral animals are ones that have escaped domestication and are established in natural ecosystems.

Feral swine, some dating back to pigs introduced by early Spanish settlers, are prevalent in temperate regions of North America and Europe. They usually don't survive in areas with long cold winters. Feral swine can carry pseudorabies, **classical swine fever, trichinosis**, porcine **brucellosis**, and **porcine reproductive and respiratory syndrome (PRRS)**. They present a constant threat to swine disease-control programs, because they occasionally commingle with domestic pig populations, particularly at breeding time. Diseases of feral animals and wildlife are difficult to control, because their free movement limits their identification or testing.

Classic Wildlife as Reservoirs of Livestock Diseases

Many livestock and human diseases have reservoirs in wild animals. **Rabies** is endemic in foxes, skunks, and raccoons in specific ecosystems in North America and is partially controlled by bait laden with oral vaccines. It is also endemic in bats in Latin America where control efforts are based on distribution of anticoagulants that are lethal to blood-sucking bats.

African malignant catarrhal fever (MCF) is permanently established in wild ruminants that roam the plains of Africa. This viral infection is usually fatal for cattle and there are periodic bovine epidemics when wild ruminants and cattle commingle. African MCF sometimes causes fatalities among cattle near zoos in non-African nations.

Sheep-associated MCF is caused by a different virus than African MCF. It is also fatal to cattle. It is carried by apparently healthy sheep and is endemic in some nations where it is controlled by segregating sheep from cattle.

Foot-and-mouth disease is established among wildlife in parts of Africa, including South Africa's Kruger National Park, and occasionally escapes its fenced borders to infect nearby cattle and small ruminants.

Viserotropic velogenic Newcastle disease (VVND), also called exotic Newcastle disease, a highly fatal poultry disease, is carried by parrots and other wild birds. In some countries it is controlled by vaccination. Other countries attempt to exclude VVND by prohibiting importation of caged birds and maintaining bird-resistant biosecurity measures at commercial poultry farms.

Commercial livestock operations are at continual risk from diseases transmitted by rodents, free-ranging and captive wildlife, or feral animals and birds. These species are beyond human control and unavailable for testing.

Countries claiming disease-free status to meet export requirements can only certify the health of commercial livestock. For purposes of the disease reporting system maintained by the **Office International des Epizooties (OIE)**, countries may claim disease-free status when commercial operations are free of a specific disease. The OIE permits disease-free claims even if the infection is present in free-ranging species that don't commingle with commercial operations. This decision was reaffirmed in the mid-1990s. At that time, some delegates felt countries should not profess freedom from classical swine fever if it is present in feral swine populations or from **highly pathogenic avian influenza (HPAI)** if it is present in wild birds. The subject was revived in 2002 when a plan of an OIE working commission included developing a new status of "disease-free with the disease present in wild populations". Several years may pass before the issue is resolved.

Livestock health requirements are increasingly employed as barriers to trade. LHP-makers will be challenged to understand the role of free ranging and captive wildlife and feral species in transmission of livestock diseases.

Globalization Movement and LHPs

Globalization is the thesis that ever-increasing populations and global shrinking in terms of real-time distances support a "one world" concept. Ideally, globalization closes gaps between production and consumption points and between ecologically distinct regions. It balances economic opportunities in a world moving toward incentive-driven economies. As expressed in the goals of the United Nations, the General Agreement on Tariffs and Trade (GATT), the International Monetary Fund (IMF), the World Bank, and the World Health Organization, free trade and investment in poorer regions by economically vibrant countries will permit the strengths of one region to counterbalance the weaknesses of others, encourage economic opportunity, increase national incomes and employment rates, reduce starvation, and increase standards of living worldwide.

Obstacles to the success of globalization include cultural objections to competitive markets or incentive-driven lifestyles; the failure of formerly socialist, newly independent nations to make the transition to free-market economies; the hopelessness of poverty stricken, virtually bankrupt countries who see little hope of rescue; and corruption and graft in some economies.

Critics of globalization represent labor interests, proponents of isolationism, and activists who stage unfocused protests at WTO, IMF, and other international meetings in opposition to free trade, capitalism, big business, racism, war, environmental degradation, AIDS-control investments, and the foreign policies of their home countries. This discord not withstanding, the globalization movement appears to be struggling forward with minimal signs of total reversal. Like other sectors of the global economy livestock industries are impacted by the implications of globalization.

Formation of the Sanitary and Phytosanitary (SPS) Agreement of the World Trade Organization (WTO)

A globalization-related turning point for the international livestock health community occurred in the mid-1990s with the development of the SPS Agreement of the WTO. It outlined principles for the development of health requirements imposed on livestock products moving in international trade. Its sanitary provisions were designed to limit the spread of livestock diseases and protect animal and human health.

In the twenty-first century, the WTO SPS Agreement will be a major reference point for every livestock health decision. Its principles are detailed in chapter 5. They must be understood by national animal health regulators, the leadership of livestock industries, the veterinary profession, and other stakeholders.

The General Agreement on Tariffs and Trade (GATT), begun in 1947, was intended to reduce trade barriers, stimulate international commerce, and increase incomes and employment throughout the world. The GATT now has over 120 signatory countries and multiple commodity agreements that occupy over 20,000 pages. Sections governing agricultural products, introduced in the 1986 Uruguay Round of the GATT, were developed to reduce tariffs, increase international trade in agricultural products, and eliminate the use of sanitary measures as artificial trade barriers. The GATT agricultural agreements were signed in 1994 and ratified by the U.S. Congress and most member countries in 1995.

Also in 1995 the WTO was established and empowered by GATT-signatory nations. It serves as the international governing body to implement and adjudicate all GATT provisions. The WTO codified the GATT agricultural agreements into the WTO SPS Agreement. This agreement respects the sovereign rights of nations and makes sanitary requirements the prerogative of recipient countries. In so doing it outlines the rights, responsibilities, and obligations of countries pursuing international trade.

The WTO SPS agreement requires that SPS measures be transparent, equitably applied without discrimination (national treatment), scientifically sound, risk-assessment based, applicable on a regional basis, undertaken in recognition of the fact that equal levels of risk mitigation can be achieved by differing sanitary measures (equivalence), and guided by international standards. These principles are discussed in detail in chapter 5.

Soon after its establishment, the WTO designated the OIE as the organization responsible for international standards for livestock health. For several decades, the OIE had published standards for the international movement of livestock and livestock products.

The SPS Agreement revolutionized global trade in animals and animal products and altered livestock production and processing practices. Some provisions of the agreement are controversial and variously interpreted by nations struggling to protect their livestock industries in a competitive free-market economy.

Scientifically Based Sanitary Measures and the Precautionary Principle

A strenuously debated provision of the GATT agricultural agreement was the requirement that import regulations be based on sound science. Some countries opposed this provision because of constant changes, multiple uncertainties, and continual debate within the scientific community as to what constitutes good science. One such issue involves proving negative hypotheses such as establishing that a drug or feed additive will not produce delayed harmful effects. The counter position, which ultimately prevailed in GATT deliberations, was that without some requirement for scientifically based requirements, nations would be free to invoke baseless trade barriers to protect non-competitive industries. Without requiring a transparent scientific basis, supporters contend, countries could invoke import restrictions that counteract the objectives of GATT and the WTO.

After ratification of the SPS Agreement, opponents of sound-science provisions sidestepped them by invoking the previously rejected **precautionary principle**. The precautionary principle evolved in Germany in the 1970s. At that time it was suggested that the dying of the trees in the Black Forest was due to acid rain from power-plant emissions. In absence of proof to the contrary, the German government regulated emissions based on *vorsorge*, translated "forecaring." Soon *vorsorgeprinzip*, the "forecaring" or precautionary principle, emerged and found other applications in food safety and public health. In international trade, the precautionary principle states that if unproven risks are suggested, the importing country can exclude a product until there is scientific proof of its safety. The precautionary principle is rejected by most countries but occasionally invoked when scientific uncertainty exists (see Discussion Topic 6).

The EU excluded U.S. beef from cattle fed growth hormone (see Discussion Topic 1). The United States is a supporter of science-based sanitary requirements and an opponent of precautionary measures. Despite this, the United States did exclude ruminant offal from livestock feeds and prohibit blood donations from people who had spent over six months in Great Britain as precautionary measures to prevent the introduction of BSE, VCJD, or other TSEs.

The WTO SPS provisions can also be sidestepped by misinterpretation, improper translation, innocent or intentional ignorance, mistaken claims of disease freedom, and a failure of higher authorities to accept agreements negotiated by veterinary authorities. These transgressions can result if trade officials are unfamiliar with animal diseases. They can also occur intentionally to achieve trade advantages or protectionist objectives. They may accomplish short-term advantages but usually damage the integrity and future trade potential of perpetrating countries (see Discussion Topic 5).

Prerogatives Surrounding the WTO SPS Principles and International Standards

The WTO SPS Agreement provides general guidelines for international trade measures. Disease-and-commodity-specific standards appear in the *OIE International Health Code* (OIE 2001). Most nations expect their trading partners to adhere to these guidelines and standards.

Nations may impose any sanitary requirements necessary to protect their livestock, poultry, wildlife, and human populations from disease as long as the principles of the WTO SPS Agreement are fulfilled without discrimination or arbitrary and unjustified differences. Countries can impose import measures exceeding OIE standards if they are justified scientifically.

The WTO SPS principles provide an equivalent of the Ten Commandments, or a "golden rule," for international trade in livestock products. Like those guidelines, they are subject to interpretation and abuse and those not complying eventually pay the price. The result of blatant disregard of the WTO SPS Agreement is loss of international credibility and of the trust of trading partners.

Success in international trade requires that LHP-makers understand and comply with these expectations, which are detailed in chapter 5.

Growing Public Concern About Animal Welfare

There was mounting public involvement in animal welfare issues toward the end of the twentieth century. These activities focused on preservation of endangered species, reduction of animal abuse, control of research on animals, and improvement of livestock management (see Discussion Topic 3). These concerns added a further dimension and new interest groups to LHPs. They involve humane care by animal owners and welfare regulations by local and national governments. More extreme proposals came from groups opposing meat consumption or supporting granting animals rights comparable to humans. In an effort to be proactive the Cattle Care Working Group of the National Cattlemen's Beef Association developed animal care guidelines (Rossman and Foster 2002). These include

- Providing basic care including adequate feed, water, and disease prevention
- Safe and humane facilities for restraint and movement of livestock
- Approved methods for euthanasia of sick or injured animals

- Training workers in proper care and handling of livestock
- Monitoring to assure that basic needs of animals are met
- Transportation that avoids undue stress
- Staying updated on advances in the industry
- Refusing to tolerate mistreatment of animals

Other livestock organizations have developed similar guidelines in response to requests by fast-food chains to undertake science-based improvements in the humane conditions for rearing food animals. This trend is expanding to international markets, some of which are considering requiring audited certifications that livestock products originate from animals produced under humane conditions.

In the United States there is some concern that welfare policies, particularly for animals used in research, may be imposing regulatory burdens without clearly benefiting the animals (Anonymous 2002). The extension of rights to animals has generated international philosophical and ethical debates that involve discussions of the natural predator-prey hierarchy, the reasoning and pain-perception abilities of the species, and laws of survival of the fittest (Pollan 2002).

Growing Consumer Concern About Food Safety

There has been a revolution in public concern about food safety. This was sparked by an expansion of the meat-packing industry and new mass-marketing strategies that permitted widespread single-source outbreaks of food-borne illnesses demanding investigation. Improved case-finding activities that permit tracing of common source epidemics have intensified the food-safety focus.

These activities were expedited by newer techniques for the identification and diagnosis of food-borne pathogens like ***Listeria monocytogenes***, ***E. coli* O157:H7**, ***Camplobacteria,*** and new ***Salmonella*** strains.

The seriousness of food-borne diseases was compounded by expanding numbers of people with suppressed immune systems resulting from aging populations, growing numbers of HIV-infected individuals, and increasing use of chemotherapy and irradiation for cancer or to prevent rejection of grafts or transplants.

In the face of increasing media coverage of food-borne outbreaks and product recalls, attention focused on the packing industry and spawned the **hazard analysis critical control point (HACCP)** meat inspection program (see chapter 2).

Later, the realization that food-borne bacteria are present when animals and poultry arrive at slaughter generated the "farm-to-fork" approach to food safety. The farm-to-fork emphasis covers meat, milk, and eggs, but it addresses the fact that fruits and vegetables also carry **pathogens** and points out the need for kitchen sanitation.

The search for a food-safety magic bullet will continue endlessly. It will provide media with finger-pointing opportunities, researchers with funds, epidemiologists with outbreaks to investigate, and LHP-makers with endless challenges. Food-borne diseases will continue, because the causative organisms not only survive in human and animal gastrointestinal tracts but almost anywhere. They adjust to changing environments and antimicrobial drugs.

People generally ignore warnings about risk reduction. Laws and regulations will not keep bacteria from multiplying and mutating or stop people, poultry, wildlife, and livestock from defecating. Throughout the farm-to-fork food chain, all possible risk-reduction measures are essential. Most importantly, homemakers and kitchen workers must

- Scrub hands with antiseptic soap before handling food
- Scrub hands, dry with paper towels, and use the towels to shut off faucets and open the door after using bathrooms.
- Cook poultry, fish, and meat, particularly patties, till very well done
- Thoroughly rinse raw produce
- Keep poultry, meat, or fish from contacting other foods
- Thoroughly wash counters, cutting boards, utensils, and dishes that contact uncooked poultry, meat, or seafood before using them again
- Immediately freeze or refrigerate leftover foods and discard them if not used within two days
- Discard any food that has been at room temperature for more than three hours or over 80 degrees Fahrenheit for 90 minutes

The subject of food safety comes up in almost every aspect of LHP. It is mentioned in a slightly different context in every chapter of this book (see Discussion Topic 2).

Growing Concern About the Environment

The global movement to restore the environment that humankind has ravaged for centuries attained crisis proportions at the end of the twentieth century. The environmental movement has impacted every economic sector and the history of environmental issues indicates that every future LHP action must consider potential environmental impacts.

Concerns about the environmental impact of livestock operations arose from housing developments moving into rural areas, farm size expanding, livestock numbers increasing, and forests and prairies being replaced with crops, livestock, and human densities comparable to the industrially polluted urban areas new homeowners had hoped to escape.

The expanding livestock industries were increasingly forced to address environmental issues like manure handling, carcass disposal, odors, and the pollution of ground water with nitrates, phosphorous, ammonia, pesticides, pathogenic microorganisms, and antimicrobial compounds.

Pressures on livestock industries came from environmental groups who sometimes joined forces with animal welfare or food-safety interests. Most of these groups raised legitimate issues, but some have a long-term hidden agenda such as achieving a vegetarian society.

The increased focus on agricultural damage to the environment shifted the focus away from industrial pollution, overextended municipal sewerage systems, malfunctioning septic tanks, goose droppings, and tobacco smoke. The chemical, microbial, and toxic contamination of lakes and rivers comes from the collective contributions of industrial emissions, ineffective human-sewerage disposal systems, burgeoning solid waste problems, fertilizer runoffs, and wildlife, bird, and livestock excrement. Solving these challenges will require comprehensive approaches like the farm-to-fork food-safety movement.

Application of Epidemiology and Risk Analysis to Livestock Health Disciplines

The dynamics of globalization and the focus on population medicine, public health, and changing public perceptions of risk set the stage for epidemiology and risk analysis to emerge as livestock health disciplines. Policy makers need a basic understanding of epidemiology if they are to function effectively in the livestock health sector.

Epidemiology is a branch of medical science that records the distribution of diseases, infections, test results, or other health-related attributes in populations. It explains the observed patterns and applies the conclusions to disease-control strategies (Last 1983). In literal interpretation of its Greek root words, *epi* (upon), *demos* (people), and *ology* (the study of), epidemiology means the study of that which falls upon the people.

Epidemiology has been used in medicine since the mid 1800s. In the first half of the twentieth century the term "epizootiology," which replaces *demos* (people) with *zoo* (animal), was promoted to distinguish veterinary epidemiology from medical epidemiology. The term **epizootiology** was not widely accepted and the term "veterinary epidemiology" is commonly used instead. The terms **epizootic,** for an outbreak of disease in animals, and **enzootic,** for an entrenched disease in animal populations, persist and are frequently used.

In the early twentieth century livestock owners and veterinarians focused on treatment of individual animals. As herd and flock sizes increased emphasis on individuals gave way to group concerns, and herd and flock health became a major part of food-animal medical practice and management. Today academic and regulatory veterinarians utilize epidemiology, and livestock practitioners function as field epidemiologists. Epidemiology was introduced into U.S. veterinary college curricula in the early 1960s.

In livestock medicine, epidemiologic approaches are used to evaluate sickness, infections, deaths, abortions, positive test results, or production data. These attributes are evaluated in terms of time (temporal distribution), place (spatial or geographic distribution), and individual characteristics of affected and unaffected individuals or populations. Epidemiologic analysis involves comparing affected and unaffected groups with each other and with exposure to potential risk factors to determine the basis for disease. In simpler terms, recording and analyzing who has a disease, when they had the disease, and where they had the disease will reveal why they had the disease and identify measures needed to prevent recurrences.

Applications of epidemiologic strategies to livestock health include field investigations of herd problems, statistically designed surveys, and long-term population studies. Epidemiologic analyses must be conducted systematically and without predetermined conclusions.

Outbreak investigations combine the knowledge of veterinary epidemiologists, experienced clinicians, and skilled laboratory workers to determine the cause, source, and extent of livestock disease outbreaks or production shortfalls.

Long-term epidemiological methods include **serological** surveys, risk analyses, vaccine field trials, cohort studies, case control studies, and longitudinal population studies. These are usually conducted by academic or regulatory personnel to evaluate preventive strategies or seek causal relationships between potential risk factors and disease prevalence.

The results of epidemiological studies are used to prioritize livestock disease-control and research expenditures, determine efficiency of production practices, and evaluate the effectiveness of drugs and vaccines and the accuracy of claims of disease freedom. They require elaborate preplanning to assure efficient resource utilization, appropriate sample sizes, and unbiased sampling procedures. Statisticians must be involved initially and throughout these projects to clarify hypotheses, determine appropriate statistical methods, and analyze data.

Statistically designed long-term epidemiological studies are sometimes more applicable to human medicine than livestock health. In animals hypothesized associations between risk factors and diseases can be evaluated by controlled experiments. These experiments are not possible in human studies and are discouraged in many countries where animal-rights groups wield influence.

Descriptive, or qualitative, and analytic, or quantitative, epidemiological methods are applicable to livestock diseases. They have broad utility in private practice, regulatory medicine, diagnostic services, academic research, and trade activities.

In contrast to human medicine, where the focus is on individuals thus leaving population medicine to public health authorities, livestock medicine focuses on herds and flocks. The USDA, recognizing the need for institutionalizing this approach, established a **Center for Epidemiology and Animal Health**

(CEAH) at Fort Collins, Colorado, in the 1980s. The CEAH conducts epidemiological studies, interprets animal-disease monitoring and surveillance data, evaluates and plans disease-control programs and conducts analytical risk assessments.

Epidemiological methods are used in regulatory programs to maintain healthy domestic populations, exclude exotic diseases, investigate livestock health emergencies, and conduct **monitoring, surveillance, and reporting (MS&R)** activities. MS&R systems are needed to prioritize resource utilization and fulfill expectations of domestic stakeholders and the international community (Kahrs 1999).

In food-animal practice herd or flock population considerations overshadow the diagnosis and treatment of individual animals. Veterinary practitioners increasingly focus on preventive medicine and use epidemiologic questioning techniques and data analysis to customize livestock health programs, management, and feeding practices.

Veterinary diagnostic laboratories support epidemiologic activities of practitioners, regulators, and academicians by providing specific diagnoses. Diagnostic laboratories can be most helpful and conduct the most appropriate tests when a thorough epidemiologic history accompanies each specimen. In academic research epidemiological data provide focused questions for experimental studies.

MS&R systems and risk analysis apply epidemiologic techniques to livestock health. They are crucial to the success of domestic disease-control programs and international trade.

Monitoring implies general observation of the total health status of populations and the programs that oversee them.

Surveillance focuses on inspection, testing, and reporting activity for specific diseases. Active surveillance involves regular summarization of test results and inspection reports for programs like brucellosis and tuberculosis eradication. Passive surveillance is less focused and involves testing of specimens collected for other purposes and follow-up on suspected cases.

Reporting involves summarization and transmission of health and disease information to multiple stakeholders, the international community, and everyone involved in the data generation, collection, and funding. In participatory societies the reporting function is a key determinant of support for animal health programs. Transparent disease reporting assures international credibility.

The importance of any livestock disease depends on its economic impact, **zoonotic** potential, geographic distribution, and prevalence. The estimated incidence of livestock diseases is often proportional to the intensity of case-finding activities. This means that countries aggressively seeking a disease will often find it.

Epidemiologists strive to avoid the drawing of false conclusions by reducing bias and standardizing terminology. For example, they distinguish between incidence, that is the number of new cases in a measured population in a given time period, and prevalence, or total existing cases or positive tests, both old and new, at a given point in time. Epidemiologists also distinguish between mortality rates, which express proportions of a given population dying from a specific disease over time, and fatality rates, which express the proportion of affected individuals succumbing from a specific disease, epidemic, or disaster.

Fundamental Concepts in the Epidemiology of Livestock Diseases

Other epidemiologic concepts expand on the who, when, and where equation. Livestock disease is frequently explained in terms of simple cause-and-effect relationships, diseases of multifactorial **etiology**, the "disease iceberg analogy," and agent-host-environment interactions.

Simple cause-and-effect relationships between animals and pathogenic agents explain only a few diseases. Others follow intricate pathways involving several causative influences.

The concept of multifactorial etiology says diseases result from complex interactions of host characteristics, pathogenic agents, and environmental influences.

The disease iceberg analogy compares infectious diseases to icebergs. The submerged portion of an iceberg supports the visible iceberg. Similarly there are unobserved agent-host-environment interactions that push infections to a point where there are observed signs, symptoms, or deaths. In this analogy the water's surface represents the clinical threshold, and the observed disease is just the tip of the iceberg. Monitoring and surveillance can lower the clinical threshold by exposing otherwise unobserved disease factors.

Agent-host-environment interactions are challenging to sort out, as is the case when attempting to analyze the ecological requirements of vectors of insect-borne infections. The agent characteristics that influence infectious diseases are pathogenicity, transmissibility, and the ability to establish **persistent infections.** Pathogenicity is the ability to produce detectable disease or **lesions**. The comparative degree of pathogenicity is called virulence.

Transmissibility is the capacity to spread. Communicable diseases transmitted by direct or indirect contact are called contagious diseases. Vector-borne diseases require an intermediate host, usually insects, to transmit infection, a susceptible population, and threshold levels of competent vectors. The survival of disease-producing agents in nature influences the transmissibility of the disease and is a function of their resistance to disinfectants and environmental conditions.

Host characteristics reflect those of populations and individuals including age, breed, sex, and immune status. Aside from immune status, age is probably the most important host factor influencing the outcome of infections. For example, in the protected uterine environment the fetus is vulnerable to transplacental infections. Little data are available on the effect of breed and gender on the outcome of livestock infections. However, the environment imposed on certain breeds can be a factor as with the aggregation of animals in feedlots.

Use of age, gender, and breed distribution in the investigation of disease outbreaks to compare the characteristics of sick versus unaffected animals provides clues to the source of problems and suggests control strategies. Age, gender, and breed often dictate modes of housing and lead to identification of spatial differences in disease distribution. When combined with environmental factors the tabulation of these traits among affected and unaffected animals provides a template for a systematic investigation of outbreaks (Kahrs 1978) and for developing regulatory strategies.

Immunity and susceptibility are key determinants of the outcome of exposure or infection. There is a relationship between age and susceptibility to infections. Age often differentiates between **active immunity**, imparted by vaccination or natural exposure, and **passive immunity**, acquired by injection of immune serum or by nursing the first milk, or colostrum, of an immune mother. Passive immunity dissipates, and passively immune individuals soon revert to susceptibility unless exposed or vaccinated.

Population immunity, expressed as the percentage of individuals possessing some degree of protection from previous exposure or vaccination, can be measured by serologic surveys. As immunity waxes and wanes in populations the probability of the successful reintroduction of infections rises and falls as does the likelihood of infections causing clinical signs. Population immunity is influenced by the stresses of aggregation and the rate of new entries into a herd or flock.

Environmental factors are significant determinants of the outcome of infections in both individuals and populations. They include weather, stress levels, quality and quantity of available feed and water, and population density.

Stress results from foul weather, immigration, socialization, pecking order realignment, and adjusting to new environments. Aggregation of animals enhances the pathogenic effects of infections that could be insignificant in healthy, well-nourished, unstressed animals in established social systems.

Management practices also influence economic losses associated with infectious diseases. Drainage, moisture levels in areas where animals are housed, timely removal of manure and uneaten feed, and activities to eliminate crowding of animals all influence the incidence of disease in livestock.

Availability of feed and water and nutritional status directly impact the outcome of exposure to infections. Central feeding and watering areas expedite animal-to-animal transmission. Anxiety and apprehension associated with competition for water and feed contribute to infectious diseases. Introduction of new animals into populations, regardless of the size or density of those populations, results in stress and the incidence of new infections.

Population size and density and associated stresses help determine the outcome of infections. Extreme crowding increases the mortality rates from infectious diseases.

The complexity of the agent-host-environment interactions influencing livestock diseases complicates their diagnosis, control, prevention, and the assessment of associated risks. These complexities require that livestock diseases be addressed on a population basis. Investigation of outbreaks and the development of control strategies are best undertaken using tested epidemiologic approaches.

Risk Analysis

Risk analysis originated as a statistical engineering approach to construction standards. It compares the strength of materials to estimated possible stresses. It functions effectively where quantitative measures of risks and risk-mitigating procedures are available to permit the calculation of the likelihood of failure.

Risk analysis loses precision when applied to biological systems, because they are hard to quantify and subject to unpredictable variability. Nonetheless, biologic risk analysis is a far superior alternative than its antithesis, which is either a total lack of standards or the routine application of the precautionary principle.

Risk analysis gained LHP prominence in the 1990s when the WTO SPS Agreement decreed that sanitary measures imposed on imports must follow international standards or be based on scientifically sound risk analyses. In animal health circles, risk analysis comprises risk assessment, risk management, and risk communication.

Risk assessment is an epidemiological approach to livestock health decision making, disease-control programs, and import regulations. It can be very simple or very complex depending on the method selected and the political sensitivity of the issue involved.

Import risk assessments are used to justify import measures that are more stringent than international standards. At a minimum, import risk assessments should:

- Define acceptable levels of quantitative or qualitative risk before proceeding
- Identify the risks, or diseases, potentially associated with commodities proposed for importation
- Estimate the likelihood that the proposed import can introduce each disease in question

- Estimate the likelihood that the exporting country has each disease in question
- Estimate the likelihood that the proposed import can introduce each disease in question given conditions in the exporting country
- Identify and estimate the chances that once introduced the disease in question can become established in the recipient country

Because zero risk is unattainable, past strategies of attempting to eliminate all risk are being replaced by determinations of acceptable levels of disease-specific risk. Acceptable level of risk is sometimes called acceptable level of protection. Countries have sovereign rights to unilaterally establish acceptable levels of protection, but the international community has yet to agree on the definition of an acceptable level.

Import risk assessments also outline risk-management or risk-mitigating measures such as processing, testing, or quarantines that can permit the import to occur safely and at the same time meet the importing country's acceptable level of protection.

When **quantitative risk assessments** are conducted, acceptable levels of risk can be expressed numerically. For example, a 1:1,000,000 likelihood of introducing and establishing one disease agent may be acceptable to an importing country while a 1:100,000,000 risk may be deemed the minimum acceptable risk for a second disease.

Acceptable levels of risk may also be expressed non-numerically. For example, a country may choose to accept an import if it determines qualitatively that the risk is negligible. For **qualitative risk assessments**, it is necessary to establish a continuum of risk levels. For any proposed import risk, levels can be rated as maximum risk, high risk, moderate risk, low risk, slight risk, or negligible risk. The criteria for each category should be defined in terms of origin factors, destination factors, and disease factors.

Origin factors include the disease prevalence and characteristics of the animal health infrastructure including the monitoring and surveillance systems, diagnostic capacity, and border security in the exporting country. Destination factors include the intended use and distribution of the import, which determines the potential for entry, establishment, and eradication of a disease in the recipient country. Disease factors include pathogenicity, transmissibility, and economic impact of a disease. Risk communication involves documentation and transparency of formal risk analyses and the application of risk management procedures in domestic livestock populations.

LHP-makers need some understanding of epidemiology and risk analysis. Disease prevention and exclusion strategies require proactive population-based approaches, because individual animal treatments are frequently impractical, inefficient, ineffective, or too late.

The Age of Information Technology (IT)

In the early and mid 1990s, LHPs were hampered by the paperwork required to develop, implement, oversee, and disseminate transparent regulations in a complex livestock health environment. The paperwork challenge offered excuses for regulatory agencies with non-communicative cultures to limit the transparency of controversial activities.

The development of computers and wireless communications in the closing decades of the 1900s brought visions of IT miracles. The age of IT permitted rapid collection, analysis, storage, and dissemination of data and information. The advent of the Internet, and ready availability of web sites, provided opportunities for anyone wishing to communicate. It suggested the mountain of paperwork would disappear. Previously non-communicative individuals and organizations could now reach out. But would they?

The IT age presents an opportunity for rapid and simplified collection, sorting, storage, and dissemination of clinical and diagnostic information, regulations, standards, and certificates for the interstate and international movement of livestock and products.

The vision of an immediate communication miracle faces major challenges. These challenges were underestimated until efforts were made to coordinate the use of IT. This has required cooperation among multiple organizations using different hardware, software, vocabularies, and programs. In cultures where non-communication is ingrained, the fighting of turf wars over regulatory authorities, conflicting goals, and funding has compounded communication problems.

Emergence of **Genetically Modified Organisms (GMOs)**

GMOs entered the LHP arena in recent decades. This innovation represented a significant upgrade in technologic sophistication and introduced challenging and controversial new issues.

GMOs are plants, animals, or microorganisms altered by genetic intervention, or genetic engineering. These procedures adjust the genetic sequences that control inheritance, protein synthesis, metabolism, reproduction, growth, and disease, drug, or insecticide resistance.

Strictly speaking, GMOs and new species appear continually in nature via the long-known processes of mutation, environmental adaptation, breeding, inbreeding, and cross breeding. However, conventional usage confines the term to indicate alterations achieved by human manipulation of genes.

Molecular techniques for genetic intervention, such as gene insertions or deletions, gene splicing, *in vitro* fertilization, cloning, and others appeared rapidly toward the end of the century. They became entrenched in agricultural technology before concerned individuals, interest groups, and regulatory officials knew what happened. Animals have been used for all these processes, but the most widespread applications and vehement controversies have involved plant products. When plant GMOs are fed to animals, LHPs enter the mix.

Supporters of GMOs consider them the greatest advance in food production the world has ever known and as offering hope in feeding its starving people. Opponents, mostly European, who apply the precautionary principle and strive to preserve non-competitive small-farm economies, believe GMOs could possibly induce health or environmental problems.

The advent of, and controversy surrounding, GMOs has widened trade gaps between the United States and the EU, and is symptomatic of the challenges presented by the pivotal events of the past three decades. These are the events that will mold LHPs in the new millennium (see chapter 7).

Bibliography

Anonymous. 2002. Resolved, to Help Prevent Imposition of Needless Regulatory Burdens. *Am Jour Vet Research* 63(9):1217-1218.

CDC. 1998. *Emerging Infectious Diseases: A Strategy for the Twenty-first Century*. Atlanta, GA: National Center for Infectious Diseases, National Center for Disease Control and Prevention. www.cdc.gov

CDC. 2002. *Emerging Infectious Diseases: A Peer Reviewed Journal Tracking and Analyzing Disease Trends*. Atlanta, GA: National Center for Infectious Diseases, National Center for Disease Control and Prevention. www.cdc.gov

Kahrs, R. F. 1978. Techniques for Investigating Outbreaks of Livestock Disease. *J Am Vet Med Assoc.* 173:101–103.

Kahrs, R. F. 1999. The International Animal Health Community's Expectations of the U.S. National Animal Health Reporting System (NAHRS). *Proc U.S. Anim Health Assoc.* 103:100-109.

Last, J. M., ed. 1983. *A Dictionary of Epidemiology*. New York: Oxford University Press.

Marsh, R. F. 1990. Bovine Spongiform Encephalopathy in the United States. *J. Am. Vet Med Assoc.* 196:1677.

OIE 2001. *The OIE International Animal Health Code.* 9th ed. Paris: Office International des Epizooties.

Pollan, M. 2002. The Unnatural Idea of Animal Rights: An Animal's Place. *New York Times Magazine* (November 14):58-66.

Rossman, M. and H. Foster. 2002. Who's To Say? Corporate America, Worried About Consumer Reaction, Is Paying More Attention to How You Raise Your Livestock. *Beef Today* (August):13-16.

Wrathrall, A. E., K. D. F. Brown, A. R. Sayers, et al. 2002. Studies of Embryo Transfer from Cattle Clinically Affected by Bovine Spongiform Encephalopathy (BSE). *Veterinary Record* (150): 365-378.

Chapter 4

Components of Effective Livestock Health Infrastructures

INTRODUCTION

Every nation needs a **livestock health infrastructure** as a permanent basis and cohesive guiding force for livestock health, food-safety, and international marketing programs. An infrastructure is a crucial element in the livestock health policies (LHPs) of every country.

In most countries national veterinary services oversee domestic livestock health activities, international livestock trade, and some food-safety matters. Subnational agencies, livestock and veterinary organizations, the academic and diagnostic communities, and individual stakeholders are indispensable players in these programs.

Food-safety agencies inspect food-processing facilities and test foods for contaminating organisms and residues. Food-inspection activities are often administered by the same organizations that oversee livestock health programs and these two functions must be integrated.

International marketing activities are divided among livestock brokers, food processors, representatives of national and subnational governments, and animal and plant health officials who establish import and export requirements. Livestock health infrastructures are crucial to international marketing success.

Livestock health infrastructures are most successful when they involve **stakeholders** in decision making. Stakeholders, that is parties with vested interests, include livestock producers, industries that process livestock products, and producers of veterinary pharmaceuticals, **antimicrobials**, and vaccines. They also include subnational animal health officials, the academic and diagnostic communities, ancillary special interest groups, trading partners, and national and international veterinary and food-safety organizations.

National livestock health agencies usually operate on restricted budgets and compete for funding with other critical national needs. Even if they have limited capacity to implement the activities involved in maintaining livestock health, they need to understand them.

It is crucial for national veterinary services and food-safety agencies to have clearly defined missions, logically organized operational structures, adequate funding, and legal authority to promulgate and enforce regulations. These resources are needed to protect the country's livestock, exclude **exotic diseases**, shield the public from food-borne and zoonotic diseases, and maintain foreign markets for livestock products.

Functional livestock health infrastructures face many challenges. They must:

- Gain the support of livestock owners and veterinary professionals who comprise the first line of defense against livestock diseases
- Provide a network of diagnostic laboratories with personnel and facilities capable of determining the exact cause of disease outbreaks in time to prevent economic disasters
- Maintain national eradication or control programs for selected domestic diseases
- Establish disease **monitoring, surveillance, and reporting (MS&R) systems**
- Maintain a national animal identification (ID) system
- Provide border security, emergency disease programs, and information management systems
- Provide regulatory oversight of animal drugs and **biologicals**
- Support a network of subnational livestock health programs that cooperate in national endeavors

The infrastructure should be a cooperative, closely knit partnership among livestock producers, processors, sustaining industries, the academic and diagnostic communities, and the nation's veterinary profession.

Animal health infrastructures establish the credibility of national governments within domestic and international animal health communities. They determine the success of each nation's livestock health and food-safety programs. The strength and integrity of a country's livestock health infrastructure are primary criteria for decision-making by domestic consumers and importers of livestock products.

It is the responsibility of LHP-makers to provide resources and authority to permit successful program implementation and management by knowledgeable professionals with communication skills and leadership abilities. There should be periodic external reviews of livestock health programs.

Regulatory Organization, Authority, and Responsibility

Regulatory agencies and other governmental divisions responsible for livestock health and food safety must interact effectively with the political leaders of the home country. They must have authority, personnel, resources, and the desire to:

- Implement disease-control and eradication programs
- Oversee domestic movement of animals and enforce border control
- Levy user-fees needed for the administration of livestock-based **sanitary measures**
- Interact successfully with multiple stakeholders, interest groups, and the media
- Lead in management of livestock disease emergencies
- Maintain good relations with the livestock health and academic communities
- Maintain close affiliation with the local and subnational diagnostic laboratories
- Maintain control over high-security laboratories approved to handle exotic disease agents

In exchange for authority and resources, both national and subnational livestock health agencies must be held responsible for the health and security of the country's animals and the credibility of the nation's livestock products in the international marketplace. National and subnational livestock health agencies should be administered by veterinarians, biologists, and agriculturists that are experienced with livestock production practices and the complexities of animal health and disease.

Establishing a Permanent Presence of Vigilant Livestock Owners and Veterinarians

National livestock health infrastructures need the capacity to rapidly recognize and respond to livestock health emergencies. This capability will exist if livestock owners and their employees are imbued with an obligation to recognize and promptly report sickness in their flocks and herds. Livestock health officials and producer organizations need to offer continual reminders about danger signals and the necessity of obtaining prompt assistance. These reminders can emanate from educational programs, posters, flyers, or radio and television alerts. They need to be emphasized in courses in agriculture and veterinary medicine.

The first line of defense is activated when livestock workers contact veterinarians upon the appearance of sickness among animals. Many livestock diseases look alike. It is easy to mistake **foot-and-mouth-disease (FMD), rinderpest, classical swine fever, or viscerotrophic velogenic Newcastle disease** for common maladies in the early stages of outbreaks. At first glance FMD is identical in appearance to **vesicular stomatitis**, rinderpest is identical to **bovine viral diarrhea**, and classical swine fever mimics **African swine fever**. Veterinary practitioners may not initially suspect exotic conditions. It is easy to consider them common diseases until they fail to respond to initial treatments or spread more rapidly than expected. Such delays cause loss of valuable time.

Most exotic-disease investigations produce negative results. Livestock health officials must continually urge veterinarians to request help in suspicious situations. LHP-makers must make all possible efforts to stimulate vigilance.

Reporting incentives can include prompt return of results of laboratory tests and epidemiological investigations, awards for disease reporting, and official statements of support even if episodes are eventually determined to be non-emergency conditions.

Multijurisdictional National Authority for Livestock Health and Food Safety

The allocation of authority and responsibility for livestock health infrastructures is a function of the governmental style of each nation, the relationships between national and subnational governing bodies, the relationships of government agencies to the animal health community, and the degree to which public input is considered in each nation's legislative process.

It is essential to maintain a balance between two possible extremes of livestock health authority. At one extreme is a monocratic system with all authority vested in a single agency or individual. At the other extreme are widespread multiple authorities in which responsibilities are so dispersed that it is difficult to determine who is responsible.

Ideas regarding the extent of authority vested in national livestock health agencies will vary among regulators, academicians, and privately employed individuals. The challenge is to achieve a workable balance that fits the nation's style of governance and public participation in policy development. There are many regulations designed to protect the health of U.S. livestock, wildlife, and human populations. Federal jurisdiction over these responsibilities is shared among the United States Department of Agriculture (USDA) and other branches of the federal government. In some areas, these agencies have limited authority over states or territories.

The U.S. **Food and Drug Administration (FDA)** regulates pharmaceuticals, medical devices, and non-meat human edibles. The USDA **Food Safety and Inspection Service (FSIS)** controls the human health aspects of processing animal products, and the USDA **Animal and Plant Health Inspection Service (APHIS)** provides regulatory oversight of animal health. The jurisdiction over fish and fish products is divided among the FDA, the **U.S. Fish and Wildlife Service** and APHIS. In instances where missions overlap, the involved agencies must cooperate closely.

This division of labor gives agencies clearly defined missions, responsibilities, and authority, which enable them to focus their activities. It provides extensive checks and balances and minimizes the opportunity for corruption and graft.

Overlapping responsibilities can cause confusion over priorities, accountability, and limits of authority. Some bureaucratic confusion results from lack of inter-agency communication. Stakeholders and trading partners become frustrated when conflicting regulations are imposed, duplicative requirements must be met, or requests for information are repeatedly referred to other offices. Overlapping authorities can occasionally result in turf wars over jurisdictions or budget allocations.

Some countries grant authority for livestock health and food safety to a single agency or individual. These authorities can speak with one voice and respond rapidly to queries and emergencies. In such systems there is limited scientific debate, little room for dissent within the bureaucracy, and far more opportunity for corruption or graft.

Mutual Dependence of Food-Safety and Livestock Health Infrastructures

Food-safety infrastructures are inexorably linked to livestock health programs. In most countries meat inspection programs are supervised by an agriculture department that also regulates livestock health. In some countries, the director of agriculture or the **chief veterinary officer (CVO)** administers both food-safety and livestock health programs. In other countries these programs are distinct. There are advantages and disadvantages to both arrangements, as discussed above in the section on multijurisdictional authorities.

Meat inspection systems examine livestock carcasses in packing plants. The safety, quality, and wholesomeness of meat products is assured by checking for bacterial contamination, residues of hormones, antimicrobial drugs, feed additives, injection site blemishes, or lesions of diseases or injuries.

Meat inspection officials must work in synchrony with livestock health agencies. The meat inspection system is an integral part of each nation's livestock disease MS&R systems.

Tracing problem carcasses to the herd of origin requires an effective national **animal identification (ID)** system. Conditions recognized at slaughter by meat inspectors are key to national livestock disease-control and eradication programs. In the United States tuberculosis lesions recognized at slaughter support the **bovine tuberculosis** eradication effort, and blood specimens collected from cattle at slaughter are vital to the bovine **brucellosis** eradication program. Histopathological and histochemical examinations of brains, collected at slaughter or at diagnostic laboratories, are the basis of U.S. surveillance for **transmissible spongiform encephalopathies (TSEs).**

In the United States, multiple governmental agencies, each with a slightly different scientific perspective and legal authority, share responsibility for the safety of human foods. These include the health departments of individual states and federal departments such as USDA's FSIS and APHIS, the FDA, the Centers for Disease Control and Prevention (CDC) and the Environmental Protection Agency (EPA). There are discussions about forming a single agency to oversee all U.S. national food-safety programs. This suggestion has emerged because of concern over food-borne illness, most of which could be controlled by adequate refrigeration, proper cooking, and kitchen hygiene. There are an estimated 70 million human cases of food poisoning annually. These result in about 5000 fatalities, largely in aged people and those with impaired immune systems due to AIDS, chemotherapy, or neoplastic diseases. There seems to be a media-fed public and legislative frustration with the multiple agencies that seek funds for food-safety programs. Few agencies want full responsibility for the slow progress with a problem that exhausts over $30 billion of health care expenses annually and requires repetitive ongoing public education programs for consumers and food handlers. The reported high incidence of human food-borne illnesses in the United States as compared to other countries may be due to advanced diagnostic technology, high levels of reporting, media coverage, or lack of immunity that accompanies the constant exposure in many countries.

Food-borne disease results from ingestion of inadequately cooked foods that have been contaminated somewhere in the food chain. These organisms require specific conditions of temperature, moisture, and a nutrient environment to multiply into numbers adequate to produce illness. Most food-borne disease organisms have been known for decades. They are carried in the intestinal tracts of livestock and people. Mutants, variants, and newly emerged strains such as ***Camplobacteria, E. coli* O157:H7, *Listeria***, and drug-resistant ***Salmonella*** and ***Staphylococcus*** continue to appear. LHP-makers should be able to integrate the livestock health infrastructure with a "farm-to-fork" food-safety program that includes public education, improved food-handling methods, and cooperative regulatory programs.

Leadership of National and Subnational Livestock Health Agencies

Qualified leaders are essential for the successful development and implementation of LHPs. The leaders, whether appointed or elected, should be veterinarians or agricultural scientists who understand livestock management practices and have regulatory experience. As described in chapter 9, they also need interpersonal and communication skills to successfully interact with the livestock industry, local and national legislators, the general public, and the media.

Diagnostic Capacity

Diagnostic capacity is essential to operating disease-control and eradication programs, supporting livestock disease MS&R programs, and fulfilling the expectations of trading partners.

A functional diagnostic system can rapidly determine the cause and extent of livestock diseases. This requires facilities and personnel to perform:

- Tests to isolate and identify pathogenic agents including bacteria, fungi, viruses, and toxins
- Serologic tests to estimate the prevalence and geographic distribution of infectious diseases, certify animals for international movement, and evaluate the effectiveness of vaccines
- Post-mortem examinations on animals
- Microscopic examinations of tissues

Few laboratories have expertise and reagents to perform all known tests for all livestock diseases. Many prefer that veterinarians call for instructions about the availability of tests and the selection, collection, handling, packaging, and transportation of specimens.

Accredited diagnostic laboratories have trained scientists and technologists, support personnel, facilities, and resources to identify both common conditions and emerging diseases. These labs are monitored by laboratory accreditation boards, must pass proficiency tests, and can conduct validated tests in harmony with international standards. Such laboratories are crucial for the recognition of exotic diseases.

Diagnostic Laboratory Accreditation

Accrediting agencies monitor and evaluate diagnostic laboratories operated by universities, national or subnational governments, private contractors, or corporations. Accreditation assures that they meet minimal standards needed to:

- Accurately diagnose diseases

- Participate in disease-control or eradication programs
- Support national MS&R systems
- Conduct tests required for exports

Laboratory accreditation can be done by government agencies, independent organizations like the **American Association of Veterinary Laboratory Diagnosticians (AAVLD)**, or national veterinary medical associations. The accreditation process requires clearly documented standards, assay proficiency testing, and inspection procedures. Ideally, all animal disease diagnostic laboratories should be accredited. Sometimes corporate laboratories that use test results for internal purposes will forego accreditation.

Countries vary in the extent to which laboratory accreditation is required. Some countries merely mimic test procedures of other nations. Diagnostic services, reagents, and facilities need national oversight if test results are to be used in disease-control programs, food-safety activities, or international commerce. Some countries accept diagnostic test results for export certifications only if they are from nationally supervised laboratories.

The U.S. Animal Disease Diagnostic Laboratory Network

The United States has a network of APHIS-approved federal, state, and university laboratories including the National Veterinary Services Laboratories (NVSL) at Ames, Iowa; the Foreign Animal Disease Diagnostic Laboratory at Plum Island, NY; and state-operated facilities and laboratories at most colleges of veterinary medicine. This network provides diagnostic services for most livestock producers. College laboratories also provide training for veterinary students.

After the 2001 terrorist attacks and **anthrax** mailings, efforts were undertaken to strengthen the diagnostic network. The AAVLD urged a strengthening of the system by:

- Improving the security, reporting, and alert systems
- Standardizing the rapid diagnostic procedures at the state and national levels
- Upgrading laboratory equipment
- Training personnel in diagnosis of exotic, emerging, and zoonotic diseases
- Improving quality-assurance training and evaluation in laboratories
- Upgrading biocontainment capacities of taxpayer-supported laboratories
- Periodically running test exercises to sharpen the diagnostic, reporting, and response capacities of the laboratory network

Many laboratories accept samples only from veterinarians. This helps control the volume and quality of specimens and improves descriptions of the clinical signs exhibited by affected animals.

Most U.S. laboratories are partially supported by public funds but charge for diagnostic services requested by private veterinarians.

Validation of Diagnostic Tests

Test validations estimate the performance of laboratory procedures and determine their fitness for the detection and identification of infectious agents, toxins, antibodies, or DNA.

Antibodies indicate animals have responded immunologically to an agent. Antibodies take time to develop. They can be absent in the early stages of a disease but persist for months or years afterward. They are usually regarded as evidence of past exposure to infections or toxins. The presence of specific DNA indicates the organism was present in the animal when the specimen was collected.

There are many variables regarding test validation and many validation methods. These were detailed in a workshop on diagnostic test validation held at the 2002 AAVLD meeting (Elvinger and Thurman 2002). There is a lack of unanimity on the precise definition of a validated test. The scientific community considers a test validated if it is commonly used and generally accepted as producing consistent results in detecting the presence or absence of the **analate** in specimens. (Analates are substances detected by laboratory analysis.) Test validation is usually a two-step process involving bench and field determinations.

The Office International des Epizootices (OIE) publishes the *OIE Manual of Diagnostic Tests and Vaccines* (OIE 2000). Chapter 1.1.3 (OIE 2000) details five steps in test validation:

- Feasibility studies involving controls
- Development and standardization of reagent concentrations, protocol parameters, and repeatability
- Determining performance parameters, sensitivity and specificity, and selecting a gold-standard test for comparison
- Monitoring the validity of assay performance
- Continued maintenance and enhancement of the validation criteria

The **Association of Analytic Chemists (AOAC International),** a not-for-profit organization, works to standardize methods in chemistry and microbiology through validation of analytical methods, laboratory proficiency testing, training programs, and distribution of reference materials. The OIE and AOAC International strive to improve public trust in analytic methods used in disease diagnosis and food safety.

In 2001 the USDA FSIS and the AOAC International initiated a secure database of methods used in food analyses. This electronic compilation of analytic methods (e-CAM) contains details of methods for foods, feeds, drugs, and related international standards and regulatory methods. It is available by subscription.

In domestic diagnostic situations, there are a variety of tests and modifications used for local diseases. When countries require laboratory tests for international movement of livestock they frequently request validated tests described in the OIE manual.

Proficiency Testing for Accuracy of Laboratory Results

Diagnostic test results can become flawed amidst busy work schedules. External systems of checks and balances are valuable components of diagnostic laboratory networks.

Proficiency testing is an expensive and exacting procedure and is generally conducted by national laboratories. The central laboratory prepares a battery of coded specimens, sends them to laboratories, and requests results within a specified time. The submitting laboratory receives a report of test accuracy and suggestions for improvement. When substandard results are reported the laboratory staff is retrained in the procedure. Repeated failing evaluations can cause laboratories to lose the approval to perform certain tests or to lose accreditation.

The OIE has reference laboratories throughout the world. The national veterinary services of member countries can obtain test protocols, reagents, and advice from OIE reference laboratories and send staff to them for training.

Standardization and Harmonization of Diagnostic Tests

It is challenging to standardize diagnostic tests among veterinary laboratories because of variations in laboratory procedures and reagents. Some reagents are developed in laboratories and others are purchased from commercial firms whose products vary slightly from batch to batch. This variation can be reduced by proficiency testing, the use of validated diagnostic tests, sending specimens to other laboratories for confirmation, and the training of laboratory personnel.

Some livestock corporations own and operate their own diagnostic laboratories, thus reducing shipping time, turnaround time, and expenses. Corporate-owned laboratories aren't held to quotas on numbers of samples and they offer proprietary confidentiality not available at government or university laboratories, which are bound by freedom of information requirements.

In the international livestock health arena, standardization and harmonization of laboratory test procedures is challenging, because individual countries use different tests for the same disease. When several countries use the same test, there are often major differences in protocols, reagents, and results.

The OIE has made progress in standardizing and harmonizing tests used for international movement of livestock products. The OIE manual (OIE

2000) and reference laboratories offer hope for the gradual standardization of laboratory tests used in international trade.

Diagnostic Laboratories in Exotic-Disease Exclusion

Diagnostic laboratories play a crucial role in the detection and response to introductions of exotic diseases. If tests for common diseases prove negative, laboratory workers may be the first to sense the presence exotic diseases not suspected by livestock owners or their veterinarians. As discussed later in this chapter the diagnostic community is key to prompt emergency response.

Disease-Control and Eradication Systems

Disease-control and eradication programs can be undertaken on an individual site or at the state, provincial, regional, or national levels.

Programs undertaken at farms, ranches, feedlots, or poultry-rearing facilities are usually based on managerial practices and vaccinations. They focus on diseases of local importance, are free of government oversight, and may change from month to month.

Some livestock enterprises have well-coordinated management, health, and nutrition programs designed by professionals. Others have few such provisions. Often, local disease-control activities are initiated retrospectively in response to problems and rely on treatment rather than prevention. Herd or flock health programs based on prevention-oriented managerial practices or carefully chosen vaccination programs can be very effective.

Disease-control programs undertaken by subnational or national governments focus on infections of economic or public health significance. They require tax-supported resources, legal authority, and public cooperation. To be successful they require careful planning, participatory execution, effective administration, and adequate funding. They can be disrupted by insufficient oversight, lack of cooperation, or communication shortfalls.

Traditionally the most successful and most widely recognized livestock disease-control programs are undertaken by national governments. Their chances of success are greater if they are initiated at the urging of livestock producers who perceive a disease problem that cannot be successfully addressed locally. Diseases meeting in this category are usually contagious and difficult to control by individual livestock owners.

Before a national veterinary service attempts to force livestock producers into control or eradication programs, there are certain questions that must be addressed about the disease, the ecosystem, and the suggested program. These include financial implications, the level of support by the livestock industry and the general public, the level of authority possessed by the agencies involved, and the availability of domestic and wild species for testing.

Most livestock disease-control or eradication programs are conducted within national boundaries and overseen by veterinary officials of the involved country. There are provisions for establishing disease-free areas that deviate from national borders using a process called **regionalization**. The **World Trade Organization (WTO) Sanitary and Phytosanitary (SPS) Agreement** espouses trade-oriented regionalization by establishing disease-free areas comprising areas or groups of countries sharing common ecosystems (see chapter 5). To date this concept has had limited global application.

Characteristics of Controllable and Eradicable Diseases

Livestock diseases are candidates for control or eradication when they cause serious economic losses, are transmissible to people, or impact trade. Control programs try to reduce diseases to manageable and economically acceptable levels. Eradication implies total elimination of the disease and its causative agent from a territory.

In establishing national livestock health programs an initial goal of control is often more realistic than eradication, because unpredictable obstacles can surface after programs are initiated. When control efforts have been successful in reducing disease prevalence, and eradication appears feasible, the lessons learned can be applied to advance the program. National control programs require support and the active participation of subnational livestock health agencies and producer and processor organizations.

The United States has successfully eradicated **African horse sickness, contagious bovine pleuropneumonia, cattle tick fever, FMD, glanders, Venezuelan equine encephalomyelitis (VEE), screwworms,** classical swine fever, **swine vesicular disease, vesicular exanthema of swine, sheep scabies, highly pathogenic avian influenza (HPAI),** and velogenic viscerotrophic Newcastle disease. These diseases are now considered exotic.

The USDA has been working for almost 50 years to control bovine tuberculosis and bovine brucellosis but has not yet accomplished their eradication.

Some pathogenic organisms are more easily controlled and eradicated than others. The characteristics of diseases amenable to control efforts include manageable incubation periods, readily recognizable symptoms, the availability of diagnostic tests to identify the causative agent, and a lack of persistent infections in individual animals.

Before committing to eradication or control programs, policy makers and national veterinary services must carefully explore numerous criteria. The following questions should be answered:

- Is the disease endemic or exotic
- Is the disease economically important
- Is the disease transmissible to humans

- Does the disease infect multiple species of domestic animals
- Does the disease have reservoirs in free-ranging wild animals or birds
- Can the causative organism establish persistent infections that permit animals to serve as prolonged sources of infection
- Is there a simple, inexpensive, and reliable live animal or food-product test for detection of the disease agent
- Does the country have the capacity to conduct large-scale testing for the disease
- Do national and subnational livestock health agencies have adequate infrastructure, resources, and authority to undertake control or eradication along with current programs
- Does the proposed control or eradication program have the support of livestock producers
- Is there an effective vaccine for the disease that consistently induces a prolonged protective immunity
- Can inexpensive tests distinguish vaccine-induced immunity from antibodies produced in response to natural infections
- Is there a credible MS&R system in place for the disease
- Is there reasonable assurance of cooperation by subnational livestock health authorities
- Does the national veterinary service have adequate authority and resources to place restrictions on the movement of animals, products, and vehicles; to establish and enforce quarantines; to undertake seizure of infected animals; and to pay indemnities
- Are there clearly defined criteria for lifting quarantines from herds, flock, or areas

These questions should be addressed in public forums with a wide variety of interested parties before commitments for eradication or control programs are undertaken.

Monitoring, Surveillance, and Reporting (MS&R) Systems

Animal disease MS&R systems are essential for the maintenance of healthy and competitive livestock industries. They form the basis of **national animal health reporting systems (NAHRS)** and are essential for prioritizing livestock health, research, and regulatory programs.

Monitoring involves general oversight and awareness based on reports from diagnostic laboratories, investigation of suspicious outbreaks, and anecdotal reports.

Surveillance can be general oversight of the health of populations but usually focuses on specific diseases. Active surveillance is ongoing and aggressive. It follows standard protocols for identifying and tracking a disease using on-the-farm tests or analysis of specimens collected at slaughter. Some active surveillance involves searching for evidence, such as tubercles indicative of tuberculosis, in abattoirs. There is a fine line between active and passive surveillance.

Passive surveillance is disease-specific but less intense than active surveillance. It usually involves designating a condition as a reportable disease and investigating suspected outbreaks. The name passive is unfortunate, because it incorrectly implies officials are relaxing and waiting for something to happen.

Reporting is an indispensable component of monitoring and surveillance. Without transparent dissemination of disease information it can lie veiled in secrecy. This can undermine control efforts and the nation's credibility among domestic stakeholders, trading partners, and the global community.

Workable MS&R systems require a solid national infrastructure and reliable diagnostic capacity. They depend on cooperation from all segments of the national livestock industry and are principal determinants of its economic success.

In free market economies countries depend on the health and competitiveness of their livestock industry. In some nations the livestock industry is the key to economic survival. Competition for foreign markets is based on globally determined prices, fragile competitive advantages, and political relationships between trading nations. These realities are driven by global market conditions that are largely beyond the control of countries, governing bodies, or industries.

In this economic scenario, globally competitive livestock industries will survive. Those unable to compete will be relegated to subsistence agriculture or part-time farming operations. National governments may choose to subsidize non-competitive industries in response to political pressures to preserve traditional lifestyles, environmentally sound land utilization, or ecosystem stabilization efforts. Non-competitive livestock industries can impose a constant drain on the resources of their mother countries.

Some importing countries may forego competitively priced products in favor of buying from countries more conscious of animal health and food-safety issues, with credible NAHRS, animal ID systems, trace-back capacity, and consumer-conscious regulatory programs.

Animal health parameters for operating in the global marketplace are set by the WTO, the OIE, and the expectations of trading partners. They are inexorably linked to animal disease reporting systems. Present MS&R systems must differ from those of previous decades due to global competitiveness, changing trade paradigms, computerized communications technology, and increasing expectations of trading partners.

These realities translate into an urgent need for LHP-makers to redefine and reorganize their countries' NAHRSs.

Essentials of MS&R Systems

MS&R systems help prioritize research and regulatory programs and support international trade. They require the cooperation of all segments of national livestock industries including the diagnostic and regulatory communities and those involved with food safety and human health.

For an NAHRS to function effectively, a responsible agency must gather information from multiple sources, consolidate it into a single report, and distribute it in a form that is understandable domestically and internationally. Therefore NAHRSs require standard vocabularies, case definitions, electronic messaging, and animal identification (Case 1998).

Disease Categorizations for NAHRSs

There are several categories of diseases to be considered in each nation's NAHRS. All **OIE List A** and **List B** diseases (see chapter 5) should be included. The country should identify diseases that are subject to active surveillance based on focused testing and those subject to passive surveillance. The system should include diseases in various stages of national disease-control or eradication programs (Salmon 1998). It is difficult to obtain accurate data about diseases for which no regulatory or surveillance programs are in place. This information is usually available from state livestock officials or the nation's diagnostic laboratories.

Disease-control authorities must recognize and communicate the differences between reportable diseases, which require regulatory action, and notifiable diseases, which are recorded for informational purposes only.

Six categories of reportable or notifiable diseases that can be included in MS&R systems are:

- Contagious animal diseases currently the subject of eradication or control programs
- Existing contagious animal diseases that are endemic and not currently the subject of eradication or control programs
- Habitat-adapted infections or parasites
- Exotic diseases
- Emerging diseases
- Spongiform encephalopathies

Each category requires a different level of monitoring or surveillance, diagnostic testing, border security, and biosecurity for research and diagnostic facilities. These categories differ from the OIE disease lists, which focus on international trade and emphasize the urgency of reporting based on the potential for global transmission, public health importance, and economic significance.

Contagious animal diseases under control or eradication programs should have disease-specific mandatory active surveillance, mandatory annual reporting, and standardized diagnostic profiles. Reports of programmed diseases should initiate regulatory action. There should be standardized quarantine or slaughter procedures and criteria for releasing herds from quarantine. Disease-free zones or subnational regions should be designated using clearly defined transparent standards. Research and vaccine production and utilization should be monitored by the national government and included in NAHRS reports.

Existing contagious livestock diseases that are endemic in the country but not subjected to control programs should also be included in NAHRS reports. Their presence is generally common knowledge and they are described in the literature. The causative agents of these diseases can be in common use in research and vaccine production. They are not subject to regulatory measures. There is a degree of population immunity against endemic contagious diseases as a result of inapparent infections, intermittent outbreaks, or vaccination. Status updates every three years are adequate for endemic contagious diseases.

Vector-borne or habitat-adapted infections and parasites are confined to certain areas by specific transmission requirements. In many cases vector-borne diseases are not subject to disease-specific MS&R requirements, testing, or quarantine procedures. They are amenable to regionalization on the basis of ecological and geographic boundaries. Reporting of vector-borne diseases can be on a three-year basis unless there are new incursions or major outbreaks.

Exotic diseases are those absent from a country or region. They are usually monitored by passive surveillance techniques, exotic-disease investigations, and diagnostic testing in high-security facilities maintained by national authorities.

Exotic-disease vaccines are for emergencies only. They are produced and stockpiled only in highly secure facilities or in other countries. Exotic-disease investigations are initiated as soon as they are suspected. The USDA investigates 200–300 suspicious outbreaks annually. Exotic diseases should be reported as soon as the diagnosis is confirmed but informal quarantines and trace backs can be initiated based on strong suspicions.

Emerging diseases are newly recognized conditions or existing diseases that appear in new forms or reemerge after periods of quiescence. Depending on their human and animal health importance, they should be reported annually or more frequently.

TSEs are prion-induced conditions with long incubation periods. They usually cannot be positively diagnosed in live animals. Territories cannot be considered TSE-free without a surveillance program that includes examination of the brains of animals dying with neurological signs. Annual reporting of **bovine spongiform encephalopathy (BSE)** and other prion-induced diseases is essential. BSE-free countries should report the condition as soon as the diagnosis is positively confirmed.

National Expectations of NAHRS

Each country's NAHRS must address the rights, obligations, and concerns of both livestock industries and representatives of animal welfare, environmental, food-safety, labor, human rights, and manufacturing interests. These groups often have contradictory and conflicting goals.

There are multiple stakeholders within each nation's livestock industries. The system should protect proprietary confidentiality by not naming affected areas, farms, or ranches unless emergencies exist and disease diagnoses are verified according to standard case definitions. The rights, obligations, and concerns of subnational livestock officials must also be respected. Their active involvement and cooperation is essential to any NAHRS.

Sometimes livestock industries object to transparent reporting systems because of past experiences with loss of foreign markets. This can occur over diseases that are globally ubiquitous, present in the recipient countries, or scientifically irrelevant to the commodity in question. Embargoes are sometimes initiated by trade officials who lack knowledge of livestock diseases. They may be imposed to protect domestic industries from competition. Diplomatic face-saving, compromises, and scientific and technical exchanges are usually required to remedy inappropriate embargoes.

International Expectations of NAHRS

Every county's NAHRS should meet the expectations of the WTO and the OIE, which have authority over international trade in livestock products and individual trading partners and trading blocs. The international community expects national governments to report diseases in an honest and timely fashion (Kahrs 1999).

WTO Reporting Expectations of Livestock Exporting Countries

International trade guidelines, outlined in the WTO SPS Agreement authorized by the General Agreement on Tariffs and Trade (GATT), have the force of international law.

The Agreement indicates that SPS measures should be scientifically sound, transparent, non-discriminatory, equitably applied, in harmony with international standards, taken in recognition that similar risk mitigation can be achieved in different ways (**equivalency**), risk-assessment based, regionally applied, and, where equal conditions prevail, no less favorable than domestic requirements.

If these principles are fulfilled without discrimination or unjustified differences, nations may impose any requirements deemed necessary to protect the health of their livestock, wildlife, and human populations. As signatories to the GATT, and members of the WTO, most countries are committed to these principles.

Import policies should address WTO expectations by evaluating proposed importations with respect to commodity-based disease-specific risk factors in exporting regions. Requests to import animals and animal products into a territory can be evaluated on a case-by-case basis. The evaluation criteria include prevalence of restricted disease agents in exporting regions and adjacent areas, vaccine use, organizational parameters such as quality and quantity of disease monitoring and surveillance, diagnostic testing, border security, and overall animal health infrastructure.

Many factors determine a country's suitability to export livestock and livestock products. The credibility of their MS&R systems is a major factor in determining the sanitary measures imposed on their exports.

OIE Expectations and Commitments in Livestock Disease Reporting

The OIE has about 160 member countries, each with one delegate and one vote. The OIE collects and disseminates global animal disease information. It encourages scientific governance of international trade in animal products by setting standards, categorizing diseases into List A and List B, and recognizing the disease-free status of countries. Member countries support these activities through financial contributions, submitting disease reports, participating in policy discussions, and providing scientific input into proposed standards.

The OIE requires each country's delegate to submit immediate reports of significant epidemiological events, monthly reports of national disease activity, and a detailed annual disease report. These are distributed in weekly *OIE Animal Disease Reports*, *Bimonthly Bulletins*, and an annual review of the global animal health situation. The annual review is prepared jointly by the Food and Agriculture Organization of the United Nations, the OIE, and the World Health Organization. These documents are distributed globally. They are used by countries to develop protective import measures and to evaluate the livestock health infrastructures of exporting countries.

The OIE develops lists of disease-free and disease-affected countries or regions as the WTO-designated international livestock disease reporting organization. However, except in the case of FMD or contagious bovine pleuropneumonia, for which OIE requires documentation, these self-proclaimed disease-free status reports are unverified and unguaranteed. Importing countries often conduct site visits to evaluate MS&R systems, the diagnostic capacity, and the animal health infrastructures of proposed trading partners.

Expectations of Trading Partners

Trading partners expect other countries to comply with WTO and OIE policies. The OIE expects livestock disease reports to be based on scientific evidence. However, science is constantly changing, subject to multiple interpretations, and can be distorted by economic objectives, political expediencies, and cultural influences.

When it comes to import measures and disease reporting, animal health authorities and other decision-making officials are subject to political and cultural pressures. While recognizing commitments to international trade agreements, they must be responsive to the concerns of their livestock industries. They must also consider issues raised by environmental, animal welfare, and consumer groups.

Regulatory functions were once the sole domain of government agencies. Today there is a global movement toward strengthening government-industry relationships. This is producing successful cooperative, or voluntary, disease control, quality assurance programs, and privatization of testing and inspection procedures. This trend is resisted by controlled economies and animal health officials of countries where governments are major sources of employment for veterinarians. The movement toward partnering between governments and industries is bringing pressures to bear on reporting systems. This comes from industry groups that want increased foreign markets but are not enthused about reporting diseases that can be used to curtail their exports.

In many countries, regulatory agencies respect certificates only if they are signed by full-time employees of national governments. They regard certifications by private veterinarians, private laboratories, and voluntary reporting systems as conflicting with impartial and independent regulatory practice. Also, national livestock health officials prefer to negotiate only with national governments. These realities require **veterinary services (VS)** of national governments to oversee livestock disease control and operate a national MS&R system.

Contrary to science, which is rapidly advancing, and political convictions, which can be ephemeral, cultural traits are slow to change. Ethnic and religious traditions and national pride profoundly impact livestock disease reporting. Cultural traditions are easily institutionalized within regulatory agencies. They adapt slowly to scientific advances and political pressures and sometimes distort disease reporting (see chapter 5).

Credible International Livestock Health Reporting

Accurate MS&R is the foundation of successful domestic livestock health programs and can have a positive or negative impact on foreign markets. Livestock disease monitoring and surveillance is often regarded as a singular freestanding activity of presumed value to livestock health infrastructures. Unless disease information is transparently disseminated to domestic and international stakeholders, it is like a boat without a rudder, or a kite without a tail. Both move wildly in the tide or wind without direction and are potentially capable of self destruction and damage to their operators.

Candid reporting of animal diseases raises issues of interpretation, proprietary confidentiality, and the potential use, misuse, or distortion of information. It begs the question of whether all countries report with equal openness. Therefore, national reporting of contagious diseases should occur on a countrywide basis. Reports should not identify subnational entities or farms except in cases of program diseases, exotic-disease incursions, or situations where habitat-adapted vector-borne conditions can be regionalized.

Most countries expect trading partners to reveal their animal disease status. They should reciprocate. They should be able to certify that their exports meet the same standards that they impose on imports when equal conditions exist. Countries should not certify freedom from diseases for which they have no surveillance system or for which they permit vaccination.

Although the urge to withhold MS&R data is understandable, secretive approaches ultimately damage trade and fly in the face of commitments to the WTO. Deceptive disease reporting can cause forfeiture of opportunities for leadership in developing equitable, open, global SPS measures. Inaccurate disease reporting also violates democratic commitments to free expression. It compromises the integrity of veterinarians and food inspectors at packing plants. Shady reporting practices hinder the efforts of national and subnational regulators, and subjugate the national livestock health infrastructure. In the international marketplace, credibility is a country's most cherished, and most fragile, possession. The long-term credibility of forthright MS&R systems will outweigh short-term market gains achieved by withholding disease data to spuriously open foreign markets.

In countries with transparent participatory governments there is need for a new global outlook and coordinated approaches to MS&R. Progress in this venture, while controversial and sometimes temporarily counterproductive, will ultimately enhance the prosperity of the national livestock industries.

The pressures of the new millennium require that each nation develop a credible NAHRS based on the up-to-date electronic distribution of livestock disease information. This will help them expand markets abroad, respond to pressures from the international community, and address the increasing worldwide emphasis on open government.

For decades, OIE, national, and subnational officials have pushed the NAHRS concept. At the national level it is usually agreed that knowledge of the nature and distribution of livestock diseases is needed to reduce the spread of infections and prioritize disease-control and research activities.

The United States and other countries with transparent participatory governments have had difficulty getting stakeholders to agree on mechanisms of data collection, levels of information distribution, and the organizations most suited for oversight of reporting systems.

In the new millennium the diagnostic community resurrected old arguments about test sensitivity and specificity, distinguishing between vaccine-induced and infection-induced **titers**, and the need for proprietary confidentiality of test results. Diagnosticians feared that candid reporting would cause reductions in sample submissions by producers fearing loss of foreign markets. Adequate samples are needed for teaching, research, and income.

Subnational regulatory officials objected to infringement on their authority by requiring reports. They feared their states would be assigned the disease status of neighbors that send specimens to their laboratories or whose livestock cross their borders. They also feared trade inequities arising from differing reporting levels from state to state.

Integrated livestock operators suggested their biosecurity measures were adequate to exclude disease so they should have less stringent reporting requirements than smaller farms.

There were voices saying that only laboratory confirmed specific diagnoses should be reported and others saying only clinical syndromes, without naming specific causative agents, should be reported. Statisticians disagreed over the best sampling scheme. Others said costs would exceed benefits.

New convincing arguments have emerged to compel nations to develop MS&R programs to preserve their livestock industries. Under the GATT, importing countries can exclude exports from regions when national governments can not provide credible animal health certifications.

In earlier decades MS&R discussions were bogged down by logistical questions. Today electronic data gathering, analysis, and transmission permit instantaneous animal health reports. Media coverage and competition to publish make it impossible to keep livestock disease information confidential. Trading partners sometimes hear about disease situations before they are known to officials of the affected nations, neighboring countries, or the OIE.

As the animal health communities of some countries debate over NAHRS and national animal ID systems, other countries are implementing programs and preparing new import measures. These will require exporting countries to have nationally verified livestock health reporting and ID systems capable of tracing any animal or carcass with evidence of disease, microbial contamination, or residues to the farm of origin.

Redefining NAHRS to Address Urgent National and Global Imperatives

Most livestock-producing countries need exports for expansion of their livestock industries. Expansion of livestock production is needed to feed a protein-starved world that offers profitable global markets for livestock products. Countries seeking these markets should immediately implement nationally supervised, cooperative, veterinarian based, livestock disease reporting systems that:

- Provide the basis for a national annual summary of livestock diseases and describe the livestock health infrastructure
- Are consistent with monthly, annual, and special reports submitted to the OIE
- Report the national disease status without mentioning states, provinces, or subnational territories except for program diseases, exotic disease incursions, or domestically regionalized situations
- Provide guidance for prioritization of animal disease-control programs
- Assist in prioritization of animal health research and vaccine-development activities
- Identifiy non-contagious vector-borne livestock diseases and parasites that can be regionalized for export purposes
- Provide a credible scientific basis for sanitary measures imposed on livestock products entering the country. This requires identification of exotic diseases, diseases for which there are nationally supervised control or eradication program, and diseases for which vaccines are produced and used in the country
- Provide a credible scientific basis for certification of exported livestock products
- Are cooperatively implemented in all states, provinces, commonwealths, territories, possessions and industries wishing national endorsement of export certificates for animals, livestock products, or germplasm

Suggested Contents of an NAHRS-driven Annual Livestock Health Status Report

In cooperation with the national veterinary service, each nation's NAHRS working group should develop and publish an annual report of the national livestock health status. It should be distributed electronically and in hard copy to national and international stakeholders. This report should contain

- A description of the animal health and food-safety infrastructures including their multijurisdictional authorities and responsibilities

- A description and progress report on each nationally sponsored animal disease-control and eradication program
- A description of exotic disease exclusion, surveillance, and diagnostic programs
- A list of OIE List A and List B diseases that are certifiable as exotic to the country
- A description and summary of exotic disease diagnostic investigations in the past year
- A summary of the country's import regulations and export certification procedures
- A list of non-contagious communicable diseases that are confined to limited parts of the country. This provides a potential basis for certifying the rest of the country as disease-free by the regionalization criteria in the ***OIE International Animal Health Code***
- A list of contagious diseases endemic in the country or diseases for which vaccines are approved for use and for which the country cannot certify disease-free status
- Criteria for prioritizing national livestock health programs
- A summary of new livestock health programs
- A description of future plans

NAHRS Leadership by National Veterinary Services

The national veterinary service is the logical choice for leadership of the NAHRS mission because:

- WTO conducts business with member countries and not subnational governments. Article 13 of the SPS Agreement holds national governments responsible for compliance by non-central governmental agencies and non-governmental bodies within their territories
- The OIE considers national veterinary services as the competent veterinary authorities for disease reporting and health certification purposes and the CVO as the delegate. OIE sends mailings only to delegates and accepts official correspondence only from delegates
- Most countries deal exclusively with national governments and won't consider proposals from subnational bodies, states, provinces, or industry groups
- Most importing countries accept international health certificates only if endorsed by officials of national governments
- For regionalization, trading partners require a competent national veterinary authority to endorse regional credentials
- Most countries accept applications and documentation of animal health status only from representatives of national governments

- National governments of most counties have the authority and responsibility to oversee national livestock health programs

These factors indicate that each country's national veterinary service has authority and responsibility to develop, administer, and enforce a NAHRS.

Challenges to MS&R Leadership

Support for expanding national MS&R activities is stifled by understandable fear of excess government controls. Many livestock producers don't directly export animals or germplasm. They are indifferent to the complexities of international trade. They don't appreciate that commodity prices are determined in a global marketplace.

The international MS&R situation is further complicated by the multiplicity of regulatory agencies involved in international trade. This multijurisdictional authority provides checks and balances. It sometimes results in miscommunication and confusion. Such confusion can result in erroneous statements about disease-free status or agreements that cannot be met by domestic industries.

Animal Health Information Systems

A national animal health information system is essential to every country. It should permit two-way communication between livestock health officials and domestic and international stakeholders. This system should provide electronic recording, verification, storage, and dissemination of data from diagnostic laboratories, inspection points, and quarantine stations. It needs to be able to summarize the distribution of each livestock disease, regularly generate MS&R information and identify animals for tracing to point of origin. It should be able to produce updated lists of accredited veterinarians, licensed veterinary biologics and pharmaceuticals, and laboratories capable of testing for each infectious and toxic agent.

This automated information management system should make existing and proposed regulations available to the public. It should be capable of electronically processing requests and delivering licenses or permits to produce, import, or export livestock products.

It must be capable of triggering active responses to outbreaks and generating disease investigation summaries suitable for media purposes.

The dream of paper-free information technology (IT) systems for national livestock databases fizzled when officials recognized the complexity of the task, the obstacles in its path, and the multiple national and subnational agencies and organizations involved.

Despite the extent of the task, available technology indicates it is possible. It requires resources, multi-agency authority, and a comprehensive master plan.

The task should begin with a carefully laid out set of general and specific goals, preferably in priority order. It will require standardized systems and vocabularies and coordination among agencies that already have individual systems and web sites in place. It must strive for consistency with selected existing national, subnational, and international databases.

After initial surveys of available databases and other information sources each nation can strive to develop a national animal health information system that is most compatible with the livestock health and food-safety needs of the country and the international community.

Animal Identification Systems

Over the years, farmers, ranchers, livestock marketers, and regulatory officials throughout the world have used various methods to identify and verify the source of individual animals. Some identification methods, like brands, can be read from afar and are used to establish ownership. Others, like ear notches and large plastic ear tags, can be seen from some distance and are used to sort animals for management procedures.

Metal ear tags and tattoos are placed in the ear or flank. Their identifying letters or numbers can be read only if the animal is restrained. They have been used in disease-control programs, quality assurance programs, herd or breed registries, or production monitoring systems. In some countries numbering systems and identification devices are standardized. In others there is minimal standardization and few coordinated searchable databases.

In recent decades there has been heightened public concern about food quality and safety and the spread of livestock diseases via international trade or bioterrorism. These concerns have provided incentives for application of electronics to remote surveillance for identification and tracing of animals as they move through the food chain. They have led to a growing emphasis on livestock identification systems as essential components of national animal health infrastructures. Effective ID systems permit regulatory agencies to rapidly determine the cause, source, and extent of outbreaks of food contamination, programmed diseases, or exotic infections.

In some countries processors package identifiable brands of meats carrying guarantees concerning the humane handling of animals and assurances they were not treated with hormones or antibiotics. These processors will pay premium prices for animals positively identified as having been raised under certain conditions on farms open to inspection and verification. Processors who package value-added meat products must be able to trace defective, blemished, or contaminated products to the farms of origin.

There is a wide variety of livestock identification devices. Technology now permits unique country codes and individual alphanumeric identifications so no two animals carry the same address.

Rapidly advancing animal identification technology provides remote reading and electronic storage of data. This permits live animals to be sorted and separated into groups by place of origin, dietary history, weight, vaccination status, or other parameters. After slaughter, reports on meat quality and consistency or the presence of blemishes or residues can be promptly reported to producers enabling them to improve management practices and be remunerated by processors. When adequate automated livestock ID mechanisms are in place, diseases recognized at slaughter can be promptly reported to the responsible regulatory agencies.

In large integrated livestock operations or in situations where direct marketing is practiced, a variety of identification devices, mostly electronic and sometimes called radio frequency identification (RFID), are currently in use (Maday 2001). One of these is an ear tag, the so-called electronic button tag, that can be securely and permanently affixed to the ear. However, on some button tags the visual identification numbers are hard to read from a distance. Another is a modification of traditional, large, flat, plastic ear tags with the last four digits visible from a distance and other digits and information electronically gathered from bar codes or other transponders.

RFID devices can be implanted by injection or administered orally as boluses that lodge permanently in the first of the four stomachs of ruminants. There is also a patented electronic, retinal imaging system that uses computers to capture unique fingerprint-like patterns of blood vessels inside the eye. These devices offer many advantages for farmers, ranchers, and marketing organizations. They also provide the trace-back capacity essential to livestock health officials.

Small producers and some livestock associations see the global movement toward compulsory national livestock identification systems as imposing additional costs, infringing on their privacy, and violating their right to proprietary confidentiality. They view them as unnecessary government intervention and resent the effort and cost devoted to them. On the other hand, automated RFID systems with remote reading capacities produce marketplace advantages for large integrated livestock production, marketing, and processing operations.

An internationally recognized standard for the data contained in **electronic identification devices (EIDs)** and a set of standards for the structures of individual unique alphanumeric EID numbers called ISO 11784 have been developed by the **International Organization for Standardization (ISO)**. Further standards, designated ISO 11785, outline protocols for communicating between electronic identification devices and reading instruments.

Ultimately, compulsory national animal ID will be needed to report quality products, trace back diseases, and meet forthcoming marketing and import requirements that are under development throughout the world. Countries with functional animal ID systems will have competitive advantages over countries without adequate national livestock identification systems. This advantage will be particularly important in countries where the public is already disenchanted with their agricultural and veterinary communities due to BSE, FMD or food-safety concerns. These programs will be most successful if they are initially voluntary and preceded by extensive discussions among interested groups.

The European Union (EU) responded to its BSE and FMD problems with compulsory use of electronic passports for livestock. They involved considerable paperwork and engendered resentment among producers (Maday 2001).

The U.S. officials are progressing more slowly. They are conducting extensive discussions with stakeholders and carrying out pilot ID programs. In 1999, the U.S. Holstein Association developed a voluntary ID system to help dairymen oversee their breeding programs (Bower-Spence 2002).

Identification of U.S. beef cattle is a major logistical challenge and the subject of considerable controversy. In January 2002, the **National Cattlemen's Beef Association (NCBA)** published minimum voluntary cattle identification standards. These include recommendations for sourcing, gathering, submission, and use of database information entered when electronic ear tags are placed in cattle at the herd of origin.

Trial voluntary national livestock identification systems are under way in many countries. Implementation of nationwide RFID systems will probably move faster if importing countries begin to embargo products from countries lacking adequate ID programs. When the United States adopts a compulsory national RFID system its livestock producers and regulatory officials will have had field experience with various technologies, data recording, and search systems. Regulatory officials will have to choose the identification devices, remote reading instruments, and databases to be employed. The decision will not be enthusiastically received in all quarters but must be the best possible compromise.

In recognition of increasing international importance of national livestock ID systems, the OIE published a special scientific and technical review paper entitled *Traceability of Animals and Animal Products* (MacDaniel and Sheridian 2001).

Biosecurity at National Borders, Subnational Boundaries, and Individual Properties

Biosecurity is defined as protecting animal or human populations from natural or malicious attack by biological agents. It is a key element in livestock health infrastructures. Biosecurity is essential to the establishment and maintenance of healthy livestock populations, the production of wholesome and safe food supplies, the support of disease-control and eradication programs, the development of MS&R systems, and the preservation of export markets.

Security measures at national and subnational borders and livestock rearing and processing facilities mitigate actual risks and create deterrents to the introduction of diseases. Prevention and control of infectious diseases are highly problematic unless national and subnational borders are secure from uncontrolled entry of livestock. Terrestrial boundaries and land border-crossings must be protected from entry of livestock and persons carrying infectious diseases.

Personnel assigned to seaports and airports must guard against passengers carrying disease organisms or vectors on their persons or in baggage. Cargoes arriving by auto, truck, airplane, or boat must be inspected to prevent the introduction of materials contaminated with animal or human pathogens. This requires careful inspection for foodstuffs, drugs, biological products, hunting trophies, or farm equipment. Farms, ranches, and food-processing plants need security to prevent the introduction of infections hazardous to the health of livestock or people.

There are varying levels of livestock health and human food-security measures throughout the world. Some countries maintain armed guards at all border crossings, while others leave their borders relatively unprotected from potential disease threats. Island nations tend to be easier to protect than countries with vast land borders. Natural obstacles such as rivers and mountain ranges can also be formidable barriers to transmission of livestock diseases.

Border security measures are most effective if supplemented by tight farm security and strict precautions in food-processing plants. The biosecurity measures outlined below have dual effects of directly preventing introduction of disease agents and reminding people that security is serious business.

Border Security

Exclusion of exotic livestock diseases is a paramount concern in all countries. Most livestock industries live with **endemic diseases** that exist in ecological equilibrium with native livestock. They persist as mild or subclinical infections with occasional serious outbreaks. Their effects are modulated by partial immunity due to natural infections or vaccination. Diseases endemic in one nation may be exotic to other countries, because they were never present or were eradicated. Some insect-borne diseases are exotic in countries where the ecosystems are unsuitable for the survival of the vectors.

Border security adequate to deter entry of infected animals or materials requires check points at land crossings, seaports, and airports. These must be manned by trained personnel who examine import permits and health certification documents accompanying importations. These individuals are usually government employees who work closely with immigration and customs officials. They inspect shipments to verify that cargoes contain the material listed on manifests and that baggage contains only legally imported materials.

Passenger baggage from destinations infected with exotic diseases must be inspected at airports and sea terminals to assure that animals, animal products, or other hazardous materials are not present. Trained dogs are effective in identifying baggage that contains foods.

The volume of passengers, cargoes, and other entries with risk of introducing exotic livestock diseases far exceeds the inspection capacities of most countries. The reporting of foods on customs declarations is not always complete. Entries are usually inspected at random or on the basis of selection procedures called profiling. Baggage identified by sniffing dogs is always examined. The baggage of people arriving from certain areas or of individuals who behave suspiciously is inspected carefully.

Farm and Ranch Security

There has been increased interest in the security of large and small livestock holdings. A variety of security measures are invoked to prevent the accidental or intentional introduction of infectious agents. These efforts are most apparent where large numbers of animals are closely confined in environments that support the rapid spread of disease.

Farms, ranches, feedlots, and poultry operations are becoming gated communities. Visitors are admitted only on official business and their contact with animals is limited. Entering vehicles must drive through wheel washes. Persons entering animal areas must walk through disinfectant foot baths and sometimes shower and don special clothing. On poultry farms there are strict rodent-control and bird-exclusion measures. Insects are controlled by spraying and screening.

Local security measures will probably remain the prerogative of individual livestock owners. Producer organizations are establishing guidelines for their membership. Some processors are considering minimal farm-security measures as requirements of their marketing process.

Security at Facilities Processing Livestock Products

Milk and meat processing plants traditionally undertake sanitary measures to protect products from contamination with food-borne pathogens. Following the terrorist attacks of September 2001, processing plants invoked additional security. These measures have included fencing facilities, posting uniformed security guards, and limiting admission to uniformed employees with picture identification. Food processors have a unique opportunity to interact with the public to enlist their support for food-security measures, disease abatement, and emergency response measures.

Emergency Livestock Disease Management

Capacity to handle emergencies is crucial to livestock health infrastructures. Livestock emergencies can be natural, intentional, or terrorist events. They exist when there are:

- Economic losses or livestock-related human diseases in excess of the usual
- Unusual occurrences or spread of endemic diseases
- Outbreaks of emerging diseases
- Introductions of exotic diseases
- Natural disasters like earthquakes, fires, floods, hurricanes, or tornadoes
- Man-made calamities such as oil spills or widespread microbial or toxic contaminations creating excessive livestock disease or death
- Conditions permitting unusual levels of transmission of livestock diseases to humans

Most developed countries have livestock emergency management programs in place and work continuously to strengthen them. These programs vary in scope and focus. The principal components of effective emergency management programs are prevention, preparedness, recognition, response, recovery, coordination, communication, and summarization.

Each component requires qualified leaders, carefully chosen spokespersons, achievable transparent standards, and adequate funding. Most livestock health agencies have dual missions of the preservation of foreign markets and simultaneously protecting livestock, poultry, and wildlife populations from exotic diseases. Emergency preparedness is an essential ingredient of both. It provides the capacity to exclude exotic diseases and respond rapidly to eradicate them if they enter the country.

Each country contends with animal diseases, accidental livestock losses, and human diseases of livestock origin. These are usually maintained at acceptably low levels by management practices, restricted animal movement, vaccinations, and prophylactic or therapeutic medications. Despite these precautions, livestock health emergencies can arise unexpectedly and cause major losses. The time, place, and nature of livestock health emergencies is largely unpredictable.

National governments and livestock health communities must maintain ongoing, coordinated, and flexible emergency management programs. These should include monitoring and surveillance programs, exotic-disease exclusion activities, diagnostic capacity, and rapid response capability. The nature of emergencies and the necessary responses will differ. They all require lists of experts and trained workers who are available, on short notice, to leave their day-to-day activities. This requires proactive planning.

National governments, in cooperation with subnational and local governments and stakeholders, need to work out arrangements to address emergencies before, not after, they arise.

Increasing concerns about exotic diseases emphasize the need for improved coordination of emergency preparedness. Until recently national livestock health agencies have not publicized this need adequately to receive necessary funding. The development and maintenance of effective national livestock emergency management systems requires constant refinement and constant review to assure that the necessary ingredients are available. These essentials are addressed individually below.

Prevention of Livestock Health Emergencies

The old adage that "an ounce of prevention of worth a pound of cure" is true for livestock health emergencies. Its antithesis, however, is that people are rarely rewarded for preventing emergencies that never happen. Regardless of the effectiveness of deterrents, the pundits can usually find deficiencies and scapegoats when emergencies occur. In most countries disease-control efforts are under way at all levels of the food chain. It is the unpredictable and unanticipated events, such as exotic diseases or acts of bioterrorism, that defy the preventive efforts of producers, processors, and regulatory officials.

Individual livestock producers take preventive measures when they practice farm or ranch biosecurity, reduce or carefully screen additions to herds, activate management practices that assure proper nutrition and stress avoidance, and practice vaccination against endemic diseases. Livestock producer organizations practice prevention when they present informational meetings, develop quality assurance programs, encourage participation in disease-control programs, and urge producers to employ veterinarians to develop herd health programs.

National and local livestock health agencies are undertaking emergency prevention through disease-control and eradication programs, MS&R systems, and meat inspection activities.

Preparation for Livestock Health Emergencies

Despite these precautions emergencies will occur and preparation is needed. Foreign animal diseases can gain access by legally imported animals or products, smuggled commodities, or intentional introductions.

Elaborate and continual preparations for livestock health emergencies must be undertaken collectively by individual producers, regulatory officials, livestock organizations, diagnostic facilities, academic institutions, and multiple local and national government agencies.

Before emergencies occur steps must be taken to acquire legal authority and sources of immediate financial support for prompt payment of emergency contractors and workers and to reimburse producers for losses associated with quarantines and embargoes. Interest-free loans should be available for restocking farms and ranches and for cleaning and disinfection operations. There should be lists of selected high-risk disease agents that require attention.

Arrangements should be made in advance for carcass disposal in the event of outbreaks of FMD, BSE, classical swine fever, highly pathogenic avian influenza, viscerotrophic velogenic Newcastle disease, or rinderpest. Contractors for carcass services should be identified and interviewed before emergencies occur. These are the diseases in which the slaughter and disposal of infected and exposed animals is a logical early approach. Eradication by test and slaughter, the so-called **stamping out method**, is a sensitive and controversial issue with environmental, ethical, and animal welfare implications. Once such diseases become established in widespread areas, alternative procedures such as vaccination, immunological enhancement procedures, or therapy must be considered (see Discussion Topic 10).

Emergency programs and test exercises must include education of the media about slaughter procedures and carcass disposal. The methods of choice depend on the disease and the species involved.

Carcass-disposal alternatives may include burial on farms or in landfills, incineration in pyres on farms or in incinerators, composting on farms, anaerobic fermentation, alkaline hydrolysis, or rendering (National Renderers Association 2002). Many of these options are unavailable in some areas. Some selection factors include:

- Costs and potential values or hazards associated with remains and residues
- Body mass of the species involved
- Environmental considerations like water tables, available space, drainage, and the potential for groundwater pollution
- Estimated numbers of dead or slaughtered animals
- Public opinion
- Views of affected industries
- Local and national ordinances or laws
- The nature of the disease involved and the vulnerability of the organism to inactivation by various procedures

Recognition of Livestock Health Emergencies

Floods, tornadoes, hurricanes, and the effects of weapons of mass destruction (WMD) are usually obvious, and the time and place where response is required is evident. Livestock may not be the most immediate public concern in these situations.

Conversely, infectious-disease emergencies may have subtle and insidious beginnings. Many livestock diseases look alike and recognition can be delayed. In some diseases animals can spread the infection before sickness is observed. In such cases immediate quarantines and cessation of movements are not always possible. When such measures are invoked hastily and the presumptive diagnosis is not confirmed apologies are essential, but "better safe than sorry" is an appropriate policy.

Farmers, ranchers, veterinarians, and animal-disease diagnostic laboratories are key components in exotic disease recognition.

Response to Livestock Health Emergencies

Advance planning for response to emergencies is complicated by the variety of potential livestock health crises, the numerous species that may be involved, and the multiple individuals, organizations, and agencies responsible. Prompt responses present many challenges. They can be planned to address infectious diseases, toxicological episodes, natural disasters, acts of bioterrorism, and attacks by WMD. For each category an outline can be written that assigns the lead agencies, support organizations, personnel, procedures, equipment, resources, and legal authorities necessary to deal with contingencies. The system can be evaluated in test exercises. Emergency actions should be undertaken immediately without waiting for federal confirmation (Nolen 2002).

Recovery From Livestock Health Emergencies

Once an animal health emergency is resolved, new challenges arise. Unanswered questions and unfulfilled commitments will remain. Recovery and follow-up procedures must

- Salve the wounds of those most directly affected
- Update supporters, critics, and the media
- Reimburse those suffering financial losses
- Provide counseling to affected individuals
- Repair consumer confidence
- Release quarantines and restrictions on livestock movement
- Clean, disinfect, and repopulate infected premises in a timely fashion
- Assure that focused surveillance is continued to identify residual flare-ups
- Continue regular news releases
- Send thank you letters to participating agencies, individuals, the media, and legislative bodies that appropriated emergency funding
- Prepare a summary of the emergency and the response

Coordination of Livestock Health Emergency Activities

The complexity of livestock health emergencies is compounded by the multiplicity of governmental agencies and private individuals involved. Operational pressures make it imperative that obligations and assignments are clearly allocated and a lead agency is assigned to each type of emergency.

Leaders should be assigned for every function during each potential event. It is crucial that the chain of command and delegation of specific responsibilities be written in advance and made public. These assignments will vary with the nature and cause of emergencies.

In the United States the Federal Bureau of Investigation (FBI) plays the lead role in acts of bioterrorism, undue violence, and use of WMD. The USDA leads in outbreaks of animal and plant diseases and the FDA leads in food-safety emergencies. This coordination must be clearly and repeatedly communicated to those involved, to the general public, and to the media.

Communication of Livestock Health Emergency Information

Communication is the most important component of emergency disease operations. It is easily overlooked. The best emergency management plans can go awry if adequate communications are not maintained throughout. LHP-makers must insist that communication protocols be part of each emergency management plan.

Good communication requires daily or weekly meetings of the leaders of the organizations and agencies involved and succinct written reports of items discussed. Clear top-to-bottom communication is essential at each link in the chain of command. All individuals and organizations holding stakes in emergency situations, the media, and the public must be updated regularly.

Livestock emergency information transmission should be an ongoing process and not reserved for times of crises. Education of the general public about potential emergencies and response plans can take place long before disasters or exotic disease incursions occur. Carefully prepared, clearly written scenario projections, position papers, and issue analyses can be distributed to media contacts as they are generated. If clearly written and interesting they will find their way into print during periods of relative calm when newsworthy activity is minimal. Media moguls are hungry for information and will accumulate this information for use when actual emergencies occur. They may request further information, clarification, and interviews. These offer opportunities for partnering with the media that keep the public and legislators alerted to the preparations for potential emergencies.

Written Summarization of Livestock Health Emergencies

A major, but often overlooked, responsibility of emergency management programs is the writing of summaries. It is essential to document successful outcomes so they can be repeated and shortcomings so they won't be repeated. The lead agency should assign a competent writer to draft a succinct detailed report of each episode. The report should contain the vital statistics about the prevention, preparedness, recognition, response, recovery, coordination, communication, personnel, and finances of the operation. It should highlight success and candidly address flaws. It should be reviewed and carefully edited, but not sanitized to disguise shortfalls.

U.S. Livestock Emergency Disease Recognition and Preparedness Programs

Although there is always need for improvement, the current emergency-response capability in the United States is based on proactive programs. These should not necessarily be emulated by other countries, but they offer thought-provoking items for discussion. These livestock disease surveillance and recognition and programs include:

- About 50,000 accredited veterinarians who are obligated to report new or unusual conditions and suspected exotic or emerging diseases
- A cadre of about 350 trained **foreign animal disease diagnosticians (FADD)** who conduct investigations of exotic diseases
- A system of Regional Emergency Animal Disease Eradication Organizations (READEOs)
- A network of federal, state, and university animal disease diagnostic laboratories, including the **National Veterinary Services Laboratory (NVSL)** at Ames, Iowa, and the **Foreign Animal Disease Diagnostic Laboratory (FADDL)** at Plum Island, NY
- Routine surveillance associated with domestic control programs for brucellosis, tuberculosis, pseudorabies, scrapie, and BSE
- Routine surveillance programs conducted at abattoirs
- The tests applied to U.S. animals to meet import requirements of trading partners
- The statistically designed surveys of key animal health parameters conducted periodically by the **Centers for Epidemiology and Animal Health (CEAH)** at Fort Collins, Colorado

These programs provide reasonable assurance that prompt recognition systems are in place for exotic diseases and that statements of disease freedom are reliable.

The animal disease emergency-response capability of the United States is rapidly being expanded and strengthened under stimulus from the European FMD and BSE disasters and the events of September 11, 2001. **Emergency Disease Guidelines** have been prepared for FMD, classical swine fever, bovine spongiform encephalopathy, African swine fever, African horse sickness, highly pathogenic avian influenza, viscerotrophic velogenic Newcastle disease, and Venezuelan equine encephalomyelitis. Periodically, the USDA conducts animal disease emergency test exercises in cooperation with state officials and producer groups to learn the strong and weak points of the emergency response system.

The USDA has conducted and documented analysis of the economic and environmental dimensions of disinfection and carcass-disposal procedures that may be feasible if infectious disease emergencies occur.

The United States has developed a National Animal Health Emergency Management System (NAHEMS) steering committee aimed at strengthening the national response to animal health emergencies. It is comprised of representatives of national organizations and federal agencies directly concerned with the management of emergencies. Its activities are outlined in the committee's annual report (NAHEMS 2002).

Recommendations for Strengthening U.S. Responses to Livestock Health Emergencies

A variety of initiatives are needed to strengthen coordinated responses to livestock health emergencies in every country. In the United States, programs outlined above and suggestions for improvements continue to emerge as post-September 11th discussions unfold and test exercises reveal areas needing attention. Some of these suggestions may also have potential applications in other countries. They include:

- Improved coordination of animal disease reporting systems
- Improved coordination of exotic disease investigations
- Re-evaluation and restructuring of the **accredited veterinarian** program
- Accelerated training of private, state, federal, and corporate veterinarians and animal health technicians in disease diagnosis and reporting techniques
- Strengthening the livestock health emergency infrastructure
- Strengthening the NAHRS and animal ID programs

It will be challenging to accomplish these suggestions with limited resources. Nonetheless, these goals are becoming more realistic each year with the unfolding of new diagnostic and information technologies and added attention to homeland security.

Livestock Health Emergency Responses at Local and Subnational Levels

The first line of defense against livestock health emergencies is immediate action by livestock producers. When things go awry farmers and ranchers must call veterinarians. The veterinarian's response involves initial examinations, preliminary clinical diagnosis, and immediate notification of local and subnational livestock health officials. The cooperation of livestock producers is essential to the process. Producers must have confidence in the local and national diagnostic system. A reward and indemnity program should be in place before emergencies occur.

Producer confidence must be such that livestock owners willingly invoke voluntary cease-movement orders and comply immediately with orders from state or national governments. This confidence can only be present if there is broad-based producer awareness and stakeholder involvement in emergency response preparation and planning. It is essential that there be participation and a sense of ownership by livestock producer organizations, local and state veterinary medical associations, the academic and diagnostic communities, and local law enforcement officials. Collectively, this team should create written local, subnational, and national emergency response plans that would include people at all levels in the chain. Emergency response plans should not be driven totally by central governments, because incidents must be addressed initially at the local level. States, neighborhoods, and communities must be prepared to relate to national governments and vice versa.

The written response plan must be rehearsed continuously. In the event of an emergency, participants must be available on the ground continually for prolonged periods. The plan should include an impact assessment, procedures for containment and security, a clearly articulated public information program using diplomatic spokespersons, clear statements of how potential environmental impacts will be addressed, and provisions for crisis management and stress counseling. It is important that there be a funding strategy to support livestock owners whose animals are quarantined or slaughtered. Subnational emergency strategies should include a regularly published newsletter that lists OIE List A and List B diseases and succinctly details strategies for dealing with each.

Oversight of Pharmaceutical and Biological Products

The maintenance of livestock health depends on judicious use of animal medicines and veterinary biologics. Oversight of the manufacture, importation, and use of these products is an essential component of livestock health infrastructures.

Livestock medicines include pharmaceutical products, antimicrobials, anti-inflammatory drugs, and a variety of natural and synthetic compounds used in animal health. The words medicines, medications, or pharmaceutical products are currently favored over the term drug to distinguish between legally and appropriately used products and illegally used or addictive drugs. In many countries, animal medicines are regulated by the same agencies that oversee veterinary biologics.

In some countries, like the United States, pharmaceutical products and biologics are regulated by separate government agencies. The USDA **Center for**

Veterinary Biologics (CVB) oversees production of biological products designed to diagnose, treat, and prevent livestock diseases through licensing, inspection, compliance, and laboratory activities.

Veterinary biologicals include vaccines, sera, and diagnostic reagents. While some are synthesized, most have biologic origins and are prepared from animals, animal cells, or disease-producing agents. They are variably effective in controlling or preventing disease.

Regulatory oversight of biologicals is required, because some can be ineffective or even counterproductive to livestock health. Their biologic origins permit them to carry contaminating pathogens or to produce disease under certain conditions.

There are differences between livestock pharmaceuticals and animal biologics. Both require regulatory oversight including:

- Licensing requirements
- Pre-release testing
- Labeling requirements
- Expiration dates
- Licensing and inspection of production facilities
- Product inspections
- Investigation of reported untoward reactions

Prerelease Testing and Licensing

Biologicals and pharmaceuticals used on livestock should be licensed by agencies of national governments in order to protect livestock and consumers from ineffective, harmful, or contaminated substances. Most countries have detailed processes for licensing livestock medicines, feed additives, and biologics. License applications request detailed descriptions of ingredients, uses, expected responses, potential toxic reactions, and contraindications. They also request the results of required laboratory and live animal testing procedures.

Labeling Requirements

Manufacturers must submit proposed labels when requesting licenses. Label requirements can be modified by regulatory agencies. The label must list all ingredients, place and date of manufacture, the serial number of the production lot, indications and contraindications, expiration dates, withdrawal times, and antidotes if toxic or allergic reactions may occur.

Inspection of Manufacturing Facilities

Regulatory agencies usually require manufacturing facilities to be approved and licensed before production begins or new product licenses are issued. Facilities are inspected intermittently while products are being produced.

Product Inspections

Most countries require manufacturers to submit samples of each serial produced. These are tested randomly and kept for detailed analysis should untoward reactions or contaminants be suspected.

Investigation of Reported Untoward Reactions

Agencies regulating pharmaceutical products and veterinary biologics seek reports of untoward reactions so problems can be investigated. Special reporting forms may be available to encourage notification and submission of essential information such as age, breed, and sex of animals treated, name and address of their owner, product name, manufacturer, serial number, mode of administration, and dosage.

When appropriate, trained officials visit premises and interview workers.

Linking the Private and Public Sectors of Livestock Health Activities

In nations with participatory governments, a key to effective livestock health infrastructures is the involvement of producers, processors, practicing veterinarians, and their organizations. Their experience in the day-to-day operational aspects of disease prevention, diagnosis, control, and eradication makes them vital to the infrastructure. It is essential to gain the understanding and support of various private and public interest groups and their representative organizations. Livestock health policy makers should encourage the interactions discussed below.

Livestock Producers in Livestock Health Infrastructures

In each country the livestock owners and producers and their employees comprise the backbone of its livestock health infrastructure. They are directly involved in the rearing, feeding, and movement of livestock. They have a financial stake in the outcome of policies imposed upon their industries. Their ideas and input are essential in policy discussions and their participation should be encouraged. Many countries have learned that imposition of livestock health programs without input from affected industries can be counterproductive.

Producer Organizations in Livestock Health Infrastructures

Input from individual and corporate livestock producers is invaluable to successful livestock health infrastructures. In countries with transparent participatory governments, producer voices, opinions, and needs are clearly presented and best received by policy makers when expressed as the views of groups whose members have debated issues and arrived at collective positions.

Livestock producer organizations that meet regularly and have articulate spokespersons are essential to national livestock health infrastructures. Full-time employees of producer organizations usually represent the viewpoints of those in daily contact with livestock. These organizations represent the vested interests of their memberships. They often raise issues never considered by policy makers and government officials. They are thoughtful balancing forces in the process of developing livestock health policies.

Livestock producer organizations should be the first groups to be consulted in the policy development process. In an ideal world they would be first to recognize the need for regulations to protect the health of national livestock industries. Realistically, however, individual livestock producers are often too deeply involved in day-to-day operations to tackle issues of national or global interest.

The reluctance of industry to be regulated, particularly without representation, is understandable. Nonetheless, their initial involvement is essential to the success of livestock health infrastructures. Even if final rules, which are the purview of government officials, are not necessarily embraced enthusiastically by affected industries, producers will be more cooperative if they have had an opportunity to participate and hear the rationales presented by livestock health officials and non-industry groups.

Veterinarians in Livestock Health Infrastructures

Food-animal veterinarians are key players in livestock health infrastructures. The veterinary profession should provide the leadership of each country's national livestock health agency. Veterinarians possess the training, knowledge, and skills to distinguish the signs of disease, to recognize the anatomic and physiological systems involved, and to develop a mental list, known as the differential diagnosis, of the potential cause of problems. They can sense the potential seriousness of livestock disease episodes. They know when government officials should be involved, when special diagnostic tests are needed, and how to collect appropriate diagnostic specimens. With appropriate training veterinarians can develop the leadership and communication skills needed to make major contributions to a country's livestock health infrastructure.

Many countries believe livestock health regulatory activities, such as animal inspections, preparation of health certificates, and collecting samples for testing, should be conducted exclusively by full-time government employees.

Other countries, like the United States, have long traditions of veterinarians working in the private sector. They have found that privately employed veterinarians can contribute to national programs by working cooperatively with publicly employed colleagues.

Accredited Veterinarian Programs

Many countries, including the United States and Canada, rely on qualified private veterinary practitioners to conduct official tests and vaccinations. In some cases these practitioners, called accredited veterinarians, prepare point-of-origin animal health certifications for live animals that produce meat, milk, fiber, or germ plasm for export. When certificates for international movement of livestock are prepared in the field, they are usually endorsed by national or subnational officials who certify signatures of accredited veterinarians indicating that they are approved government representatives.

In the United States, federally accredited practicing veterinarians and livestock producers provide the backbone of the animal health infrastructure. Accredited veterinarians are paid by farmers or brokers for whom they perform professional services. They must avoid the slightest suggestion of conflict of interest. It is difficult to convince trading partners, particularly those with highly controlled economies, that accredited veterinarians are a legitimate extension of national governments. Thus it is essential that they perform with the utmost credibility.

Before certification as accredited veterinarians, U.S. practitioners undergo an orientation program that outlines their duties and responsibilities. They have special disease reporting obligations that are codified in Title 9, Parts 160-162 of the **U.S. Code of Federal Regulations**. They must be meticulous in animal identification and sampling techniques when collecting specimens for official purposes. They know their accreditation can be revoked if abused. In this era of animal health and food-safety concerns, this obligation requires high levels of professionalism and a global outlook. The accredited veterinarian program has been in effect since 1921. It has undergone occasional updating and needs constant revision.

Individual Food Processors in Livestock Health Infrastructures

Unlike livestock owners and producers, food processors are more involved with food safety and less concerned with livestock health. They are not usually directly involved in the rearing and feeding of livestock. They are affected by transportation of animals and their condition on arrival at slaughtering and processing plants. Animal disease emergencies can limit movement to processing plants and make products unsuitable for export or unsafe for human consumption. They increase rejections by inspectors and cripple processing operations. Thus food processors have a major stake in livestock health policies.

Food processors are regulated regarding food safety and their input is essential in the development of LHPs. Unlike livestock producers, processors have a direct link to consumers and can influence public opinion through advertising and package labels. Many food-processing corporations lobby government officials and legislators. Their positions often receive more attention when presented through trade organizations.

Processor Organizations in Livestock Health Infrastructures

The organizations representing meat and milk processors can be major partners in a country's livestock health infrastructure. Their input is valuable because of their direct contacts with both livestock producers and consumers. They are concerned with the safety, price, and availability of wholesome foods. These organizations can play pivotal roles in the review of policies and initiatives. They can support livestock health by promoting risk abatement practices and emergency preparedness activities in processing facilities and on farms that supply them. Because of this influence, organizations representing food processors are vital to development of LHPs.

LHP-makers should persuade food processor organizations to form committees on the role of livestock health in food-safety and animal disease emergency preparedness. Such committees could address issues that are best attacked at the grassroots level and activate stakeholders who may be unmoved by producer issues or government programs. These committees could:

- Offer biosecurity incentives and disease-reporting recognition to producers
- Provide package label alerts on the cost of exotic diseases to consumers
- Publicize baggage restrictions for travelers
- Provide incentives for meat, poultry, and milk transportation equipment that emulates deterrent thought modes
- Encourage suppliers to report diseases promptly
- Establish private emergency endowments to help reimburse producer losses
- Support local legislation to permit rapid quarantine of exposed livestock

The ever-increasing risk of livestock health or food-safety disasters that gained prominence after the terrorist attacks of September 11, 2001, points out that it is crucial to involve food processors and their organizations in livestock health policies. Some possible contributions of food processors to LHPs are discussed below.

Biosecurity Incentives Provided to Livestock Producers by Food Processors

A wake-up call far more effective than government programs would be for food processors to offer premium prices to producers who follow security protocols involving gated premises, foot baths and wheel baths, prohibiting employees from keeping livestock at home, providing work clothes for employees, and providing shower-in-shower-out access to animal holding areas. Such measures can prevent incursions and attract attention to disease risks.

Recognition of Disease Reporting by Producers

Rapid reporting is essential to deterring incursion and spread of exotic diseases. Failure to suspect exotic diseases can result from their initial appearance in species in which they don't cause obvious symptoms, such as FMD in sheep. Delays can result from assumptions that an illness is a routine problem. Simply waiting a few days to see if affected animals will get better can be disastrous to the entire country. Addressing these shortcomings is more effectively done with incentives from processors who purchase commodities than by government programs. Recognition of livestock owners or employees who report suspicious events or diseases would help develop a mind set for vigilance.

Package Label Alerts About Exotic Diseases

For risk-abatement efforts to succeed the general public must be aware of the situation. Neither producers nor regulators have the direct line to the public that is available on the packages of dairy and meat products. A succinctly worded warning that exotic livestock diseases such as FMD, rinderpest, classical swine fever, or highly pathogenic avian influenza could result in a tripling of food prices could alert the public to their potential role in preventing or reporting problems.

Gaining Support for Baggage Restrictions for Travelers

The general public is unaware of the risks associated with meat products carried by airline passengers. FMD outbreaks often arise from swine eating meat scraps from FMD-infected regions. Thousands of tons of such meats are brought into the country annually by visitors carrying ethnic specialty meats to relatives in the United States. Nobody tells passengers when they purchase airline tickets that this is illegal and that the meat will be confiscated at U.S. ports. By the time they have lugged it for 12–24 hours they are willing to lie to custom officials when asked if baggage contains meats, fruits, or vegetables. Creative communication efforts by food-processor organizations, in cooperation with airlines, could reduce this risk considerably.

Developing Disease-deterring Transportation Equipment

Before FMD or other exotic diseases enter a country, it is essential that all livestock, poultry, and milk transportation vehicles be equipped with devices that reduce the likelihood of spreading disease. FMD and other viral infections can spread from farm to farm before animals actually show signs of sickness. Modifications to reduce this likelihood should be implemented immediately and continued indefinitely. Drivers of trucks hauling livestock or milk must be equipped with rubber boots, disinfectants and brushes. Their boots must be scrubbed before leaving every farm. They must also be equipped with individual coveralls for each farm. Trucks need wheel washers, and milk tankers should be equipped with filters for air exhaust ducts. These essentials could be implemented by meat, poultry, egg, and milk processing organizations. Most national and subnational agencies have neither the funding nor the authority to conduct these activities.

Initiating Discussions on the Environmental Impacts of Eradication Programs

Producer and processor discussions with environmental groups often begin on a contentious note. However, with time, patience, and the development of personal relations, these groups can develop the trust and understanding needed for mutually agreeable strategies. The best time for discussing the environmental and humane aspects of disease-control and eradication programs is before emergencies occur. Processor groups that interact with all segments of the population could initiate dialogue prior to the incursion of diseases like FMD that are best eradicated by slaughter of affected and exposed animals.

Encouraging Reporting Activities

Meat, poultry, egg, and milk processing companies can make major contributions by repeatedly reminding their suppliers and the public that early disease reporting is essential. The rationale for prompt reporting, the criteria for reporting, and communication routes for calling in suspected disease situations must be known in advance. The first step would be to call veterinarians and urge them to examine animals carefully, particularly the feet, teats, and nasal passages and to look inside the mouth. Veterinarians should be urged to notify subnational officials if anything looks suspicious and informally halt all movement onto and off of the farm. Involvement of processors that pay for livestock products in the crusade for alertness is vital.

Establishng Emergency Endowments to Reimburse Producer Losses

In some countries public funds may be available to reimburse producers for the fair market value of livestock dying or slaughtered due to FMD or other exotic diseases. If such commitments are stipulated in advance there will be more producer enthusiasm for prompt reporting and isolation of afflicted livestock. This support will be more easily maintained if industry groups establish endowments to supplement government reimbursements. The establishment of such funds will strengthen public support for necessary eradication and control programs. Taxpayers will be more amenable to eradication efforts if they know producers and processors are willing to contribute to support of programs from which they will benefit.

Local Legislation to Permit Quarantine and Disposal of Exposed Livestock

As essential as it seems, many subnational governments lack the authority to quarantine and dispose of infected and exposed livestock.

National governments usually have a diagnosis confirmation and authorizing interval during which quarantine or disposal actions can be delayed or challenged. During that interval, however brief, FMD and other highly transmissible diseases can spread considerably.

It is essential that local and subnational governments undertake precautionary quarantines, place restrictions on livestock and vehicular movements, and if necessary, dispose of sick or exposed animals. Passing legislation to permit subnational governments to expend funds to permit rapid action is time consuming. Legislatures will be more likely to act on the issue if the processing industry supports it.

Support for National Livestock Identification Programs

Meat processors have a unique opportunity to encourage producer support for national livestock ID programs by touting the positive aspects of such a program and using those programs to benefit producers. They can emphasize that identification permits immediate feedback on quality issues that affect prices they receive. They can also stress to producers that identified animals can greatly reduce the time required to initiate disease-control measures in the event of animal disease emergencies.

Support for National Animal Disease Reporting Systems

Both meat and milk processing organizations can encourage their members to actively support the development and implementation of NAHRS. This requires explaining the value of reporting to export markets that increase demand for their products. They could also describe the producer confidentiality provisions of NAHRS under which diseases are reported on a national basis without revealing farm names or locations.

Support for Sale Barn Security

Some countries have extensive movement of livestock through auctions and livestock sales barns en route to feedlots or slaughter facilities. Where sale barns and other livestock assembling operations are essential, strict biosecurity is essential. Efforts to improve security and disease-control measures at these facilities is a challenge that should be addressed by producer and meat-processor organizations.

In some countries there is increasing movement to direct marketing. In such programs food processors contract directly with livestock producers. This bypasses multiple middlemen and avoids the use of disease-and-residue-prone environments. Though not feasible for all classes of livestock, it provides an excellent opportunity for processors to provide feedback to producers and eliminates many opportunities for disease dissemination.

Academic and Diagnostic Communities in Livestock Health Infrastructures

Despite their vital roles in livestock health the diagnostic and academic communities are not yet integrated into livestock health infrastructures. In some countries few college curricula in agriculture or veterinary medicine emphasize organized livestock health activities, regulatory processes, or food safety. Reversing this trend requires the combined efforts of academicians, veterinary organizations, livestock producers and processors, and national and subnational animal health agencies. The task of changing animal science and veterinary medical curricula has been compared to herding cats. Nonetheless, enlightened leadership with a global perspective can move these programs in directions supportive of livestock health infrastructures.

User Fees and National Livestock Health Programs

In some countries fees are charged for portions of government programs. User fees may be levied on diagnostic tests, government-issued import or export certificates, inspection of imported products, use of quarantine facilities, or licenses for the manufacture of veterinary products. Nations applying user fees follow varied procedures.

The determination of equitable fees can be complicated. Most programs benefit all citizens to some extent. Thus, officials must identify those services that exclusively benefit producers, processors, exporters, and importers. Then they must determine a fee appropriate to those activities. Consistency and fairness in fee calculation and collection are crucial, and the fees can be constantly evaluated and adjusted as needed.

Some countries are learning that citizens evaluate and comment thoughtfully on programs that carry direct charges. Countries initiating agricultural user fees are advised to involve stakeholders in program development. While users of livestock health services usually object to fees, if given opportunities to comment as the process unfolds they are less likely to complain when fees are levied.

The question of user fees for livestock health services will eventually have to be addressed by the LHP-makers of each nation.

Skillful Negotiators

One measure of the success of livestock health infrastructures is the skill of national officials in negotiating domestic and international issues. Negotiations are discussions designed to come to terms or reach agreement. Most business, professional, and personal activities involve negotiations. There are a variety of negotiating strategies that are useful when differing views are brought to the table (Karrass 1970 and 1974).

Animal health issues are subject to intense (sometimes contentious) negotiations. Domestically, this often involves issues of the authority of national and subnational livestock health agencies, the determination of government versus private prerogatives, the requirements for safe movement of animals and animal products within a country, and the deployment of animal health personnel.

International animal health negotiations involve sanitary measures needed to expedite exportations and protect importing countries from exotic diseases. Negotiating international trade issues is an elaborate process requiring knowledge, skills, experience, wisdom, and patience. Negotiators must sensitively address political, economic, cultural, and regional differences. They must be able to distinguish between legitimate risks and spurious concerns fabricated to create obstacles to trade. This requires accurate perceptions of the motives of the other side, careful preparation, an understanding of the scientific principles involved, and conformance to international standards. Each country should consider adopting guidelines and standards for its negotiators.

General Negotiating Styles

There are a variety of negotiating styles. One is known as "principled negotiation" (Fisher and Ury 1991). It attempts to balance soft, or friendly, and hard negotiations by accepting early differences and identifying common objectives and shared goals. It involves working cooperatively to seek mutually acceptable middle-ground solutions by separating the people from the problems, focusing on interests not positions, inventing options for mutual gain, and establishing objective criteria.

There are ground rules for applying these principles in real-life situations like personal, marital, business, or professional discussions. These rules are:

- Regard the other side as counterparts, colleagues, or partners in negotiation rather than as opponents. Treat them accordingly
- Get acquainted with the other side and attempt to establish mutual trust
- Listen without interrupting
- Discuss rather than argue

- Control tempers
- Do homework
- Emphasize common interests and goals
- Offer suggestions rather than threats
- Shift gears when discussions get stalled

It is essential to make conscientious efforts to bridge cultural gaps between the parties. This requires the establishment of mutual trust, sensitive diplomacy, and extraordinary efforts to understand where the other side is coming from. These tactics are not always successful.

Some non-argumentative strategies for breaking stalemates include suggesting future meetings after study and consultations by both sides, using third party arbitrators, or suggesting mutual exchanges of scientific and technical information. Such exchanges familiarize negotiators with the programs and concerns of the other side and provide a venue for becoming personally acquainted.

Guidelines for International Livestock Health Negotiations

Negotiation of international livestock health issues can be a complicated undertaking. Sometimes, particularly in low-level technical discussions, veterinarians play major roles and serve as principal representatives of their countries.

When veterinarians are spokespersons, that is leaders of delegations, for both sides, matters are expedited by mutual understanding of livestock disease nomenclature and a collegial spirit. Often, this relationship is impeded by the presence of lawyers, trade representatives, or agricultural officials who talk themselves into a hole due to lack of background in disease transmission or food safety. Livestock health officials are often absent because livestock and food-safety issues are commingled with other trade issues and comprise a minor part of discussions. However, livestock health officials can play important roles as advisors to national trade delegations.

In international animal health or food-safety negotiations, the general guidelines listed above are keys to success. These items also merit attention:

- Observing international protocols such as spokespersons and seating arrangements
- Beginning with amiable welcomes, introductions, and statements of goals of the meeting that emphasize common interests of both parties
- Establishing negotiating guidelines including time limits, understanding of the level of authority of each delegation, and the nature of agreements. Step-by-step final agreements are less common than a complete undertaking in which nothing is agreed until everything is agreed

- Attempting to establish contemporary science as the basis of understandings while remaining fully aware that extremely different levels of technology can exist between countries and that sound science is in the eye of the beholder and can be manipulated for economic, political, or cultural purposes
- Determining the membership status of both countries in the OIE and carrying copies of the *OIE International Animal Health Code* and the *OIE Manual of Diagnostic Tests and Vaccines* for reference purposes
- Determining the membership status of both countries in the WTO. This is essential, because non-member countries are not bound by the WTO SPS Agreement
- Avoiding common shortcomings like arrogance, interruptive listening, and condescending or superior attitudes

In international livestock health discussions it is important to be aware that animal health issues are sometimes raised, when protection of domestic livestock industries from foreign competition and manipulation of prices are the actual motivations. It is important to determine, without asking directly, not only what the other side wants but why they want it. When the other side has been ordered by higher authority to stand firm on certain positions, cool-headed non-threatening strategies must be designed. This may involve future meetings or technical exchanges that involve discussions of diagnostic technology or sanitary measures and serve to improve personal relations and develop trust.

It is tempting to accuse trading partners of proposing sanitary measures that are unscientific or overly restrictive. Caution is advised. Such accusations are offensive and often counterproductive. Before criticizing proposed import measures, the following points should be clarified:

- What is the commodity at issue
- What domestic industry has requested opening this market for the commodity
- What is its estimated potential market value
- What specific risk factors (infections, toxins, or residues) may be associated with commodities from this country. For each risk factor provide literature citations regarding its global distribution, mode of transmission, sources of infection, survival times in various commodities, susceptibility to disinfectants and thermal inactivation, and disease-specific details of its epidemiology
- Prepare a written statement of the importing country's compliance with disease-specific and commodity-specific international standards in the OIE Code

- Prepare a written statement of the importing country's compliance with the provisions of the WTO SPS Agreement
- Prepare a written summary of official correspondence among the countries on the issue
- Prepare a written analysis of the strengths and weaknesses of the country's case regarding each risk associated with the commodity including each country's control programs and MS&R systems

Once these questions are answered it is often apparent that neither side is perfect, and some compromises are needed if the discussions are to be productive.

Export protocols and certificates must be negotiated with diligence and coordination among involved national agencies. They must be worded with clarity to ensure scientific and technical validity. Because memories are short and personnel change, everything must be in writing. There can be no unwritten understandings that can reemerge to haunt the parties or their successors. The capability of the exporting country's industries to meet the requirements must be verified. There must be assurances that inspectors can certify in writing the veracity of statements on health certificates and still maintain personal integrity and professional credibility.

Before undertaking negotiations, each country's representatives should have intelligence about the domestic measures in their own country and in the other country. They should also be familiar with SPS measures imposed upon other trading partners by both parties. They should be aware of their industry positions and knowledgeable about any diseases in question.

Sometimes livestock health issues arise unexpectedly when they are not on the agenda, and it is important for representatives to admit when they lack knowledge. Such admissions can serve to elevate the credibility of a delegation. Negotiators expecting to discuss livestock health issues often carry copies of the *OIE International Animal Health Code* (OIE 2001), the *OIE Manual of Diagnostic Tests and Vaccines* (OIE 2000), and the *Merck Veterinary Manual* (Aeillo 1998) as information sources and can request a break to consult them.

In order to function effectively and proactively in the global marketplace, each country's industry representatives, technical working groups, and negotiators should receive comprehensive, succinct, species-oriented livestock disease manuals. These should contain disease-by-disease referenced reviews of their country's livestock health status. They should also contain a description of the country's livestock disease diagnostic, surveillance, reporting, and animal ID systems.

These manuals, which can be annual reports from the country's veterinary services, should outline each country's standards for movement of livestock and livestock products. They should discuss the risks of transmission of various diseases to livestock or humans through movement of breeding and slaughter animals, zoo animals, animal trophies, hatching and table eggs, chicks, migratory birds, and processed meat. The national veterinary service should commission the development of these manuals by qualified authorities.

Often there are warning signs of impending trade problems, embargoes, or new sanitary barriers. These must be taken seriously. Suggestive correspondence should be answered promptly. Concerned industries must be consulted when trouble appears and given corrective opportunities via scientific and technical discussions with foreign counterparts. Foreign buyers should be advised that their purchases will receive better regulatory oversight if they buy directly from processors that have inspectors assigned to their plants rather than from brokers who might seek to unload slow-selling products from storage.

In this wildly competitive global economy, with trade monitored by the international community, the credibility of each country's infrastructure is at stake. The long-term national integrity should not be sacrificed in the interest of expediency or short-term trade advantages.

Export Certifications for Products Sold Abroad

Sanitary measures for livestock products should ensure safe movement of economically competitive commodities. The wording of health certificates for exports should be worked out in consultation with concerned industry representatives, subnational regulatory officials, and other agencies. Whenever possible they should be consummated at the technical level, that is by middle-level government officials who understand the role of livestock disease in international trade.

Export certificates and protocols should be based strictly on health issues and not manipulated for trade advantages. They should be negotiated and developed using standard guidelines. These goals can be accomplished as follows.

The negotiated requirements should have a sound scientific and technical basis and be in a format that can be honestly endorsed by national officials. They should be acceptable to concerned industries and compatible with regulations of subnational governments and other national agencies. The negotiated requirements should be compared with OIE standards. If both countries agree to follow the OIE Code, the measures are exempt from WTO challenge and from WTO notification requirements (see chapter 5).

If the importing country wishes measures more stringent than the OIE Code recommends, that country should submit a risk assessment supporting the proposed measures before formal negotiations are initiated. Negotiated agreements should conform to the principles outlined in the WTO SPS Agreement (see chapter 5).

The negotiated agreement should be written so its implementation will encourage harmonious working relationships among the parties. Future agreements should be based on the OIE Code and on the principles of the WTO SPS Agreeement.

Animal Science and Veterinary Medical Research, Education, and Outreach Programs

Informed livestock producers, trained experts in animal science and livestock health, and research and technologic advances are all vital to effective livestock health infrastructures. The nature and extent of these programs will vary between countries depending upon their ecological settings, agricultural systems, livestock populations, economic development, and national priorities.

The United States is fortunate. Its early leadership placed high priority on agriculture and established the **Land Grant System** of Agricultural Education, Research, and Extension. The Morrill Act of 1862 deeded tracts of land to states for agricultural colleges. States were charged to provide low-cost education in the agricultural sciences, to conduct ongoing research in the production and processing of agricultural products, and to establish systems for the dissemination of knowledge to producers and homemakers.

The information-dissemination component became the State-Federal Cooperative Extension Service. It is jointly supported by state, county, and federal funding. Cooperative extension provides bulletins on agricultural production, food processing, food preparation, and nutritional guidelines for people and livestock; experts who offer advice; and informational meetings. The nature of the Land Grant Program changed over the years as technology advanced and society evolved. It remains a major stimulus to progress in U.S. livestock production, animal health, food safety, and nutrition.

The U.S. Land Grant System is not suited for all countries and is not necessarily recommended for worldwide emulation. Nonetheless, its three components of teaching, research, and information dissemination comprise time-tested missions for sound livestock health infrastructures and an informed citizenry.

Broad-Based Livestock Health Partnerships

The term infrastructure suggests governmental regulations, livestock disease-control authority, and bureaucratic programs. Livestock health programs must reach beyond bureaucracies and find broad-based participatory support from many organizations, institutions, and individuals. These participants must be supportive of sanitary measures, food-safety initiatives, border security, animal identification, and MS&R systems. They should also support efforts to gain funds for livestock health research, academic institutions, and educational programs. They should work to establish and expand foreign markets and conduct exotic-disease exclusion programs. In case of emergency they must be asked to support drastic reductions in livestock populations where necessary to control rapidly spreading diseases.

If LHP-makers expect to achieve the goals outlined in this chapter, they will have to work continually to build a broad-based partnership comprised of livestock producers, livestock and breed organizations, practicing and corporate veterinarians, the diagnostic and academic communities, national and subnational veterinary officials, food-processing industry organizations, and the local, national, and international media.

Livestock Health Organizations

Livestock health organizations play vital roles in livestock health infrastructures. They bring together organizations and individuals of various persuasions that can influence livestock health policies and practices.

In many countries there are groups representing the interests of each portion of the livestock industry. Livestock producers tend to collaborate by species. Poultry producers often link up organizationally. Pharmaceutical and biological manufacturers and food processors also have their own organizations. It is easy to omit groups with peripheral interests, and one goal of policy makers should be to get input from all these interests and encourage them to listen to opposing views on livestock health and food-safety issues.

In the United States some of these needs are met by the **United States Animal Health Association (USAHA)**. It is dominated by state animal health officials. However, the USAHA membership includes breed associations, federal officials, food-safety officials, employees of drug and biologic manufacturers, and research, diagnostic, and academic interests. The USAHA meets annually. It has committees that debate issues and prepare resolutions. Resolutions that are approved by the Executive Board, comprised largely of State Veterinarians, are forwarded to the USDA or other government agencies for action. Other organizations, such as the **Coalition for Animal Agriculture** and the **National Institute for Animal Agriculture (NIAA)** provide input from slightly different perspectives. The pharmaceutical, biologicals, and food-processing industries should provide more input into U.S. LHPs.

External Reviews of National Livestock Health Infrastructures

Periodic external reviews of national livestock health programs can provide valuable information. Review panels must be carefully selected to represent a diversity of knowledge, skills, and backgrounds. Panel members should be far enough removed from bureaucracies that they can contribute impartially without having to answer to national officials or special interest groups. Extramural review panels should include subnational animal health officials; academic and diagnostic personnel; livestock producers, food processors, and their organizational leaders; and ancillary stakeholders such as consumers, environmentalists, and animal welfare and food-safety advocates. Representatives of other countries can add knowledge and experience to the deliberations of review panels. In selecting review panels, both the managers of organizations and their members who are working in the field should be represented.

It is sometimes necessary to review the nation's entire livestock infrastructure. Usually, reviews cover a particular program such as emergency management systems, diagnostic capacities, border security, food-safety systems, export certifications, domestic disease-control and eradication programs, or communication efforts.

The review panel's reports should candidly outline program strengths and weaknesses and contain succinct summaries of findings and recommendations. It is essential to avoid efforts to sanitize reports by glossing over identified suggestions for improvement. The written report, regardless of how unfavorable it sounds, must be widely distributed within government and industry circles and be made available to the media. The leadership of the national programs under examination should receive a mandate to respond with substantive changes within a year.

Positive Media Relations

Effective livestock infrastructures need public understanding and support. The media provide a direct line to the citizenry and its leaders. The power of the press cannot be underestimated. The media can be allies or adversaries of LHP-makers. The choice is in the hands of livestock health officials. Generally, when media are treated with respect and openness they will report issues fairly. Media partners can be cultivated by regular press conferences and the distribution of background information, position papers, and issue analyses. If they are to be used, these must be well thought out, clearly written, scientifically sound, forthright, and free of bureaucratic legalese, protective deception, defensiveness, and gobbledygook.

Summary

The issues discussed in this chapter can guide the development and maintenance of livestock health infrastructures in a changing world. More detailed strategies for the activation of infrastructural objectives are detailed in chapter 10. Certainly no nation can implement all the ideas described here but suggestions offered in this chapter can guide nations that wish to review, prioritize, or update their livestock health infrastructures.

Bibliography

Aiello, S. E. ed. 1998. *The Merck Veterniary Manual*. Whitehouse Station, NJ: Merck and Co. Inc.

Bower-Spence, K. 2002. Holsteins Basic ID. *Dairy Today*. (February): 22.

Case J. T. 1998. Status of Health Information Standards in Veterinary Medicine. *Proc U.S. Anim Health Assoc*. 102:71–77.

Elvinger, F. and M. Thurman. 2002. *Proceedings of the AAVLD Workshop on Validation of Diagnostic Tests*. Presented at the 2002 Annual Meeting of the AAVLD in St. Louis, MO. Davis, CA: American Association of Veterinary Laboratory Diagnosticians.

Fisher, R., W. Ury, and B. Patton. 1991. *Getting to Yes*. 2d ed. New York: Penguin Books Inc.

Kahrs, R. F. 1999. The International Animal Health Community's Expectations of the U.S. National Animal Health Reporting System (NAHRS). *Proc U.S. Anim Health Assoc* 103:100-109

Karrass, C. L. 1970. *The Negotiating Game*. New York: Thomas Y. Crowell Publishers.

Karrass, C. L. 1974. *Give and Take: The Complete Guide to Negotiating Strategies and Tactics*. New York: Thomas Y. Crowell Publishers.

MacDaniel, H. A. and M. K. Sheridan. 2001. Traceability of Animals and Animal Products. *OIE Scientific and Technical Review*. 20(2) August Paris: Office International Des Epizooties.

Maday, J. 2001. Identification Please; Like It or Not, Identification and Source Verification Are Becoming Standard Practice. *Drovers*. (March):30-33.

NAHEMS. 2002. *The 2001 Annual Report of National Animal Health Emergency Management System*. The National Animal Health Emergency Management System Steering Committee. Riverdale, MD: USDA Veterinary Services.

National Renderers Association. 2002. *Rendering: The Only Biosecure Option for Animal Mortality and By-product Disposal*. Alexandria, VA: National Renderers Association Inc. www.renderers.org

Nolen, R. S. 2002. The Network of Veterinary Diagnostic Laboratories Would Strengthen the Nation's Security. *J Am Vet Med Assoc*. 220:575-576.

OIE. 2001. *The OIE International Animal Health Code*. Paris: Office International des Epizooties.

OIE. 2000. *The OIE Manual of Diagnostic Tests and Vaccines*. Paris: Office International des Epizooties.

Salmon, M. 1998. A Monitoring System for Diseases That Are Approaching the Level of Eradication. *Proc U.S. Anim Health Assoc.* 102:64-70.

Chapter 5

International Livestock Health Standards and Standard-Setting Organizations

INTRODUCTION

Several international standard-setting bodies meet regularly to establish and update guidelines for international movement of livestock products. The **Office International des Epizooties (OIE)** sets standards for animal products. The **International Plant Protection Convention (IPPC)** sets standards for plants and plant products. The **Codex Alimentarius Commission (CODEX)** sets standards for drugs, pharmaceuticals, and foods. The **International Organization for Standardization (ISO)** sets standards for overall global commerce. These bodies have differing organizational structures, memberships, and operating rules.

The OIE, IPPC, CODEX, and ISO have been assigned standard-setting responsibilities by the **World Trade Organization (WTO)** under authority granted by the **General Agreement on Tariffs and Trade (GATT)**. These organizations provide educational materials and technical assistance to support the livestock health efforts of all nations.

In livestock health the **WTO Sanitary and Phytosanitary (SPS) Agreement** outlines the guiding principles for international trade, which are then implemented by the OIE. The livestock health standards documented in the *OIE International Animal Health Code* (OIE 2001) and the *OIE Manual of Standards for Diagnostic Tests and Vaccines* (OIE 2000) are continually updated.

The SPS provisions of the GATT and the WTO require that import–export measures be scientifically and technically sound, transparent, and based on harmonized international standards. They urge importing countries to apply fair national treatment to exporting countries and to strive to negotiate equivalency agreements. They require that **sanitary measures** be based on risk assessments and the principle of **regionalization.** It is expected that countries negotiate in good faith and make all efforts to resolve disputes at the lowest possible levels.

The North American Free Trade Agreement (NAFTA) involves Canada, Mexico, and the United States and may expand into a Free Trade Area of the Americas (FTAA). It includes sanitary guidelines similar to the WTO SPS Agreement and the animal health standards established by the OIE.

This chapter lays out guidelines for **livestock health policies (LHPs)** that govern international trade and serve as templates for domestic regulatory practices. It also describes the international organizations responsible for these standards and outlines the processes by which they develop, disseminate, and monitor the standards.

Knowledge of international standards and the organizations that promulgate them is essential for effective LHP-making in an era of expanding international trade.

International Treaties, Trade Agreements, and Trading Blocs

Most of the world's countries are signatories to treaties or multilateral trade agreements that shape their regulations and guide the sanitary measures they impose on importations of livestock and livestock products. The United States, Canada, and Mexico comprise the NAFTA and all participate in the GATT, the WTO, and the OIE.

General Agreement on Tariffs and Trade (GATT)

The GATT is an ad hoc international organization without firm legal foundation. It was originated in 1947 by 23 countries to try to stabilize a world in turmoil following World War II. Its purpose was to stimulate international commerce, increase incomes and employment rates throughout the world, and reduce tariffs, quotas, and **technical barriers to trade (TBTs).** The GATT now has over 100 member countries and multiple commodity agreements spelled out in thousands of pages of documentation. Agricultural products and intellectual properties were introduced into the GATT in 1987 in a round of talks in Uruguay. The resulting agricultural provisions were finalized in April 1994 in Marakesh, Morocco, and are known as the Marakesh Accords. They were ratified shortly thereafter by most GATT member countries.

The livestock health authorities of participating countries have both rights and obligations under the GATT. These are outlined in the *GATT Agricultural Agreement,* which contains several annexes and detailed dispute resolution procedures. After its ratification, the responsibility for implementation of the GATT was assigned to the WTO, which has power of international law. The GATT agricultural provisions became the WTO SPS Agreement.

For the most part the SPS provisions of the NAFTA mimic those of the GATT and the WTO. Participating countries consider compliance with the WTO SPS Agreement to fulfill the general conditions of the GATT and the NAFTA. The SPS provisions of the three accords are usually discussed collectively. The NAFTA, however, contains references to many commodity-specific issues, such as cheese, pork, poultry, and citrus products in more specific terms than found in the WTO SPS Agreement.

Subsequent rounds of GATT negotiations will undoubtedly strengthen the working mechanisms, logistical details, and scientific soundness of the GATT and the WTO.

The North American Free Trade Agreement (NAFTA)

The agricultural agreements in the NAFTA and the GATT and the resultant WTO SPS Agreement are intended to gradually reduce tariffs, quotas, TBT, and export subsidies. These goals should increase international trade in agricultural products and eliminate the use of sanitary measures as artificial trade barriers.

The NAFTA was initiated in 1989 by the inclusion of Mexico in the Canadian-United States Trade Agreement. It provides incentives for these countries to purchase products of North American origin and reduces trade barriers in accord with the provisions of the WTO SPS Agreement. It has expanded the export markets of all three countries.

Canada and the United States have almost identical livestock health status. The addition of Mexico provided new challenges, because Mexico has different geography, ecology, and prevalence and distribution of diseases and animal parasites, some of which serve as vectors of insect-borne infections. Mexico has a different animal health infrastructure and communication style from its northern neighbors. The three countries have worked to open and expand markets and reduce the risk of spreading livestock diseases. Their geographic proximity and good relations have increased trade for all three countries. The potential addition of all Western Hemisphere countries to the NAFTA, to form the FTAA, will add further challenges.

Canadian, Mexican, and U.S. livestock health officials meet regularly as a Tripartite Animal Health Group. They discuss common goals, develop joint programs, and preempt potential problems. They also cooperate as leaders in the OIE Regional Commission of the Americas to shape international standards that are equitable, scientifically sound, and support legitimate interests of NAFTA countries.

Proposed Free Trade Area of the Americas (FTAA)

Since the early 1990s there has been an ongoing movement to expand the NAFTA to include all Western Hemisphere countries except Cuba. The proposed FTAA would expedite trade; reduce tariffs, quotas, and restrictions on commerce; enhance market access for member countries; and provide a unified hemispheric voice to address the EU, the Commonwealth of Independent States (the countries of the former Soviet Union), and other multinational trading blocs that negotiate collectively.

Early FTAA negotiations began in Miami in late 1994 at the first Summit of the Americas. They continued in Santiago, Chile, at the Second Summit of the Americas in 1998. In preparation for the 2002 Summit the Bush administration sought and eventually gained **Fast Track Authority**. Fast Track Authority, now called **Trade Promotion Authority (TPA)**, permits the Administration to negotiate with one voice and forces Congress to vote either yes or no, without amendment privileges, on ratification of trade agreements. TPA permits knowledgeable trade officials to spend full-time on proposed agreements and interact authoritatively with U.S. stakeholders, administration officials, and Congress. In granting TPA, Congress insisted on being updated on trade issues. Congress was understandably reluctant to abandon its constitutional right to amend treaties, but they were aware that negotiators lack credibility when they speak with limited authority and if their tentative commitments are subject to reversal by diverse political bodies. Informed negotiators understand the ramifications of proposals and compromises essential to reaching agreement among thirty-four nations, each with its own trade objectives and political and cultural constraints. TPA was resisted by interests opposing **globalization**.

Early drafts indicate that the FTAA will probably mimic the WTO SPS Agreement except in areas where experience indicates that unique Western Hemisphere clarifications are needed. Some divergence from the WTO SPS Agreement in the areas of **harmonization** with international standards, **equivalency**, and the rights of importing countries is expected (Bowman and Desrosiers 2001). Harmonization involves adjusting national policies to global standards; equivalence involves treating nations similarly when comparable conditions exist with respect to trade issues.

The World Trade Organization (WTO)

The WTO was established in January 1995 as a successor to the GATT to implement and oversee international trade rules. The WTO is headquartered in Geneva, Switzerland, where diplomats from all nations participate in its governance. Designated international standard-setting organizations and the trade guidelines outlined in the SPS Agreement, along with its dispute resolution authority, implement the LHPs of the WTO.

Upon formation of the WTO, some minor alterations to the GATT agricultural provisions evolved into the WTO SPS Agreement. The Agreement states each country may establish whatever measures are needed to protect its animal, plant, and human health. To qualify for this right, the 150 WTO member countries have multiple obligations. They are obligated to:

- Minimize restrictions to trade
- Refrain from using SPS requirements as trade barriers
- Deal equitably with all nations without discrimination
- Invoke only those sanitary requirements deemed necessary
- Base SPS measures on sound science
- Harmonize SPS procedures with international standards
- Participate in the OIE, the IPPC, and the CODEX
- Provide access to programs, procedures, and test results
- Consult freely with other countries on requirements and procedures
- Base SPS procedures on internationally acceptable contemporary risk-assessment procedures
- Adopt internationally acceptable regionalization criteria for assessing the point-of-origin livestock health status of potential imports
- Render transparent all SPS measures by prompt publication of regulations and changing requirements
- Provide inspection privileges, prompt and clear explanations, and accurate information about their animal disease status and livestock health infrastructures
- Limit animal disease-control programs and test requirements to the essentials
- Make import requirements no more stringent than subnational regulations (in situations where equal conditions prevail)
- Strive to recognize when trading partners have achieved equivalent animal health measures. Equivalency is achieved if an exporting member objectively demonstrates that its products achieve the importing country's appropriate level of protection, even if different measures are employed to achieve this status. Countries are also urged to expedite trade through formal equivalence agreements

- Provide technical assistance to other countries
- Support and encourage the efforts of developing nations and regions
- Cooperate with the GATT and the WTO Committees on SPS procedures
- Participate actively in administration of the SPS provisions of the GATT and the WTO
- Work actively to implement these provisions in international trade
- Participate in good faith in dispute resolution procedures

These expectations are largely accomplished when countries conform to established international standards. This conformance is referred to as harmonization with international standards.

The WTO general meetings are attended by high-level agricultural and trade officials and some representatives of non-governmental organizations (NGOs) from member countries. WTO meetings are sometimes picketed by protesters representing groups that oppose the globalization movement as a threat to jobs, the environment, and human rights.

Animal health officials rarely attend WTO meetings but sometimes participate in meetings of the SPS Committee. Meetings on SPS issues often involve both plant and animal health issues, and countries may decide to send plant or animal experts or both.

International Standard-Setting Organizations

Animal health policy makers should be familiar with OIE, CODEX, and IPPC. Several international standard-setting organizations operate transparently to assist countries in developing policies for the maintenance of healthy livestock populations. Most national **veterinary services (VS)** relate to the OIE, the CODEX, and to a lesser extent, the IPPC. These organizations were all in operation before the development of the agricultural provisions of the GATT and the NAFTA. They were assigned standard-setting authority by the WTO after its establishment in 1995.

These standard-setting organizations are gradually achieving global consistency of import requirements. They try to achieve consensus by representing the concerns of the various regions of the world and those of the developed, developing, and less-developed nations as they promulgate and periodically review SPS standards.

WTO member countries are obligated to participate in the development of international SPS standards, strive for harmonization by using them as a guide in developing their own requirements, and conform to them if possible.

As long as they are able to justify them scientifically, any nation can develop whatever SPS measures it deems necessary to protect the health of its animal, plant, and human populations. Countries must be prepared to be challenged by trading partners if their import requirements differ significantly from international standards. They must have documented risk analyses to scientifically justify the measures, prove that they are essential to meet their acceptable level of protection, and demonstrate that they are applied consistently to all trading partners of equal livestock health status.

Office International des Epizooties (OIE)

The OIE is the world's oldest international veterinary organization. Formed in 1924, it is headquartered in Paris, France, and includes about 160 member countries. Its goals are to develop and maintain a worldwide animal disease-reporting network and to facilitate world trade by minimizing the risk of spreading livestock diseases.

The OIE is the WTO-designated international standard-setting organization for livestock health. It maintains an international animal disease reporting system, prepares criteria for disease-free status of countries, and recommends sanitary measures such as testing, quarantine, and health certification procedures for the safe international trade in livestock.

The OIE publishes the ***International Animal Health Code*** (the Code) (OIE 2001). The Code describes livestock diseases and recommended testing, vaccination, health certification, and quarantine measures for the international movement of livestock germplasm and related commodities. The OIE also publishes a similar *International Aquatic Animal Health Code* for fish, mollusks, and crustaceans; the *OIE Manual of Standards for Diagnostic Tests and Vaccines* (the Manual); and a similar volume for aquatic animals. The manuals lay out validated diagnostic tests and vaccine production protocols.

The Annual OIE Meeting is attended by **chief veterinary officers (CVOs)** and accompanying delegations from all over the world. Each country's CVO is the sole voting delegate. National delegations include national and subnational veterinary officials and representatives of some non-governmental organizations (NGOs). The U.S. delegation usually includes representatives from the **United States Animal Health Association (USAHA)**, the **American Veterinary Medical Association (AVMA),** the academic and diagnostic communities, the **United States Department of Agriculture (USDA),** and state veterinary officials. The annual OIE meeting provides opportunities for veterinary officials from around the world to meet formally as well as to network informally.

During the OIE meeting there are breakout sessions at which delegates from five geographic regions meet to develop positions and discuss agenda items. The regional commissions represent Asia, the Far East and Oceania, Europe, the Americas, and the Middle East. They assemble to strengthen regional cooperation, review regional animal health status, and focus on technical issues of regional importance.

Future OIE work plans will address animal welfare and trade, food safety and animal production, harmonization of the terrestrial and aquatic codes, and the upgrading of existing standards.

Relationships developed at OIE meetings help establish trust and lay the groundwork for international cooperation in livestock disease control and trade.

International Standards Set by the OIE

The OIE uses regionally balanced expert working groups to develop draft standards that are then circulated for comment prior to adoption. Comments are only accepted from delegates. Most delegates involve their scientific, regulatory, and agricultural communities, which strengthens the delegates' effectiveness. Despite occasional efforts to politicize them, OIE standards are usually based on sound science. LHP-makers should be familiar with the nature, authority, magnitude, and format of OIE standards.

Countries may apply import measures more stringent than OIE standards if they are transparent, science-based, and supported by **risk analyses**. SPS measures founded on OIE standards are exempt from reporting regulation changes and conducting risk analyses. They won't be challenged beyond consultation, a preliminary step in the WTO dispute-resolution process. Most countries try to conform to OIE reporting requirements and international standards. Those that cheat gradually begin to conform as the benefits of conforming become evident and international pressures prevail.

Reference laboratories and member countries review OIE standards. They are adopted, usually by consensus, by the General Assembly at annual meetings. If there is a call for a vote, there is one vote per country. The CVO is the voting delegate from each country.

The OIE international standards include general guidelines and specific procedures published and regularly updated in the Code (OIE 2001). The 500-page Code contains guidelines for the maintenance of livestock health and the operation of national veterinary services. It includes sections on definitions, risk analysis, import-export procedures, disease notification and reporting, and guidelines for the safe use of veterinary biologicals. There are also sections on disease-control procedures at artificial insemination centers and in poultry breeding flocks, hatcheries, apiaries, and equine centers.

There is a section on procedures for destroying pathogens and insect vectors, which includes guidelines for the disinfecting and inactivation of **foot-and-mouth disease (FMD)** virus and the causative agents of the **transmissible spongiform encephalopathies (TSEs)**. There are also sections on transport of animals, epidemiological surveillance systems, and notifiable diseases. The Code recommendations are intended to be trade-neutral, which means sanitary measures should be the same for both importers and exporters.

The disease-specific standards in the Code vary in length and complexity depending on each disease's seriousness, mode of transmission, and the number of susceptible species. Disease chapters define each malady, list the conditions required for disease-free status, and list specific conditions for international trade.

The chapter on FMD is lengthy and complex. It outlines the conditions required for a country or zone to be considered FMD-free, with or without vaccination. It outlines criteria to be met for the importation of livestock commodities from FMD-free and not-free nations into both free and affected countries. There are detailed FMD-specific guidelines for the importation or exportation of live domestic and wild ruminants; of semen, ova and embryos of swine and ruminants; of the fresh meat of swine and ruminants; of meat products of domestic and wild swine and ruminants; and of hunting trophies from FMD-susceptible wildlife. There are also guidelines for the importation of milk, cheese, and other products of animal origin intended for human food or for the manufacture of pharmaceuticals, biologicals, or vaccines.

Because of the complexity, political sensitivity, long incubation period, and scientific uncertainty surrounding **bovine spongiform encephalopathy (BSE)**, that chapter is also extensive. It outlines the risk-management strategies required to establish a country as BSE-free. These strategies include monitoring and surveillance, clinical examination of suspect cases, microscopic examination of cow brains, and restrictions on feeding of ruminant offal. The BSE chapter also outlines detailed requirements to be applied when importing cattle, meat and meat products, bovine embryos or ova, meat and bone meal, and other specified bovine offal from countries with BSE.

Diseases for which similar, though less complex, guidelines are presented are discussed in eight groupings. These include the diseases of multiple species (such as rabies and **anthrax**), cattle, sheep and goats, equines, swine, birds, lagomorphs (rabbits), and bees.

Countries may impose import measures that exceed Code standards if they are justified scientifically and are not discriminatory. Importation requirements based on OIE standards are exempt from the requirement to notify the WTO of regulation changes, provide detailed **risk assessments**, and cannot be extensively challenged beyond early consultation in the dispute resolution process. OIE standards also include descriptions of diagnostic test methodology and procedures for vaccine production and usage. These are published and regularly updated in the Manual (OIE 2000).

The Codex Alimentarius Commission (CODEX)

The CODEX is a subsidiary of the United Nations **Food and Agriculture Organization (FAO).** It works in cooperation with the World Health Organization (WHO). The CODEX facilitates safe trade in food, biological materials, and pharmaceuticals by establishing science-based international standards. The CODEX addresses food safety by setting trade standards for food additives, pesticide residues, and food labeling. It seeks to protect the health of consumers and to ensure fair-trade practices by encouraging governments to adopt and implement food standards, codes of practice, and other guidelines developed by CODEX committees.

The CODEX meets annually and has multiple delegations representing governmental agencies with regulatory responsibility for foods. The meetings also include NGOs representing food industries and consumer interests. The CODEX committees are composed of representatives from government, regulatory agencies, the scientific community, and food industries. They draft codes and operating principles through a time-consuming, transparent, eight-step process that includes the circulation of working papers for comment by stakeholders in member countries.

The U.S. government's CODEX delegation includes officials of the USDA **Food Safety and Inspection Service (FSIS),** the Food and Drug Administration (FDA), and the **Environmental Protection Agency (EPA)**. These agencies hold public meetings to receive comments on agenda items prior to the CODEX meetings.

Animal health policy makers need to be in constant communication with their country's representatives to CODEX to ensure interagency communication and stakeholder participation.

International Plant Protection Commission (IPPC)

The IPPC is also a subsidiary of the FAO. The IPPC focuses on preventing the spread of plant-borne diseases and pests and on developing model plant quarantine and inspection requirements for international trade. It develops pest-specific inspection and quarantine procedures to prevent the spread of plant pests in international commerce.

The IPPC was formed in the 1950s and has over ninety member countries. It receives recommendations from its Regional Plant Protection Organizations. The United States is well represented among the officers and panels of the **North American Plant Protection Organization (NAPPO)**, whose membership also includes Canada and Mexico.

Animal health policy makers need an understanding of the IPPC, because many countries regulate animal and plant health activities under the same agency. Both animal and plant health issues frequently surface in international meetings and trade negotiations. Representatives of departments of agriculture stationed at foreign embassies must often address both plant and animal health issues. This is the situation in the **Animal and Plant Health Inspection Service (APHIS)** of the USDA.

The WTO SPS Agreement

The adoption of the WTO SPS Agreement caused many national veterinary services to reevaluate the scientific and technical credibility of their policies. Ratification of the SPS Agreement provided regulatory professionals with new opportunities to develop foreign markets.

Developed countries are emerging as world leaders in animal health, and other nations sometimes mimic their sanitary measures. Their export certifications and sanitary measures are ultimately imposed upon their own products and determine the extent of their international markets.

The WTO SPS Agreement encourages countries to address SPS issues on their own merits. It discourages "linkages" that involve tradeoffs on unrelated commodities. Such bargaining often involves permitting one violation of the Agreement to offset another and can diminish the stature of the WTO SPS Principles. Sometimes linkages occur by mutual agreement as a means of breaking stalemates in negotiations.

The WTO SPS Agreement reflects the directions in which many national veterinary services are moving. These adjustments have occurred in response to:

- Advancing animal health and communications technology
- Progress in the eradication and control of major livestock plagues
- A worldwide movement toward privatization of regulatory responsibilities
- Changing national boundaries
- Formation of trading blocs
- The movement toward transparent, participatory, and open governments
- Demands of trading partners

In upcoming years, nations will evaluate livestock importations with respect to health hazards, or risks, based on the **animal health infrastructure** and disease-free status of exporting countries.

Rights, Responsibilities, and Provisions of the WTO SPS Agreement

The wording of the WTO SPS Agreement resembles the GATT and the NAFTA. It essentially supersedes them in many ways. It provides rights, and imposes obligations, on signatory countries. These are spelled out in provisions on harmonization, equivalence, risk assessment, regionalization, **transparency**, technical assistance, differential treatment of developing nations, dispute resolution, administration, and implementation.

The national animal health authorities of each country can exercise these rights if they accept the obligations of the WTO SPS Agreement.

Understanding these rights and responsibilities is essential in effectively representing their industries and governments in international forums and discussions with trading partners.

The WTO SPS Agreement has both general guidelines and specific provisions that guide trade in animals and animal products and control livestock disease.

General Provisions of the WTO SPS Agreement

The WTO SPS Agreement applies to all sanitary measures invoked in international trade. It defines terms used in animal, plant, and human health. Its general guidelines recommend that signatory nations treat other countries fairly and equitably; participate in governance of the WTO, the setting of standards, and the resolution of disputes; help developing nations comply with international standards; and exercise transparency and scientific judgment in dealing with the international community. In practice the principles of transparency and sound science also translate into specific actions.

The agreement provides a template for the discussion of trade issues. Countries that permit freedom of speech, freedom of the press, transparent governance, and similar traditions are already in partial compliance with the general guidelines. This presents opportunities for global leadership in international livestock health.

It will take time for the international community to implement the WTO SPS principles. During this interval, countries, their industries, and their national veterinary services must realize that all nations may not apply these ideals. WTO-compliant nations may experience some trade disadvantages by adherence. By exemplifying the best in international conduct they should gain in the long run.

The provisions for scientifically based transparent import requirements are imposing including the presentation, upon request, of documentation on the basis of sanitary measures. In cases where import requirements exceed international standards a risk assessment must also be available.

Specific Provisions of the WTO SPS Agreement

In addition to the general principles of international behavior just discussed, the WTO SPS Agreement carries specific provisions applicable to sanitary measures used in international trade. They apply to import measures, disease reporting, health certifications, inspections, testing procedures, **quarantines**, and border-security.

The specific provisions of the WTO SPS Agreement are scientific and technical validity, transparency, **equal national treatment**, equivalency, risk assessment, and regionalization. If these requirements are fulfilled without discrimination or arbitrary and unjustified differences, importing countries may impose whatever sanitary measures they deem necessary to protect their livestock, wildlife, and human populations from disease. However, they must adhere to the SPS agreement and present documentation that the measures imposed are essential to meet their acceptable level of protection.

Import Measures Should Be Science-Based

Articles 2.2, 3.3, and 5.2 of the WTO SPS Agreement state that import measures must be based on sound science. This may appear self-evident, but the role of science in international trade is controversial and subject to many interpretations. Published data can be distorted by economic objectives, political expediencies, and cultural traditions. Science is constantly changing and some scientific facts are ephemeral. The changing scientific basis of livestock health programs has many components including:

- Advancing diagnostic technology that permits recognition and differentiation among types, subtypes, and strains of animal-borne organisms
- The continuing recognition of new diseases and pathogenic agents
- The shifting global importance of existing diseases
- Advancing surveillance techniques that permit the pinpointing of the source of epidemics and **epizootics**
- Emergence of the science of risk analysis
- Emergence of TSEs as animal pathogens with **zoonotic** potential
- Improved transportation permitting rapid distribution of perishable products to areas where table scraps are fed to backyard livestock and where wildlife and birds have access to uneaten foods
- **Integrated production-management systems** resulting in animal concentrations that predispose to stress-related diseases
- Emphasis on molecular biology and animal welfare thus diminishing animal experimentation needed to evaluate risks of disease introduction by specific commodities

In many countries the interaction of science, politics, and culture is currently tilted toward protectionism, partnering with industry, and succumbing to pressures from special interest groups. These forces can bias the interpretation of scientific inquiry, risk analyses, and international standards.

For these reasons inferences that sanitary measures are based on sound science can be questioned. Speakers must be prepared to explain the details of the scientific inquiry upon which their statements are based. They should also be prepared to have their evidence countered with equally convincing and contradictory scientific information.

Import Measures Should Be Transparent

WTO SPS Article 7 requires that importing countries clearly articulate the scientific basis of SPS measures imposed on livestock products entering their territories. Transparency is accomplished by openly discussing import requirements; notifying trading partners and the WTO of new rules 60 days before enactment; promptly publishing regulatory changes; providing information, inspection privileges, and clear explanations of import measures; and providing documentation of equal national treatment to countries or regions with comparable animal health status.

Transparency involves the distribution of proposed sanitary measures to domestic stakeholders and trading partners and the solicitation of comments with the expectation that they will receive careful consideration.

Transparent governments inform domestic and foreign stakeholders about requests for importations, regionalization, or changes in sanitary measures. They provide access to information submitted by other countries or regions. If, after reviewing risk factors, the government believes the importation can safely be allowed, it publishes a proposed rule specifying the conditions for importation and a discussion of how the decision was reached. During the comment period the public is permitted access to the information and methodology upon which the risk analysis is based. Once all comments have been received, a decision is made as to the conditions under which the importation can be allowed and the final decision is then published in a public record.

WTO signatory countries each name a contact point to whom trading partners can direct questions. The United States named the National Institute of Standards and Technology of the Department of Commerce as the national inquiry point. They have delegated responsibility for agricultural notifications to the USDA's **Foreign Agricultural Service (FAS),** which informs the WTO and involved trading partners of new or changing import regulations.

Import Measures Should Harmonize with International Standards

Harmonization implies replacing national regulatory policies with global standards. This involves merging sanitary policies, regulations, and diagnostic methods into common acceptable standards attained by compromise within the international community.

Article 3 of the WTO SPS Agreement says nations should strive cooperatively for international standardization of diagnostic tests, surveillance systems, import requirements, quarantine procedures, animal-identification policies, vaccine standards, and risk-assessment and risk-management systems.

Opponents of globalization feel that harmonization replaces good regulations and policies with less effective global guidelines, thus introducing a lowest common denominator.

The OIE is the WTO-designated international standard-setting organization for animal health. It develops sanitary regulations, testing, quarantine, and health certification procedures to encourage world trade while at the same time minimizing the risk of spreading diseases. Within the OIE, international standards are proposed by regional commissions and developed by technical working groups comprised of experts representing each of five geographic regions. Proposed standards are circulated to each country's delegate for comment and are then revised by working groups before being presented to the assembly where they are either approved by consensus and finalized, unless a vote is requested, or returned to the working group for modification.

The OIE publishes the *International Animal Health Code* (the Code), which contains guidelines for safe trade in animals and animal products and the *OIE Manual of Standards for Diagnostic Tests and Vaccines* (the Manual). Both provide minimal standards that will usually go unchallenged when applied as import requirements.

Nations are free to impose measures more stringent than OIE standards if they can be justified scientifically and are not discriminatory. Countries that appropriately apply OIE standards as import requirements are exempt from notifying the WTO of regulation changes, having their import requirements challenged beyond WTO consultation, and having to conduct detailed risk assessments when establishing import requirements. These exemptions make OIE standards attractive and therefore subject to abuse. Countries establishing import measures based on OIE standards may conduct site visits to verify disease-free status and examine surveillance data, diagnostic facilities, and livestock health infrastructures of the exporting country. This emphasis on international standards requires side-by-side comparisons of national regulations with OIE guidelines.

Most countries permit the use of OIE standards as sanitary measures in lieu of risk analysis but require risk assessments when countries propose restrictions more stringent than Code recommendations.

Import Measures Should Apply Equal National Treatment

The concept of non-discrimination, or equal national treatment, is spelled out in WTO SPS Article 2.3. It requires importing countries to apply equal SPS measures to exporting nations if similar conditions prevail. It implies that once imports clear customs, they must be treated, taxed, and distributed in the same manner as domestic products. This component of equal national treatment is sometimes interpreted to mean that countries should treat imports no less favorably than domestic products if equal conditions prevail. This interpretation has limited use as it applies only when the disease-free status and livestock health infrastructures of both countries are virtually identical for the commodity in question.

Import Measures Should Recognize Equivalency of Sanitary Measures

WTO signatory countries agree to acknowledge similar sanitary status of commodities even if different methods were used to achieve parity. This means that if two products come from animals raised, fed, slaughtered, and processed differently they can still be considered equivalent if they are similar with respect to product quality, food safety, and the health risks associated with their importation.

Countries are encouraged to develop equivalency agreements with trading partners. Such agreements acknowledge that domestic sanitary measures in each country produce equivalent results while differing in details. Bilateral or multilateral equivalency agreements permit free movement of identified commodities between the countries if they are accompanied by point-of-origin certifications signed by government officials.

The negotiation of veterinary equivalency agreements is a complicated process that can get mired in details or stalled by national pride and turf wars. Equivalency agreements require trust between countries with comparable animal health infrastructures, long-standing good relationships, and a sincere desire for free trade. Unless these conditions exist equivalency discussions can be futile and damaging to relationships.

Equivalency agreements must clearly identify the commodities and diseases covered and must be made transparent to stakeholders and citizens of signatory countries. Equivalency agreements must be explicit in detailing the health certifications and border controls imposed on imported commodities.

The 2001 FTAA negotiations raised fears that encouraging equivalency agreements would reduce border controls between signatory nations. This could open countries to incursions by exotic pathogens and vectors. Livestock health and food-safety officials of most countries consider border controls essential for effective disease-control programs and national security and they are reluctant to compromise this prerogative.

The terms of equivalency agreements for specific commodities are negotiated by individual countries or trading blocs. Treaties like the FTAA usually define equivalency and encourage its use by countries with similar livestock health and food-safety measures. The first requirement for application of equivalency is mutual trust between the involved nations.

Import Measures Should Be Based on Risk Analysis/Risk Assessment

The terms risk analysis and risk assessment are frequently used interchangeably. In animal health parlance risk analysis connotes the collective notions of risk assessment, **risk communication**, and risk management. Most LHP risk assessments are used to assess the dangers of imported products.

Risk assessment is the identification, classification, and estimation of the seriousness and possible consequences of risks. Import risk assessment occupies Section 1.4 of the *OIE International Animal Health Code* (OIE 2000). The Code says importing countries should base sanitary measures that exceed international standards on objective and defensible risk assessments. To fulfill these criteria, risk assessments should be transparent, documented as to methodologies, and include citations from the scientific literature.

Risk assessments identify risk factors, like diseases or parasites, and take into account the probability, based on country-of-origin factors and mode of transmission, of the agent entering the importing country.

The level of sophistication and methodologies of risk assessments run the gamut from gut reactions and educated guesses to extensive detailed quantitative evaluations of the risks and potential consequences of imported commodities.

Qualitative risk assessments utilize the knowledge, experience, and background of livestock health import-export staff regarding:

- Transmission and global distribution of animal diseases
- **Livestock health infrastructure** of exporting countries
- Final destination and use of imported commodities
- Risk-mitigating status achieved by point-of-origin health certifications and post-entry restrictions
- Perceptions of the credibility of the certifying authority of exporting countries

Decisions based on qualitative risk assessments take minutes or weeks to complete. Summaries of qualitative risk assessments are reported verbally or spelled out in correspondence and import permits.

The international community expects risk assessments to be transparent, scientifically sound, and non-discriminatory. Countries can demand documentation of any import decision. Sometimes the documentation and its storage in retrievable formats take more resources than the risk analysis and decision-making process. This increases work loads for importing countries.

Quantitative risk assessments are undertaken to evaluate proposed regulations, requests for recognition of disease-free status, and import requests from newly identified exporting regions. They are also applied to requests for importations that are economically or politically sensitive or require reevaluation due to advancing technology or changing distribution of disease-producing agents.

Quantitative risk assessments are more complicated than qualitative. They are extensively detailed and include probabilistic numerical estimates of unmitigated risks. They may describe the effects of various risk-mitigating measures and evaluate their acceptability. Quantitative risk assessments may take six to twelve months to complete.

The documentation attached to quantitative risk assessments details the methodology and mathematical models employed. It states the assumptions used to ascertain probabilities of various outcomes and cites scientific or professional literature.

Various methodologies are appropriate to different situations. There are a number of scenario-tree models or spreadsheet methods for risk assessment. Some are available as software packages. Experts on quantitative risk assessment often differ on the approaches used and the results obtained. Thus, if countries have differing trade objectives, quantitative risk assessments can stimulate controversy.

Theoretically, risk assessments are designed to determine scientifically sound courses of action. They are conducted in advance of decisions on sanitary measures. It is an abuse of the wording and intent of the WTO SPS Agreement to conduct risk assessments to support predetermined decisions or regulations. Risk assessments predetermined by political or protectionist interests compromise the scientific credibility of risk analysis personnel and damage the international credibility of the perpetrating countries.

Qualitative and quantitative risk analysis were detailed in chapter 3.

Regionalization

The concept of globalization, outlined in chapter 3, has led to a specific trade process called regionalization. **Regionalization** is the division of countries into regions for import/export purposes by designating disease-free and infected areas.

Regionalization is based on the notion that diseases do not respect political boundaries. It implies that sanitary measures are most logical when based on areas that are homogeneous geographically, ecologically, and with respect to disease status and livestock health infrastructure. The process of regionalization is used for localizing and containing existing or emerging diseases, containing newly introduced exotic diseases, providing a geographic basis for SPS measures to exclude the importation of exotic diseases, and for facilitating exportations from areas with definable natural or political boundaries and common livestock health status.

For purposes of regionalization, countries, parts of countries, groups of countries, or groups of parts of countries may be defined as regions. Ideally regions have insurmountable natural boundaries such as oceans, rivers, or mountain ranges. Political boundaries can be used to delineate regions if there is adequate border security.

The United States has applied the concept of regionalization for decades in programs for controlling **brucellosis, tuberculosis**, and **pseudorabies** by establishing disease-free designations and gradations of levels of infection for states, parts of states, and counties. They have also used regionalization to circumscribe introductions of exotic diseases such as **highly pathogenic avian influenza (HPAI)**.

Regionalization of the United States for **bluetongue** was used to expedite livestock exports. For several decades the northeastern United States was regionalized for cattle export purposes. The process used political, in this case state, boundaries to designate a ten- to twelve-state area where the insect vector of bluetongue could not survive the winters. A bluetongue-free area was based on a random sample of bovine blood samples that tested negative, thus permitting cattle to be exported during vector-free winter months.

Where there is a responsible infrastructure to represent a region, that is a competent veterinary authority, regionalization allows importing nations to evaluate point-of-origin animal health status of proposed importations with respect to political and geographic boundaries. It provides an ecologically rational basis for applying risk assessments to import decisions.

International regionalization expectations outlined in the WTO SPS Agreement have the force of international law and are endorsed by the OIE.

Scientifically Based Risk Assessment Using Regional Approaches

The requirement that sanitary measures more stringent than OIE standards be based upon scientific risk assessment using regional approaches (WTO SPS Articles 5 and 6) encourages countries to utilize international standards as much as possible and alter traditional ways of doing business.

As indicated in chapter 3, the realization that zero **risk** is unattainable has forced the livestock health community to select disease-specific risk levels they can tolerate. This acceptable level of risk can be defined qualitatively or quantitatively.

As long as the criteria for each category are defined, it is possible to establish a qualitative continuum of risk levels using terms such as negligible risk, slight risk, low risk, moderate risk, and high risk. Under such a scheme commodities from regions deemed to have negligible disease-specific risk levels (the gold standard) can be imported with a certificate of origin verified at ports of entry. The importing country still has inspection privileges. Increasingly stringent sanitary measures can be applied to commodities determined to present higher levels of disease-specific risks.

Acceptable risk can also be defined quantitatively as the mathematical probability of introducing a specific disease by a given commodity from a country or region. After the importing country establishes the disease-specific quantitative acceptable level of risk, a quantitative risk assessment can determine if the unmitigated risk of the importation is above or below that predetermined level. When the calculated risk exceeds the acceptable level, sanitary measures such as negative test results or quarantines can be imposed to mitigate the risk. Imposing cooking, pickling, aging, or other processing requirements to render potentially infectious agents harmless can also reduce the risk.

Both qualitative and quantitative risk assessments are based on numerous assumptions, estimates, and arbitrary determinations. These include the disease status of exporting regions and the likelihood of the entry and establishment of the disease in recipient countries. Critics of this process say risk assessments are based on insufficient data. These contentions are compounded when dealing with regions rather than with individual countries. The mutual acceptance of a risk analysis requires understanding and trust between involved parties.

There are two essential components for determining the feasibility for importations from regions rather than from individual nations. Secure boundaries of regions must be identified, and there must be an effective infrastructure (i.e., a competent veterinary authority) to represent the region and certify the origin and nature of exported commodities.

LHP-makers need to be familiar with the concept, applications, and potential hazards of regionalization. Likewise, they should be aware of the multiple assumptions, variables, and potentials for skullduggery that are implicit in the conduct and interpretation of risk analyses.

WTO Dispute Resolution Procedures

The dispute resolution procedures of the NAFTA and the GATT offer mechanisms for adjudicating contentious international issues. These procedures have largely been superseded by those of the WTO SPS Agreement, which protects the rights of member nations and assures that they fulfill their obligations. They are administered by WTO dispute resolution panels.

Signatory countries are urged to strive for solutions at the technical level before bringing issues to the WTO. The WTO encourages importing countries to withdraw sanitary measures that are not consistent with WTO SPS provisions or OIE standards. The WTO has the authority to order compensation to aggrieved nations through the use of consultation, good offices, conciliation and mediation, arbitration, expert panels, and a standing appellate body. The dispute procedures contain most provisions of international due process. These include judgment by peers and the rights to be faced by accusers, the right to view the evidence, and the right to appeal decisions. The details of the dispute resolution process become relevant when disagreements become so contentious and drawn out that they go to the WTO. Prior to that, livestock health officials need a general knowledge of dispute resolution procedures and an awareness that sanitary measures based on international standards are not likely to be challenged.

Apprehensions About the NAFTA, the GATT, the WTO, and Trade Agreements

The treaties and agreements discussed in this chapter raise concerns. Some come from groups that oppose globalization and free market economies. Less-developed nations feel the globalization movement favors developed and rich countries. They feel it is a device to force mercenary, overindulgent, and entertainment-seeking values of western societies on proud but less-developed nations with long-standing cultural and religious traditions. There are also concerns that globalization threatens the environment, human rights, workers rights, food safety, and livestock health. Some of these concerns may provide rationalizations for the use of bioterrorism to achieve international competitiveness.

Some individuals within the livestock industries and regulatory communities of developed countries are concerned that the NAFTA, the GATT, and the

WTO will decrease the competitiveness of their livestock industries or lead to the demise of the family farm. Others respond that the movement from family farms to integrated livestock enterprises is a consequence of social, economic, and cultural changes dating from the industrial revolution and enhanced by the information age. Those supportive of global free market economies feel that increased international movement of livestock products will not impact these trends.

There is a feeling in livestock and regulatory circles that free trade will increase the risk of the introduction of exotic livestock diseases and that the requirement for harmonizing sanitary measures and diagnostic procedures will lower livestock health standards. However the SPS provisions clearly indicate countries may establish whatever sanitary measures they deem necessary as long as they are transparent and equitably applied to all trading partners.

Harmonization provisions require standardized minimal procedures but do not exclude individual countries from maintaining higher standards if they are transparent and can be justified by scientific risk assessments.

Most experts agree that vibrant and stable economies are usually open, outward looking, and export-oriented rather than inward-looking, protective and restrictive. As developing nations improve their economies and raise *per capita* incomes, dietary improvement is often the first effect. Improved diets create a demand for agricultural products and benefit the economies of many countries.

Few regions can profitably produce all crops and every livestock product. The movement toward a global livestock economy permits countries to become internationally competitive by producing commodities most suited to their ecosystems. The long-term advantages of the NAFTA, the GATT, the WTO, and the formation of trading blocs should be increased global availability of food and decreased human starvation.

National Responses to the WTO SPS Agreement

To achieve compliance with the WTO SPS Agreement, many countries have rewritten their import regulations to incorporate regionalization, risk assessment, and transparency. The WTO SPS Agreement provides opportunities for national livestock health communities to revise their import-export policies, enhance trade, and simultaneously protect their livestock populations from exotic diseases.

In response to these challenges, some national veterinary services are reorganizing to emphasize trade enhancement. This often requires rewriting sanitary regulations to incorporate provisions of the WTO SPS Agreement and OIE standards. These changes will improve their competitive positions in the global free market economy. Nations recognizing that future growth of their livestock industries depends on foreign markets have emphasized export enhancement goals that are compatible with traditional missions of protecting domestic livestock populations from disease.

The challenges presented by the WTO SPS Agreement and its possible inconsistent application provide opportunities for world leadership in formulating scientifically sound international policies. These policies can be supportive of national interests while presenting opportunities for developing international credibility in the certification of livestock health situations and the sanitary status of their exports.

Developed democratic countries have emerged as world leaders in livestock health. Other nations sometimes mimic their sanitary measures and regulatory styles. When written policies are available, other countries can adopt them. This should be considered a compliment.

The credibility of animal disease reporting systems and the evenhandedness of their disease exclusion policies set the tone for requirements ultimately imposed on each nation's exports. The tendency of trading partners and competitors to invoke reciprocal measures requires that policies and negotiating styles be based on fairness, consideration of the rights of others, and sensitivity to cultural heritage and national pride. Understanding the need for international trustworthiness and respect should be a major theme of working partnerships between livestock producers, food processors, exporters, private and public veterinarians, subnational and national animal health officials, and the free press.

Guidelines for WTO-consistent Import Regulations

Sanitary measures imposed on imports must be scientifically and technically sound; be consistent with trade agreements and international standards; and protect the health of domestic livestock, wildlife, and human populations. The disease risk from imported livestock products varies from country to country. Many nations have established lists of factors for assessing disease-specific risk. These lists provide templates for accessing general items and specific risks presented by regions proposing importations.

The factors for assessing risk include the organization, authority, and infrastructure of the veterinary services that sign health certificates for exported commodities, livestock demographics and marketing practices, and emergency response capabilities. Lists of disease-specific risk factors can include:

- The disease status in the region and the date of the most recent diagnosis
- The disease status of adjacent regions
- The nature of disease-control programs for the agent in question
- The vaccination status of the region, date of the last vaccination, current extent of vaccination, and which vaccines are in use
- The degree to which the region is separated from areas of higher risk by physical or other barriers

- The extent of control over movement of livestock products into the region from areas of higher risk and the level of border security
- The type and extent of disease surveillance, whether passive or active; the quantity and quality of sampling, testing, and disease reporting
- Diagnostic capacities

Of these infrastructure elements, livestock health is the most critical and most difficult to evaluate (see chapter 4). It involves regulatory authority, resources invested in disease diagnosis and surveillance, and the credibility of disease reporting and health certification.

To assure consistency and systematic non-discriminatory treatment of regions and countries, livestock policy leaders can prepare a standard list of specific questions to be answered when addressing each of the above factors.

Transparency in Development of Import Requirements

Throughout the review of import requests, countries should inform domestic and foreign stakeholders of proposals under consideration and allow access to information received. If after analyzing a request and conducting a risk analysis they believe the importation can be safely allowed, they publish a proposed rule specifying the conditions for importation and how the decision was reached. During the comment period the public can access comments received as well as the basis for decisions. Once all comments have been reviewed, the national authority determines conditions under which the importation can be allowed and this information is published in a public record.

Risk Management Options and Biosecurity Measures for Importation of Livestock Products

Risk management options or risk mitigating procedures are applied to reduce risks to acceptable levels. Acceptable levels of risk, or acceptable levels of protection, are elusive and controversial issues. Experienced animal health officials can readily identify the components of acceptability for importations of livestock products. They can devise standard criteria for determining the comparative risk of specific diseases based on the livestock health status of exporting regions and the nature of the importation.

One method is to set a goal of achieving **negligible risk**. The circular definition is that negligible risk is the disease-by-disease risk accompanying commodities from countries or regions presenting negligible risk. This determination requires strict criteria for categorizing the disease-specific risk status of regions.

The notion of negligible risk is derived by devising a risk continuum, ranging from negligible to high risk, with clearly defined bench marks assignable to potential importing regions. For any given disease, this continuum can categorize regions as presenting negligible risk, slight risk, low risk, moderate risk, or high risk. The criteria for placing exporting countries or regions in each risk category must be defined. For example, the criteria for categorizing regions as having negligible risk for a disease could be:

- The disease agent has not been identified in the region for an appropriate time interval
- The restricted agent is not known to exist in adjacent regions
- Vaccination for the restricted agent is prohibited in the region
- Border controls between the region and adjacent areas of greater risk are equivalent to those imposed for control programs and import requirements in the recipient country
- The region maintains adequate passive surveillance systems
- The region maintains adequate policies and infrastructure for responding to occurrences of restricted agents.

Each incremental risk level in the continuum can be spelled out in similar terms. By virtue of originating in regions characterized as presenting negligible risk, or by the imposition of documented verifiable risk-mitigation measures adequate to achieve negligible risk status, the national government can consider that the commodity meets its acceptable level of protection.

Risk management procedures include testing and inspecting premises or herds of origin; point-of-origin inspections or quarantines, sometimes known as pre-clearance procedures; testing, inspection, or quarantine of animals or products at ports of entry in recipient countries; and restricted movement of imported livestock or products within the recipient country.

Requests for importations should be processed in the order received to avoid creating ill feelings among trading partners.

Evaluating Requests for Importations

Countries should establish a unit within their national veterinary services to process and evaluate requests for importations of livestock and livestock products. The unit should receive, acknowledge, log in, store, and track applications for recognition of the disease status of countries seeking importations. They should make applications available for public inspection, establish review panels, conduct risk assessments, and submit recommended risk mitigation measures to livestock health decision makers for approval.

Application of Regionalization and Risk Assessment to Domestic Disease Situations

Regionalization is a strategy to permit exportations from portions of areas demonstrably free of diseases that are present elsewhere in a territory. Countries can attempt to maintain trade through regionalization strategies on a case-by-case basis depending on the disease, its mode of transmission, its location, and disease-specific OIE standards.

Recipient countries have the prerogative to accept or reject regionalization proposals. They may also request further data or perform site visits to verify claims of disease freedom, diagnostic capacity, and border security in a region. Countries hope trading partners will afford equivalent consideration to their domestic regionalization efforts.

Dealing with Livestock Health Standards and Standard-Setting Organizations

Successfully dealing with standard-setting organizations is essential to effective import and export programs. Some approaches include

- Bringing LHPs into conformance with trade agreements and international standards
- Actively participating in the WTO and its designated standard-setting organizations, the CODEX, IPPC, and OIE
- Establishing leadership positions in the OIE
- Developing a cooperative participatory animal health infrastructure with partnerships based on two-way communication with stakeholders and the media (see chapter 4)
- Establishing high levels of credibility among domestic stakeholders and foreign counterparts
- Developing equitable transparent regulations in cooperation with stakeholders
- Emphasizing communication with domestic and international livestock health communities

These strategies are detailed below.

Active Participation in the WTO

Depending on their rank within national governments, LHP- makers need different levels of participation in the WTO. A few officials in high positions need to understand WTO goals, structure, and charter in order to represent the best interests of their countries effectively in deliberations of WTO Commissions. Livestock health officials who are usually of lower rank need detailed knowledge of the functioning of the WTO, the rights and obligations of membership, and the provisions of the SPS Agreement. They need to be able to fluently quote the goals and objectives of the WTO to people at all levels in the livestock health community and to represent their country's relationship with the WTO to groups supporting globalization as well as to those opposing their country's involvement with the WTO.

Active Participation in the WTO-Designated Standard-Setting Organizations

Knowledge of the WTO SPS Agreement is vital to LHP-makers who are active in standard-setting organizations. Standards set by CODEX and IPPC are less crucial to LHPs than OIE standards, which apply directly to the international movement of livestock products. Conformance with OIE sanitary guidelines greatly simplifies international trade and expedites negotiations with countries and trading blocs.

The OIE standards, spelled out in the Code and the Manual, are best learned when considering disease-specific sanitary measures. Using these references requires knowledge of the disease risks associated with any potential export. This knowledge is acquired from training in veterinary medicine and experience in import-export activities. Officials with this combination of skills are hard to find.

Active Participation in the Programs of the OIE

Countries with passive roles in OIE activities are quickly becoming aware that their interests need to be actively represented in OIE administration, commissions, and working groups. This participation is imperative because of the OIE standard-setting authority, the contacts and global status gained from this activity, and the opportunities it provides for networking and establishing international credibility.

Strategies for dealing with the OIE are important to nations hoping to expand foreign markets for livestock products. OIE standards and positions are adopted on one-vote-per-country majorities. Thus, each country's vote must be used effectively to support issues that are scientifically sound, technically acceptable to domestic industries, in agreement with the WTO SPS Agreement, and consistent with national interests.

Achieving those goals requires participation at each step in the standard-setting process. It involves working to nominate and elect competent communicative individuals to OIE commissions and working groups. Perhaps more importantly, effective national participation in the standard-setting process requires the expertise from academia, industry, and state and federal regulatory, diagnostic, and epidemiologic programs. This input is essential to ensure that thoughtful, scientifically sound national positions are submitted in a timely manner when proposed standards are circulated for comment. Active OIE participation also requires working closely with trading partners who share a goal of assuring that persuasive, diplomatically acceptable arguments are presented at OIE General Sessions and at meetings of OIE Regional Commissions.

Accomplishing these goals requires conscious effort from each nation's chief veterinary officer (CVO) and LHP-makers.

Success in OIE participation requires dedication, cooperation, coordination, communication, international networking, and appropriate resource allocation.

Establishing Leadership Roles in the OIE

In the deliberations of the OIE, the national veterinary services of member countries are usually represented by the nation's CVO. They have the opportunity to support their country's best interests in discussions on international policies, international standards, and the selection of officers and members of OIE committees and commissions.

In the OIE, the interests of member countries are served to the extent that their CVOs study upcoming issues, judiciously exercise their vote, and successfully network with other delegates sharing their nation's interests. Exercise of leadership in the OIE provides contacts and confidants who can strengthen each nation's credibility in the international trade arena.

Bibliography

Bowman, J. and D. Desrosiers. 2001. Free Trade Area of the Americas. In *Harmonization Alert* 2(7): 1–7.

OIE. 2000. *The OIE Manual of Standards for Diagnostic Tests and Vaccines.* 4th ed. Paris: Office International des Epizooties.

OIE. 2001. *The OIE International Animal Health Code.* 9th ed. Paris: Office International des Epizooties.

Chapter 6

Issues Surrounding Equitable Livestock Health Policies

INTRODUCTION

The development and characterization of equitable **livestock health policies (LHPs)** is complicated. They comprise a broad array of practices, guidelines, rules, regulations, laws, and edicts. They impact the health of domestic animals, consumers of livestock products, and societies at large. LHPs touch upon food safety, **zoonotic** diseases (those transmissible from animals to humans), agricultural prosperity, and global markets.

LHPs are most effective when developed by transparent participatory processes involving people at all levels of the policy-making chain. Policies and regulations should be flexible, well written, and equitably administered. Around the world and within countries, policies, laws, and regulations differ in details, degree of oversight, and levels of authority.

The establishment of competitive and equitable LHPs is a challenge for all nations. Private citizens, organizations, and state, national, regional, and international governing bodies all play a role in their development.

Once codified, LHPs can be masterpieces of intergovernmental and public cooperation. On the other hand, they can be complicated by ambiguities, entangled in interagency turf wars, and stifled by tensions.

The development and oversight of LHPs require cooperation, participation, and the understanding of many segments of society. Cooperation is needed from livestock producers and processors; public interest groups; trade and professional organizations; local, state, and national government agencies; the executive and legislative branches of national governments; and numerous international bodies and tribunals.

The strategies for building competitive and equitable LHPs vary greatly among nations. All require participation by multiple stakeholders; the cooperation of national, subnational, and local agencies; and input from groups with conflicting agendas. It would be ideal if the industries to be regulated would recognize issues that need governmental oversight and initiate voluntary quality-assurance programs before there are public calls for action, but this does not always happen.

Animal health organizations such as the **U.S. Animal Health Association (USAHA)** often recognize and publicly acknowledge the need for new policies or programs. They serve as effective intermediaries between producers and processors and their governments. Providing an opportunity for public feedback expedites regulatory processes.

Satisfactory outcomes of LHP-development processes emerge when discussions of differing positions produce compromises that ultimately lead to cooperation. The LHP-building process is becoming increasingly complex due to advancing technology, the rising expectations of society, changing political and economic behaviors, increasing global demands of expanding free-market economies, and shifting national boundaries. These factors complicate and dilute the effectiveness of livestock health measures and influence their development. This chapter discusses some considerations for developing workable and equitable LHPs.

Objectives of LHPs

The objectives of LHPs are to protect the health and welfare of consumers, improve and protect the health of livestock, advance the prosperity of livestock producers and associated industries, and maintain and expand foreign and domestic markets. Each of these objectives has several components and multiple stakeholders. With thoughtful effort, each component can be addressed in an honorable, transparent manner that considers the opinions of widely divided public interests. Meeting these objectives at the local, national, and international levels requires concerted efforts and clearly defined criteria.

The following sections can serve as a template for national or subnational governments. LHP-makers from different countries may choose to alter the pattern to accommodate national livestock industries, economies, politics, and cultures.

LHPs and the Welfare of Consumers

Protecting the health and welfare of consumers is a first priority of LHPs. Health is a principal component of human welfare. LHPs impact the availability, variety, nutritional value, and price of food. Health and welfare can be at odds when health measures raise food prices by increasing production costs or imposing tax-supported regulatory oversight. The cost-benefit ratios of LHPs require economic calculations that must ultimately put a price on human life. This book does not address that challenge. It does tackle LHPs and the sometimes-fatal human consequences of food-borne or livestock-borne diseases.

Protecting human health requires policy makers to address issues of food safety and the risks of zoonoses. The two overlap, because many food-borne infections are caused by zoonotic agents. Some livestock-borne diseases are transmitted by insect vectors or by direct contact with the livestock rather than through food. However, food is the most common vehicle of zoonoses, making food safety the principal human-welfare component of LHPs.

Livestock Health and Food Safety

Food safety is a complex and challenging issue for most countries. It cannot stand alone among challenges facing LHP-making bodies, because livestock health and food safety are inexorably linked throughout the food chain. In many countries the same governmental agency oversees both issues. The veterinary profession is involved with both, and in some countries food safety and meat hygiene are the major activities of veterinarians. Food-safety policies consider diseases transmissible by foods of plant and animal origin.

Fruits and vegetables, if they are contaminated with human, animal, or bird excrement, can carry some bacterial, and occasionally viral, diseases transmitted by meat, milk, and poultry products. Contaminated fruits and vegetables can also result from the fertilization of crops with the manure of livestock, pets, wild animals, birds or waterfowl; the pollution of fields during floods; or from random defecation by birds, animals, or farm workers.

Most LHPs focus on human diseases transmissible by foods of animal origin, namely meat, milk, poultry, and eggs. These are mostly bacterial or protozoan infections acquired by eating contaminated products that have been inadequately refrigerated or incompletely cooked.

The principal food-borne bacterial diseases come from infection with ***Salmonella, E. coli, Camplobacteria, Listeria, Clostridia, Shigella,*** or toxins produced by ***Staphlococcus***. These organisms and others produce gastroenteritis of variable severity. They occasionally cause serious disease and are sometimes fatal. Their severity, symptoms, and side effects vary, but they have relatively similar chains of infection.

Human food-borne bacterial diseases only develop when acquired in infective doses, usually by mouth, by susceptible individuals. Susceptibility frequently implies lack of previous exposure. It is exacerbated by immunological malfunction. Immune capacity can be compromised by stress; age (very young or very old); and immunosuppressive therapies like irradiation and chemotherapy, either for cancer treatment or to prevent the rejection of transplants. Immune function is also reduced by preexisting immunosuppressive conditions such as AIDS or certain cancers. People with diabetes mellitus, chronic kidney or liver diseases, and congenital immunodeficiencies are also at risk (Carithers 2002).

Contaminated meat, poultry, vegetables, and seafood are covered with microscopic organisms invisible to the naked eye. An infective dose involves numbers of actively dividing pathogens sufficient to overrun the harmless organisms present in the gastrointestinal tracts of susceptible persons. Infective numbers of organisms usually result from prior rapid bacterial multiplication in foods that provide suitable temperature, moisture, and nutrients. Successful infection is likely to occur if the infecting organism is acquired while it is actively multiplying. Viruses are unable to multiply outside living host cells and are less common agents of food-borne diseases than bacteria.

Meat-borne diseases most often are caused by bacteria of fecal origin. These can contaminate products during slaughter and processing operations, despite all efforts to sanitize carcasses and equipment. These organisms are more prevalent in ground meats. They are uniformly distributed through patties by grinding and blending, and they multiply rapidly if meat is not frozen or refrigerated. In muscle cuts they tend to be present on surfaces where they are killed by cooking temperatures. However, bacteria-killing temperatures don't penetrate meat patties unless they are thoroughly cooked.

Most bacteria in or on meats come from contact with feces, often in amounts undetectable to the naked eye. In restaurants, products relatively free of fecal-borne bacteria when purchased can be contaminated in the kitchen by workers failing to wash their hands after using bathrooms. Contamination can also result from trimming foods on cutting boards or counters previously touched by contaminated products or utensils.

No laws or regulations will stop animals from defecating or prohibit bacteria from setting up housekeeping in animal and human intestinal tracts. Nor will LHPs prevent bacteria from reproducing logarithmically and continually mutating into forms pathogenic to humans and resistant to antimicrobial drugs.

Bacterial multiplication occurs most rapidly at body temperature when there is adequate moisture and nutrients. These conditions exist in animal and human gastrointestinal tracts, unrefrigerated poultry, meat patties, or potato salad sunbathing at Fourth of July picnics. Bacteria don't read rules, and man has yet to devise methods of reversing nature. Therefore the thrust of food-safety policies must be to minimize the risks of human exposure to known sources of infection.

Food-safety measures must be carefully focused on risk-reduction activities. They must attack selected points in the food chain that have high probabilities of playing significant roles in the transmission cycle. For this approach to be effective, such points must be vulnerable to sanitary measures that are economically and mechanically feasible and can be practically applied and enforced industry wide. Most of these points are in kitchens or slaughtering-processing operations, where **hazard analysis and critical control point (HACCP)** programs are in place. Nonetheless, the entire food chain must be addressed. The complete food chain approach is the basis of farm-to-fork food-safety initiatives.

Diseases transmitted by poultry meat often result from *Salmonella* or other bacteria on the skin. They are somewhat reduced, because people in most cultures insist on eating well-cooked poultry meat, and rare chicken burgers are uncommon. One exception is mechanically deboned meat (MDM). MDM is the residue scraped from poultry skeletons after standard cuts have been removed. It provides a bacterial haven comparable to beef or pork burgers. It has been alleged to cause salmonellosis and other infections among Russian consumers of raw or partially cooked MDM of U.S. origin (see Discussion Topic 4).

Poultry-meat sausages are uncommon and, as with beef and pork sausage, are usually partially sterilized when cooked during processing. Their capacity to support rampant bacterial growth is often further reduced by the addition of spices. *Listeria* are capable of surviving these processes and withstanding refrigeration, thus expediting the transmission of listeriosis by cold-sliced sandwich meats.

Diseases transmitted by consumption of milk have been minimized by the widespread use of pasteurization. These diseases include **brucellosis**, camplobacteriosis, *E.coli* infections, **diphtheria**, listeriosis, **Q-fever** (rarely) and staphylococcal poisoning. They still occur among individuals drinking raw milk. In the United States this includes farm workers, fad dieters, and diners preferring imported specialty cheeses that are sometimes prepared from unpasteurized milk. Pasteurized milk, if contaminated and allowed to sit without refrigeration for suitable time periods, can support human-to-human transmission of **shigellosis** (bacillary dysentery) and **typhoid fever**.

Diseases caused by the consumption of eggs are partially controlled by cooking. Eggs that are incompletely cooked or eaten raw can produce the same gastrointestinal infections as meat and poultry.

LHPs and the Well-Being of Livestock

From the perspective of livestock producers, farmers, ranchers, and corporations that produce and process food animals, the improvement and protection of livestock health should be the primary objective of LHPs. However, life is not that simple. Many proposed policies originate from the ideals and agendas that are distant from livestock health and more concerned with consumers, who are actually 100% of each nation's citizens. This forces livestock producers and processors, who represent a small proportion of most populations, to respond to proposed policies or regulations that appear contrary to their best interests.

A strong argument can be made that consumers, not producers and processors, are the primary benefactors of healthy livestock populations, because interruptions in animal growth or reproduction cause increased prices, decreased availability, and sometimes increased risks to human health.

Consumers clearly benefit from healthy livestock populations, but even healthy animals can carry hidden infections that constitute food-safety risks. Measures proposed to reduce these risks are often costly to industry, difficult to implement, vague in their outcomes, and of questionable value when compared to kitchen sanitation, refrigeration, and thorough cooking of foods.

After the consumer and industry benefits of LHPs are considered, it becomes evident that effective LHPs benefit consumers, producers, and processors. Sound LHPs are crucial to the survival of domestic economies and the competitiveness of livestock-rearing countries in the global market place. Thus all segments of society have a stake in their particulars.

LHPs should strive to maximize food safety, minimize the spread of domestic livestock diseases and zoonotic infections, exclude the introduction of exotic livestock diseases, maximize production efficiency, and assure the safe and effective use of vaccines, hormones, **antimicrobials**, and other substances injected into livestock or added to their feed or water. In practice these broad objectives sometimes conflict.

Policies to Minimize the Impact of Domestic Livestock Diseases

Policies, laws, or regulations that minimize the spread of domestic livestock diseases create a delicate balance between protecting the collective interests of livestock producers and processors and infringing on their rights as individuals. Diseases and infections that are important in one component of the industry or one part of a country can be irrelevant elsewhere. The need for specific disease-control or eradication programs arises when economic losses, transmission to humans, market considerations, impediments to trade, agendas of interest groups, or media coverage signal that action is needed.

Before embarking on legislation or regulations, several questions must be answered. First, in light of existing priorities, is the disease or infection important enough to address with public funding and programs, or is it adequately controlled at present by management practices and vaccination? Second, is the disease endemic and widely distributed, or does it occur sporadically? Third, does current scientific knowledge indicate the disease is a good candidate for a control or eradication program according to the criteria listed in chapter 4?

Once these questions are answered the attitude of affected industries and interest groups must be explored. Is the affected industry concerned enough to initiate a voluntary pilot project or quality assurance program to address the condition?

It is often difficult to gain support for public policies that would deal with long-standing, relatively non-dramatic diseases unless new information appears or a crisis occurs.

Policies to Exclude Exotic Diseases

Proposals to exclude the introduction of exotic livestock diseases are usually less controversial than programs to control existing endemic diseases. The high susceptibility of domestic populations to exotic diseases sets the stage for major disasters.

Exotic disease exclusion requires an infrastructure with all the components detailed in chapter 4, including vigilant livestock owners and veterinarians; diagnostic services; regulatory organization and authority, disease-control and eradication programs; **monitoring, surveillance, and reporting (MS&R) systems**; and emergency response capabilities.

The stringent measures needed to exclude **foot-and-mouth disease (FMD)** are usually adequate to protect against the introduction of most exotic contagious diseases of livestock (see chapter 3). FMD-free countries impose strict inspections on passenger baggage and freight. They prohibit importations of live ruminants and swine and related products from infected areas. These measures, along with procedures to exclude plant pests, can create the impression that FMD-free nations are pushing to export but are unwilling to offer reciprocal import privileges. Perceptions of a trade-restrictive attitude discourage FMD-infected countries from engaging in dialogue with FMD-free nations on other issues. These perceptions can frustrate efforts to open markets for manufactured goods, communications equipment, and intellectual properties. Corporate interests and trade officials who are unfamiliar with the livestock industry and the wide-ranging ramifications of exotic diseases are often impatient with livestock health programs.

The **World Trade Organization (WTO) Sanitary and Phytosanitary (SPS) Agreement** discourages linkages of sanitary measures to unrelated commodities or non-agricultural trade. Nonetheless, the international community generally regards trade as a two-way street and tends to expect tradeoffs in exchange for importation privileges. This aspect of exotic disease exclusion adds challenging dimensions requiring that trade officials at all levels be familiar with the implications of LHPs. It also demands that livestock health officials be amenable to compromise as long as the risks are clearly understood.

Assuring Safe and Effective Use of Livestock Drugs and Biologicals

Controversy surrounds programs designed to assure the safe and effective use of vaccines, hormones, antimicrobials and other substances administered to livestock. Many products are shrouded in disagreements about their potential risks to consumers and their potential role in the development of antimicrobial resistance among zoonotic agents.

Interest groups have promoted a general fear of injectables and feed additives. There is a lack of public understanding of these products, how they work, and their potential for producing residues. These concerns are exacerbated by the complexity of enforcing appropriate withdrawal times before treated animals are marketed, and the challenges encountered in regulating the licensing, manufacture, and use of products.

The use of livestock drugs and biologicals has been a major factor in the exclusion of U.S. products from countries of the European Union (EU).

Equitable LHPs require that an understanding of cultures and national attitudes balance scientific inquiry and perceptions of risk (see Discussion Topics 1 and 6).

LHPs and the Prosperity of Livestock Owners and Associated Industries

The improvement of the agricultural economy and the prosperity of individual farmers, ranchers, food processors, and their employees and dependent industries should be major considerations in the development and implementation of LHPs. Some policies will cut into the profits of individual producers, but the long-term effects of these policies must benefit the larger industry.

Programs that reduce abortions, death, disease, and disability among livestock populations are profitable to all livestock producers. It is difficult to evaluate preventive practices or to determine if the absence of disease results from programs or natural factors. When policies are proposed that are costly to producers, processors, and associated industries, their merits will soon come into question.

Policies that exclude foreign commodities usually reduce competition and are therefore supported by domestic producers and processors. These same groups strenuously object when other countries impose similar measures. LHPs must recognize and account for these inconsistencies in an effort to be equitable to domestic interests and still maintain international markets.

LHPs and Maintenance and Expansion of Global Markets

Most LHPs produce effects that serve both domestic and foreign markets. Exports must be internationally competitive in price and quality and meet the sanitary requirements of prospective importing nations.

Most countries that import livestock products establish sanitary measures to protect the health of their livestock and human populations. Exporters assure these requirements are met by accompanying shipments with health certificates. These are developed through negotiations with officials of the importing countries. They are signed by inspectors at packing plants or by veterinarians conducting physical examinations or other tests on live animals. These export certifications include testimony, endorsed by national officials of exporting countries, that the sanitary conditions of production and processing procedures meet the importing nation's requirements (see Discussion Topic 4). They also contain detailed statements of the livestock health status of the locality from which the animals originated. Extensive MS&R activities are often required to generate accurate information for certification of covered conditions. Export certifications may be well founded and essential to protect livestock and human health in the importing countries. They are sometimes suspected as being an alternate way of protecting the industries of importing countries from outside competition, in lieu of imposing tariffs or quotas.

To equitably address the rights of importing countries, and to remain simultaneously internationally competitive, officials of exporting countries need to be sure that export certificates contain valid information and that all aspects of their livestock health infrastructure are credible.

Characteristics of Competitive and Equitable LHPs

In developing LHPs, the framers should strive for measures that are transparent, flexible, well written, and capable of being equitably administered.

Transparency is a fundamental principle of international standards. It is also a desirable characteristic of domestic policies. For a policy or regulation to be transparent, its proponents must explain the reasons for its existence; clarify its objectives; outline the means of achieving those objectives; detail the authority under which it is promulgated, implemented, and overseen; and describe the public consequences and potential penalties for violation. These details must be available for examination, be widely disseminated among concerned parties, and be clearly articulated by responsible authorities.

Flexibility is a highly desirable characteristic of LHPs and regulations. It is challenging to design policies that accomplish both *bona fide* livestock health and food-safety objectives without being so rigid that stakeholders rebel. Opponents claim they are excessively burdensome and too impractical to be accomplished without dire economic consequences that ultimately amount to increased costs to consumers and loss of foreign markets. An important function of LHPs is the deterrent effect produced by their presence. If they can be reasonably accomplished and are adaptable to changing situations, policies and regulations can have a positive impact on livestock and human health. If not, groups and individuals will be tempted to defy or test them, and successful violations may defeat the purpose of a rule or regulation. For these reasons, efforts to impart a level of flexibility are essential in the development of LHPs.

Well-written LHPs expedite the accomplishment of their objectives. Policies and regulations should be outlined to identify essential points and then organized, written, and repeatedly revised by qualified writers and editors. They must be reviewed by scientific and legal experts to assure that their intent and wording are clear and unambiguous. They should be readable by audiences at all levels of the food chain and easily translated into other languages.

Equitable administration of LHPs is essential if they are to be effective. Once enacted, it is crucial that LHPs be administered fairly. They should be uniformly applied to all segments of domestic industries and to all countries where similar conditions exist.

In international trade parlance, this non-discriminatory application is called equal national treatment and is one of the principles of the WTO SPS Agreement (see chapter 5).

Developing Competitive and Equitable LHPs

Competitive and equitable LHPs are best achieved through transparent participatory processes involving people at all levels. Ideally, they should be flexible, well written, readily implemented, well communicated, and equitably applied. The methodology for attaining these goals varies from country to country. The greatest differences are evident between monarchies or dictatorships and countries with democratic, transparent, participatory governments.

In order to function effectively, the democratic approach requires conscientious efforts to attain the input of multiple stakeholders. The need for regulation is usually recognized and flagged by people outside of affected segments of the livestock industry. Unless there is an obvious problem, like an outbreak of food poisoning, large-scale mortality among livestock, or incursion by an exotic livestock disease, the affected industry initially resists proposed laws or regulations. They will cite added cost to consumers, lack of need for regulations, and possibly discrimination. An initial determination is needed to estimate if cooperatively developed guidelines could be superior to regulations. There are usually conflicting opinions, and it is often not possible to satisfy everyone.

In the United States and other democratic countries, new ideas need significant supportive voices. The lengthy process of LHP development involves recognition of the need for policies; participatory decisions on how best to address the need; drafting of laws, rules or regulations; their presentation for discussion; revisions; finalization of the policies; and their communication to all **stakeholders**. All of these efforts require time and clear documentation that permits uniform interpretation, equitable enforcement, and translation into multiple languages (see chapter 10). The sequential process of LHP development undergoes constant changes both within and between countries.

Recognition of the need for policies can arise in numerous ways. *The Jungle* by Upton Sinclair (Sinclair 1906), a 1904 novel, aroused the American public to the horrendous corruption, graft, and unsanitary conditions in the meat packing industry so the U.S. Congress passed the Pure Food and Drug Act and the Meat Inspection Act within a year of the book's publication. Some people say the legislation was already in the works when the book was published.

The book was actually fiction directed at arousing public support for a socialist worker movement in the United States. Upton Sinclair, its author, expressed surprise that people took it so seriously. He admitted he had never actually seen the conditions he described in packing plants. He said he aimed at America's heart and hit it in the stomach. This episode is used by some as an example of how the power of the press can be used to perpetuate lies, but others say it demonstrates the value of the free press to address the needs of society. Other stimulants to policy development have been less dramatic but often involve media exposure of areas needing legislative or regulatory action.

Choosing the best methods for addressing policy needs requires thought and participatory discussions. What appears to some groups to be the best solution is often viewed as counterproductive to others. Debate will often raise thoughtful questions about the validity of the need and the best method of addressing it. These answers frequently don't surface until a potential policy, law, or regulation has been drafted, at which point several alternatives may emerge. Often the best initial approach is for affected industries to propose programs and test them in pilot projects. This alerts potential opponents and supporters of the issue and provides time for mental adjustment and a study of the scientific ramifications of the issue.

The process of drafting laws, rules, or regulations varies from country to country. It usually begins with legislative approval of the concept, a search for the legal details, and possibly a presentation of enabling legislation. During this process affected industries can study the potential costs and other aspects of implementation and mount arguments in support of, or in opposition to, various components of the proposal. Once authorized legislatively, the task is delegated to officials of the national government's agricultural, veterinary, or food-safety agencies. This procedure involves writers, editors, and lawyers.

Initial drafts are often wordy and tend to say more than is necessary. Their presentation for discussion may precipitate protests and controversy. Often, previously unheard voices surface and sometimes represent thoughtful viewpoints.

The transparency of the process is improved when officials give due consideration to all opinions and explore them to extract each bit of wisdom. The presentation of draft proposals at public meetings and their publication for study by interested parties is a valuable and essential step in bringing forth competitive and equitable LHPs. Though sometimes difficult, revisions of draft proposals to accommodate all viewpoints is an important step. With patience, greatly improved policies can emerge. Final versions of laws, regulations, or program standards constitute a major accomplishment, but still require complex implementation procedures and concerted communication efforts. The communication of LHPs is a never-ending process that ultimately determines the success of the policies.

The Ever-Increasing Complexity of LHPs

Rapidly advancing technology has made LHPs increasingly complex. Technological progress has provided sophisticated diagnostic tools for the identification of new diseases. It has permitted the production of new vaccines, antimicrobials, disinfectants, and feed additives and provided for advanced reproductive technology.

This technology has not been equally distributed among countries and regions of the world. Livestock health gaps between developed and undeveloped nations have widened, making international standards too stringent for some nations and too lax for others. This disparity makes a discussion of international standards fruitless and frustrating for some national representatives.

Rising expectations of advanced societies have imposed sometimes onerous and unrealistic burdens upon livestock health officials and policy makers. Many of these expectations arise from concerns peripheral to the actual production and processing of livestock and poultry. Some of these deal with hypothetical risks that are easily denied but difficult to convincingly disprove scientifically. Such expectations underlie the arguments involving the so-called **precautionary principle** (see Discussion Topic 6).

The movement from controlled economies to democratic free-market societies by countries with firmly entrenched non-incentive-based cultures has created further problems for nations that have supported non-competitive industries.

The increasing global demands of expanding free-market economies have made incentive-based countries even more competitive and have encouraged less-competitive nations to seek further measures to protect segments of their livestock economies losing market share. They sometimes devise questionable stalling tactics to exclude products that threaten domestic industries.

Constantly changing national boundaries and the formation of new countries and trading blocs further complicate international trade in livestock products.

Governmental Administration of LHPs

The state, provincial, or other subnational responsibility for LHPs varies throughout the world. Even in countries where the jurisdiction of subnational governments is subordinate to national authority, these agencies provide significant contributions to the health of human and livestock populations. They effectively balance national and subnational authorities, prevent federal domination, recognize geographic differences, and address local concerns.

In the United States, national LHPs are largely, but not exclusively, implemented by the **Animal and Plant Health Inspection Service (APHIS)** and the **Food Safety and Inspection Service (FSIS)** of the United States Department of Agriculture (USDA). The U.S. **Food and Drug Administration (FDA)**, the **Environmental Protection Agency**, and the **U.S. Fish and Wildlife Service** are also involved.

Intergovernmental LHP interactions are delicate, often trying, and occasionally contentious. Policy disagreements between subnational governments within a country can be readily resolved if patience and mutual trust are allowed to prevail. Disputes between national and subnational governments can usually be resolved by studying constitutional prerogatives and legal authorities. Disagreements between different branches of national governments can become turf wars and long-standing misunderstandings unless they are promptly resolved by the leadership of the disputant agencies or by higher authorities.

Administration of State or Subnational LHPs

State or subnational LHPs play significant roles in the balance of power, authority, and responsibility over livestock health issues. Regional authorities can best recognize geographic and ecological differences in disease distribution. These differences reflect the thesis that local people are in a better position to understand area conditions and can play significant roles in conducting the business of the livestock industries. Granting local policy prerogatives helps balance the influence of central governments on matters of local significance. There are, however, issues that are best addressed by national governments.

Administration of National LHPs

Subnational officials look to national leadership on issues for which central governments are usually responsible. These include monitoring of domestic diseases easily spread by movement of animals and people; exclusion of exotic diseases; licensing of animal drugs and biologicals; and dealing with issues involving international bodies, governments of other countries, trading blocs, or international organizations.

In most parts of the world national sovereignty is recognized as the primary and predominant LHP authority. National LHPs often yield to thoughtful input from subnational authorities and must cooperate with state or provincial officials if programs are to succeed. They also recognize the international prerogatives of trading blocs, multinational trade agreements, and international standard-setting bodies.

National LHPs need to be scientifically sound, transparent, easy to use by affected industries, and compatible with both subnational needs and international policies. To achieve scientific credibility, national policies and regulations must be reviewed by credible experts and constantly revised to adapt to advancing technology. It is essential that national policies work for the industries affected. This involves constant communication with those being asked to conform to the policies. Most of these requirements are met when there is a transparent policy-development procedure.

The expectation of transparency of LHPs is met to varying degrees and by various methods in different countries. In the United States, an increasingly ponderous and complex process offering opportunity for public scrutiny and comment during the development of regulations addresses an ever-expanding public interest in LHPs. While average citizens may be unaware of this activity, stakeholders, lobbyists, and others with vested interests constantly monitor government activities. They have regular conversations with colleagues, legislators, and government officials and they study the **Federal Register**.

The U.S. Federal Register, published on each regular business day, contains notices of decisions and rulings by government agencies; discussions of organizational matters including changing responsibilities and authorities; notices of petitions and applications filed with government agencies; and notices of investigations, meetings, and public hearings relevant to LHPs and other issues. It contains drafts, called dockets, that outline proposed rules, regulations, or international standards.

The Federal Register provides an opportunity for public viewing and comment. The term "proposed rule" indicates the need and desire for public comment. The comment period, usually lasting sixty to ninety days, permits organizations or individuals to submit written opinions on proposed regulations. These comments are reviewed by staff of APHIS or the sponsoring agency and are acknowledged with a letter indicating the suggestion was incorporated or explaining the basis for its rejection.

When ultimately finalized, regulations are codified and published in the Code of Federal Regulations, which is available electronically at www.access.gpo.gov/nara.

Section 92 of the **U.S. Code of Federal Regulations** (9 **CFR** 92) deals with animals and animal products. It is updated as changes occur and published annually as a complete volume. It defines the regulations, standards, and rules for animals and animal products in legally correct terms. Activities that are overseen by APHIS are detailed in 9 CFR 92 including

- Descriptions of federal livestock disease-control and eradication programs
- Rules for interstate transportation of animals, poultry, and related products
- Requirements for importation and exportation of animals and animal products
- Regulations for licensing and production of vaccines, serums, toxins, and other biological products used on animals
- Requirements for accreditation of veterinarians
- Scope and authority of the **National Poultry Improvement Program**
- Other pertinent matters including definitions applicable to each section

Specific diseases are mentioned in 9 CFR 92 if they are subjected to legislation and disease-specific regulations or are objects of federally supported programs or import-export measures.

Import regulations are imposed on exotic and poultry diseases like foot-and-mouth disease, **contagious bovine pleuropneumonia, rinderpest, cattle tick fever, scabies** in cattle, **tuberculosis**, brucellosis, **scrapie, Johne's disease, highly pathogenic avian influenza (HPAI), Newcastle disease, psittacosis, African swine fever, classical swine fever (hog cholera)**, and **bovine spongiform encephalopathy (BSE).**

Many sections of 9 CFR 92 broaden its authority by use of the all-inclusive term "any other contagious or infectious disease of animals or poultry." The Code of Federal Regulations is an excellent reference on U.S. LHPs. However, it is phrased in legalese and is not easy reading.

To expedite transparent participation in international policies, U.S. law requires the publication of agendas of the meetings of international standard-setting bodies such as the **Office International des Epizooties (OIE)** and the **Codex Alimentarius Commission (CODEX)**. The daily Federal Register lists meeting dates, places, and agendas of meetings where international standards are under consideration so that interested parties can express their opinions to U.S. delegates.

Administration of International LHPs and Standards

The international component of LHPs involves relationships with trading blocs such as the North American Free Trade Agreement (NAFTA), international alliances like the EU, international standards setting organizations like the OIE and the CODEX, international health organizations such as the World

Health Organization (WHO) and global financial institutions like the World Bank and the International Monetary Fund.

International standards are largely, but not exclusively, implemented by the OIE. The U.S. government defines international standards relating to livestock health as any standard, guideline, or recommendation adopted by the CODEX regarding food safety, by the OIE regarding animal health and zoonoses, or by the member countries of the NAFTA or the WTO. International standards usually stand more as recommendations and guidelines than as laws due to the limits on international authority and the recognition of the sovereignty of individual nations.

As described in chapter 5, international standards deal largely with global trade. They are usually less specific, less binding, and less rigorously enforced than the laws and regulations governing livestock health within individual countries. They do, however, play prominent roles in negotiations between countries and trading blocs when one party is seeking markets for products that present threats to the health of the proposed importer's livestock population or to its domestic markets.

Legislative and Executive Authority Over LHPs

State, or subnational, and federal, or national, governing bodies are key players in the implementation of LHPs. Legislative and executive bodies delegate responsibility and grant authority to agricultural, livestock health, and public health officials to create detailed regulations and procedures for fulfilling public needs for livestock health, food-safety, and competitive trade policies.

High-level officials are occupied with multiple issues and generally are unfamiliar with the specifics of livestock production or processing. They leave the details to others to formulate and administer as regulations. The actual policy makers are usually career agricultural officials. They often seek expert advice and consider the voices of all possible stakeholders. They must be non-discriminatory and politically correct, stay within legal bounds, avoid infringing on the prerogatives of state or other subnational governments, be consistent with existing laws or regulations, and avoid loopholes that can lead to major calamities.

Role of Special Interests

Special interests are individuals, organizations, or corporations having concerns with a particular local, national, or governmental issue. Special interest groups apply political pressure or use other means to achieve change in ongoing policies or procedures. They urge the election of officials who pledge to support their agendas. Because of the broad range of areas impacted by LHPs, they attract the attention of a variety of special interest groups. This extends beyond livestock health into related areas like animal welfare, food safety, human health, the environment, a broad range of private and corporate interests, and international trade with its many economic and cultural implications. Chapter 1 detailed the LHP-development roles of major stakeholders, such as farmers, ranchers, feedlot operators, veterinarians, and meat and poultry processors whose livelihoods depend on livestock health.

In addition to these classic stakeholders, the principal special interest groups that influence LHPs are food-safety, animal welfare, environmental, small-farm ecosystem preservation, and fair labor practice organizations. Groups representing these interests are increasingly active in LHP matters and offer thoughtful opinions that are often conflicting but nonetheless deserve to be heard.

Food-safety issues are an inseparable part of LHPs that involve concerted education and effort throughout the food chain. In the United States, federal, state, or local laws mandate meat and poultry inspections. Inspection requirements are implemented in the kitchens of institutional and public eating places.

Despite these regulatory activities, food-borne illness continues to be a problem. It can largely, but not entirely, be controlled by thorough cooking, adequate refrigeration, and sanitary measures to prevent cross-contamination from the sequential use of facilities and utensils for foods. The sale of irradiated prepackaged meat is a positive step. Innovations such as irradiation have encountered considerable opposition mainly from public fears of anything involving radioactivity.

Although the entire food chain, from farm to fork, offers an opportunity for food-safety improvements, the slaughter-processing-packaging step, which has been traditionally addressed by regulations and inspections, and the food preparation link, which has been addressed by inspections and education, remain most vulnerable to intervention.

The application of fluorescent real-time **polymerase chain reactions (PCRs)** to identify specific pathogenic bacteria and viruses in milk, water, or manure on farms is a recent innovation, but it will undoubtedly encounter public opposition similar to the opposition to irradiation. The feasibility, logistics, selection of organisms for screening, and testing sites remain to be developed. The choices are sure to raise objections and cries of discrimination when implemented at the farm level. Food-safety advocates often present positions considered extreme by livestock producers or processors, so care is needed to assure that the regulatory application of these technologies is conducted in a transparent, non-discriminatory fashion.

Other issues raised by food-safety advocates involve the prohibition of medications, growth promotants, and various feed additives. These substances are suspected, often with little proof, of producing health-threatening residues or of contributing to the emergence of drug resistance among pathogenic bacteria. These issues deserve regulatory action such as mandated **withdrawal times** and careful controls on the manufacture, importation, distribution, and use of medications in food-producing animals. Such regulations need a sound scientific basis and must be carefully and transparently promulgated, equitably administered, and constantly evaluated for their credibility and effectiveness.

In September 2002, Health Canada initiated the process of transparently developing polices directed at reducing bacterial resistance to **antimicrobial** drugs by issuing a series of recommendations. These recommendations include requiring that the antimicrobials used in food animals be obtained only by prescription, be used only to treat specific approved diseases, and be tested before being used as growth promotants to determine their effectiveness. It was also suggested that **antibiotic** use and antibiotic resistance in farm animals be monitored and that imported antibiotics be regulated. The process of implementing these recommendations will be time consuming and perhaps controversial but should result in equitable science-based regulations that serve the interests of the public at large.

The multiple groups and organizations supporting food-safety initiatives have drawn significant attention, and stimulated regulatory reforms and educational activity. It is crucial that the educational component be relentless. Educational efforts must clearly outline the risks of germs of fecal origin and the individual's responsibility in reducing their presence. This requires repetitive warnings in multiple educational formats to ensure that people get the message and don't believe that regulations alone will solve the food-safety challenge. Developing an awareness of the need for individual responsibility is essential.

Animal welfare interests in the United States have been less successful in stimulating livestock industry legislation than have the food-safety advocates. Nonetheless, they have directed public attention to the care and handling of livestock and have inspired significant legislation directed at the use of laboratory animals in medical research and education.

The Laboratory Animal Welfare Act of 1966, now the Animal Welfare Act, is frequently amended. It continues to expand, despite efforts to exclude livestock from this legislation. Vocal animal welfare groups have stimulated changes in methods of animal handling, restraint, transport, and slaughter. They have stimulated renovations in facilities used for the transportation, rearing, and slaughter of livestock. These changes have partly resulted from industry responses to media coverage and efforts to forestall further national regulations.

In most areas of the United States, there are existing regulations, stimulated by groups concerned with the humane treatment of animals, to permit local prosecution of gross cruelty or neglect of companion animals or livestock. Animal welfare interests oppose confinement of swine for feeding, breeding, or farrowing; confinement of cattle in feedlots; and the use of cages for laying hens. These practices have been banned in England. Animal welfare groups are working to pressure markets to require certification that food products are produced under conditions that exclude these practices. Livestock producers have always bluntly stated that "no one is about to tell me how to raise my animals." The future portends that they, in one of the most traditionally independent of occupations, may be in for a shock when markets require certification that food-producing animals be raised under standardized humane conditions.

Many such policies and practices are in effect in Europe. In 2002, Germany changed constitutional wording that says it is the responsibility of the state to protect and respect the rights of people to include animals (Pollan 2002). In Switzerland the wording of laws is being changed to designate animals as "beings" where they were formerly referred to as "things."

Livestock stakeholders regard the more extreme animal welfare advocates, often labeled animal rightists, who seek to free domestic animals by sometimes illegal methods including violence and destruction of property, as vocal minorities attempting to force irrational and extremist policies upon the public. Many animal rights advocates are emotionally attached to the **vegan** movement and wish for the collapse of the entire livestock industry and the conversion of the population to an exclusively vegetarian diet.

Despite some violent minority components, the animal welfare movement has had positive impacts on LHPs and receives substantial support from law-abiding citizens who believe the activities of this movement are justified. They will continue to do so as pressures are applied through marketing channels and restaurant chains.

The environmental impact of modern livestock production systems receives considerable attention and frequently stirs controversy. One controversial practice is the fertilization of fields with commercial chemical fertilizers and manure, which run off into waterways in time of excess rain or flooding and create phosphorous and nitrogen pollution and microbiologic contamination. These phenomena are more problematic in operations that concentrate animals or poultry. Advocates of the legislative reduction of environmental pollution by animal populations are often asked to check on the efficiency of human sewerage disposal systems during floods before pointing fingers. Other environmental complaints about livestock involve odors from intensive operations and overgrazing by beef cattle.

In Europe, and to a lesser extent in North America, a movement to preserve the small-farm ecosystem has emerged in recent decades. Its thesis is that rural ecosystems need protection from urban and suburban sprawl and from corporate-style factory farming, changes which are considered detrimental to the environment and to the cherished family lifestyle that builds work ethics and family values. Its supporters urge governmental regulations limiting the number of livestock per acre and the banning importation of livestock and livestock products from countries exceeding these quotas. This movement is seen by some as a way of protecting non-competitive livestock industries from global competition.

Advocates of fair labor practices also participate in the development of LHPs by advocating activities that prevent companies from using illegal immigrants to work at minimal wages on farms, ranches, or slaughterhouses. They also tend to oppose measures favorable to globalization in so far as it permits goods produced abroad, often with child labor or at substandard wages, to compete with domestic products.

Use of Expert Panels

Organizations and governments often impanel experts to analyze issues relevant to LHP changes. In the early 1980s, the USDA's FSIS requested that the National Academy of Sciences conduct a scientific evaluation of its meat and poultry inspection programs and present recommendations for improvements needed in light of changing technology. These programs had functioned with minor changes since the early 1900s. As processing mechanisms accelerated, national controversies arose over the effectiveness of inspections. The resulting reports on comprehensive inspection programs (Wassermann et al. 1985), poultry inspection (Rodricks 1987), and cattle inspection (Kahrs et al. 1990), along with a report from the American Veterinary Medical Association (AVMA 1989), helped set the stage and prepare the public and the processing industry for the Hazardous Analysis and Critical Control Point (HACCP) program, which revolutionized the meat inspection process. HACCP is still being refined.

In 2001 the National Association of State Departments of Agriculture Research Foundation, in cooperation with APHIS, sponsored an Animal Health Safeguarding Review. The review recommended that APHIS activities be strengthened to address escalated disease risks due to increasing international travel and the importation of animal products. It suggested integrating surveillance programs into a national system, recruiting additional qualified personnel, developing an integrated agricultural inspection and quarantine service, and improving its gathering of international animal health information (National Association of State Departments of Agriculture Research Foundation 2001).

An expert panel convened by the National Academy of Science (National Academy of Science 2002) has also addressed the current controversy over the possible hazards of eating products from cloned or transgenic animals. While suggesting that further studies are needed, the panel indicated meat and milk from cloned animals is probably safe, while questions remain about the potential dangers of producing transgenic animals by incorporating DNA from one species into another.

The USAHA serves as an ongoing panel of experts. It reports annually through resolutions published in its annual proceedings book (USAHA 2001). The USAHA represents the livestock industries and the veterinary profession with a sprinkling of academicians and is spearheaded by U.S. State Veterinarians. Its deliberations cover livestock disease-control issues, food safety, and zoonotic diseases. It meets in conjunction with the **American Association of Veterinary Laboratory Diagnosticians (AAVLD)**, which publishes abstracts of discussions of diagnostic procedures presented at its annual meetings.

The **National Institute for Animal Agriculture (NIAA),** another deliberative LHP assemblage, also prepares resolutions for presentation to legislators and government agencies (NIAA 2002). The **Council for Agricultural Science and Technology** (CAST 2000) prepares scientific analyses of current issues such as the transmissible spongiform encephalopathies (TSEs) (CAST 2000).

The impact of these efforts is far reaching. The scientific nature of their recommendations dilutes vested interests and biases, thereby strengthening the credibility, transparency, and impartiality of U.S. LHPs.

Positioning, Compromise, and Cooperation in Development of LHPs

The complexity of LHPs is magnified by the multijurisdictional authority existing within most countries and the heterogeneity of the international oversight with respect to trade in livestock products. This morass is complicated by international posturing in support of national agendas that are often founded on cultural, political, or economic factors. The result is that most countries achieve their goals through diplomatic compromises founded on mutual trust and ultimately on cooperation with trading partners, even if they are adversaries on broader global issues.

Bibliography

AVMA. 1989. *Veterinary Perspectives on Safety of Foods of Animal Origin.* Schaumburg, IL: American Veterinary Medical Association.

CAST. 2000. *Transmissable Spongiform Encephalopathies in the United States.* Ames, IA: Council for Agricultural Science and Technology.

Kahrs, R. F., H. M. Acland, R. G. Breeze et al. 1990. *Cattle Inspection: Report of the Committee on Evaluation of USDA Streamlined Inspection System for Cattle.* Washington, D.C.: National Academy Press.

National Academy of Sciences. 2002. *Report of the Panel on the Risks of Genetic Manipulation of Animals to the Environment and Potentially to Human Health.* Washington, D.C.: National Academy Press.

The National Association of State Departments of Agriculture Research Foundation. 2001. *The Animal Health Safeguarding Review: Results and Recommendations.* Washington, D.C.

NIAA. 2002. *2002-2003 Resolutions and Position Statements.* Bowling Green, KY: National Institute for Animal Agriculture.

Pollan, M. 2002. The Unnatural Idea of Animal Rights: An Animals Place. *New York Times Magazine*. November 14.

Rodricks, J. 1987. *Poultry Inspection: The Basis for a Risk Assessment Approach.* Washington, D.C.: National Academy Press.

Sinclair, U. 1906. *The Jungle.* Republished as a Barnes and Noble Classic in 1995. New York: Barnes and Noble Books.

USAHA. 2001. *Proceedings: One Hundred and Fifth Annual Meeting*. Richmond, VA: The United States Animal Health Association.

Wassermann, R. H., J. C. Bailar, F. Bryan et al. 1985. *Meat and Poultry Inspection: The Scientific Basis of the National Program*. Washington, D.C.: National Academy Press.

Chapter 7

Challenges Facing Livestock Health in the Twenty-First Century

INTRODUCTION

The preceding chapters indicate twenty-first century challenges to **livestock health policy (LHP)** are complex and increasingly subject to external influences. Livestock industries, as well as the agencies that regulate them, are under pressure to improve food safety, preserve the environment, reverse losses of small-farm lifestyles, confront concerns about **genetically modified organisms (GMOs)**, and enhance animal welfare. LHP-makers are also expected to deter terrorist attacks on livestock and prevent acts of extremism that utilize **zoonotic** pathogens. These issues are linked to livestock production and processing. They require managerial improvements, new biosecurity measures, improved animal disease reporting systems, upgraded animal identification systems, and steps to overcome the stress-associated disease risks of confinement operations.

Meeting these challenges will require increased financial support for disease-control and surveillance programs, for diagnostic laboratories, and for animal health research. They demand that regulations assuring that pharmaceuticals and **biologicals** used in animals are safe, effective, available for all livestock species, and without human health hazards. The assistance of livestock producers, industry groups, and regulatory agencies will be required, and these groups must be willing to address the legitimate concerns of opposing interests as they work to upgrade livestock health expertise and build functional infrastructures.

There must be close cooperation among livestock interests, the food-consuming public, the scientific community, elected leaders, and appointed officials. LHP-makers must also interact successfully with trading partners in different languages and cultures.

Nations seeking to develop globally competitive livestock industries and credible animal health infrastructures can meet these challenges with transparent and cooperative programs. Successful countries will have to adhere to the **World Trade Organization (WTO) Sanitary and Phytosanitary (SPS) Agreement**, abide by the international standards developed by the **Office International des Epizooties (OIE)**, and maintain the respect and trust of potential trading partners.

Challenges in Food Safety

Perhaps the most pressing challenge facing LHP-makers is to effectively and candidly address the safety of foods of animal origin. Improved diagnostic technology and increased reporting of food-borne diseases have combined with media coverage to raise public expectations. The goal of a risk-free affordable food supply is a moving target requiring improvements at each link in the food chain and setting goals for food industries and regulatory agencies that are almost unachievably high. As in traffic safety, food-safety challenges are amenable to many risk-mitigating measures but cannot be totally eliminated. The current food-safety focus on farm practices and processing procedures tends to neglect the responsibility of consumers, retail outlets, and restaurants.

The public must face the reality that the feces of people and animals contain pathogens that multiply exponentially in appropriate environments. These organisms are constantly changing their disease-producing capacities, their resistance to medicines and disinfectants, and their reactions to diagnostic tests. Mankind's imperfect efforts to improve food safety must be implemented on the farm and in processing plants as well as in the kitchen.

Policy makers, therefore, without minimizing the importance of livestock-borne organisms, need to push for educational programs illustrating the multiple links in the food-safety chain and emphasizing that properly refrigerated and well-cooked foods served promptly after preparation under sanitary conditions rarely result in sickness.

It must also be emphasized that rare, raw, and improperly cooked or improperly refrigerated foods present the greatest risks. People electing to take these risks must be apprised of simple preventive measures and the potential consequences if these precautions are ignored. This requires educating food handlers and those preparing, serving, and eating meals. Without this education, all the legislation, regulations, and media hype addressing the production, processing, and packaging of foods will produce increased prices and non-competitive global marketing but little progress in food safety.

Livestock health officials must be educated and accountable through the entire food chain, because with food safety the buck stops everywhere. Without denying the farm-to-fork linkages, policy makers must be diplomatic yet firm in the assertion that education, and perhaps irradiation or electronic pasteurization, hold the greatest hopes for food safety. Like the efforts in processing plants, relentless consumer-level food-safety education is essential. Food-safety programs must focus on those areas most likely to cause problems and on those offering the best opportunities for successful intervention such as in the areas of food processing and preparation. Although slaughter and processing are the points of greatest contamination and dissemination of pathogens, food preparation areas provide the most effective and cost efficient opportunities for eliminating the pathogens.

Protecting the Environment and Preserving Ecosystems

As global populations expand and urbanization increases, rural ecosystems are disappearing. Family farms and ranches are a bastion for maintaining undeveloped lands in rural areas. Large and intensive livestock production units are highly efficient. However, in the view of environmental groups, their intensity can ravage the land, pollute the air with dust and odors, and generate manure-disposal problems and air-polluting ammonia. Manure is a source of soil nitrogen that is best preserved by promptly plowing it into the soil or piling it so there is minimal exposure to air currents.

Large feedlots and other intensive livestock production units raise water-quality issues. There is a fear that in times of flooding they can cause watershed contamination with pathogens or animal carcasses. During floods there are many sources of contamination to watersheds, including leaves and other plant materials from forests and meadows, excrement of birds and wildlife, and human sewerage from overwhelmed municipal disposal systems and septic tanks. The media frequently focus on flood pollution by livestock operations neglecting the fact that human sewerage plants release untreated waste into waterways during floods.

There are many potential solutions to manure disposal at livestock operations. One involves spreading manure in appropriate quantities on depleted soils to regenerate soil fertility and assist marginal land in holding moisture and supporting vegetation. There are a variety of manure-treatment systems. Some are monitored by state or federal regulations that require large operations to have comprehensive nutrient management systems constructed under the direction of environmental engineers or certified consultants. These use a variety of manure-biodegradation treatments and settling ponds that reduce odors and permit marketing of solids as fertilizers and soil enrichers.

Some large livestock operations have manure digesters that produce methane to power generators that make electricity for homes, industries, or desalinization plants (Mohr 2001). Some methane-producing manure digesters require relatively dry manure from facilities bedded with paper or sawdust rather than straw, which is less readily degradable. The manure is collected by dry-scraping animal housing facilities rather than by pressure-washing them. The solid residues of the digestion process, which are less odoriferous than raw manure, can be sold as garden compost or crop fertilizer. The remaining liquids are biodegraded in lagoons and can be used as farm fertilizers (Mohr 2001). In response to pressures from environmental activists, some corporate livestock industries have invested heavily in waste-disposal technology.

The future of small farms in the environmental preservation movement remains strong. Small-scale livestock producers, many with other income sources, are exempt from many environmental regulations. They can access supply chains through contracts with corporations. These agreements provide markets for farmers meeting certain product standards (Tweeden et al. 2001).

Policy makers must hear the views of divergent interest groups as they address the conflict between economically efficient integrated livestock operations that produce affordable foodstuffs and less efficient individually owned small farms that preserve rural ecosystems and family-farm lifestyles. They must seek and support compromise solutions that permit integrated operations to be sensitive to ecological considerations, while encouraging the survival of environmentally friendly small farms.

Potential Loss of the Cherished Small-Farm Lifestyle

Urbanization, mechanization, readily accessible transportation, electronic information transmission via computers and television, changing lifestyles, and competition from integrated agricultural production units have produced a steady demise of small family farms. This trend is bemoaned because it diminishes rural ecosystems, farm work ethics, and family values. Some say it has produced a reduction in worker productivity and citizens who are less responsible. This trend is a complex sociological phenomenon that cannot be altered by legislation.

The issue of the demise of small farms will surface in LHP discussions and must be placed in perspective with other societal changes. Some countries will try to protect small-farm economies by placing trade restrictions on imported products containing GMOs or basing restrictions on environmental or animal welfare issues.

The argument that small operations produce animal products less likely to cause food-borne illness is unsubstantiated. Although some control of food-borne disease can be accomplished on the farm, other key points in controlling human food poisoning include the slaughter, processing, and packaging steps and food-preparation, food-handling, and cooking procedures. However, controlling a single step is not sufficient. Food safety requires a **total quality management (TQM)** approach that involves the entire food chain. Pre-harvest food safety may become more important as we develop methods to effectively reduce and eliminate pathogen loads on the farm.

Overcoming Public Concerns About GMOs

Though the theory of evolution remains controversial, few public objections have arisen to species improvement through cross-breeding and cross-pollination. Advancing molecular and genetic technologies have bypassed the time-consuming process of selective breeding for the production of rapidly growing, disease-resistant plants and animals. This technology is based on the identification of genes, often outside the genetic pool of the species to be manipulated, that direct disease or pesticide resistance, growth rates, and other traits. These genes can then be inserted into plants, animals, or microbes to achieve desired results.

The issues of genetic engineering, recombinant DNA technology, and the production of GMOs have come under fire from groups with varying agendas. Some objections arise from legitimate scientific uncertainties. Some are based on resistance to change. Others arise from religious, ethical, ethnic, and cultural convictions.

In many cases there are inadequate data to assess the actual risks, if any, associated with genetically modified plants or animals or GMO-based products. This scientific uncertainty is often exploited to raise vocal objections or to request the labeling of GMO-based products and to impose precautionary sanitary measures to protect non-competitive industries and products.

Many experts feel the public would be more receptive to these products if they had more knowledge and a better understanding of recombinant DNA technology, GMOs, and biotechnology. Trade in animals and animal products is complicated by speculative fears that GMOs at any part of the food chain may damage the environment or human health.

In July 2001, the European Commission (EC) adopted rules requiring food labels to carry information permitting the tracing of GMOs from farm to fork. The labels must indicate if products contain GMOs or if GMOs were used in their production. This means meat labels should state if GMOs were present in livestock feed. Reportedly, labeling requirements are intended to reduce testing, which will be done to spot check products for violations. Some observers believe the rule is intended to exclude U.S. and Canadian livestock feeds, meat, poultry, and their products, which some countries cannot produce competitively in a free-market economy. These restrictions are considered by some U.S. officials to be protectionist measures that violate the WTO

SPS Agreement. The agreement says import measures must be science-based, transparent, non-discriminatory, risk assessment-based, and applied without discrimination.

Later in 2001, a European Union (EU) report summarizing eighty-one EU-supported research projects indicated biotech products and foods made from GMOs present no evidence of new risks to human health.

Policy makers and animal health officials face a dilemma on the issue of the dangers of genetically engineered animal feeds, human foods, pharmaceuticals, vaccines, and feed additives. As with the objections to embryonic stem-cell research, which are growing, these are issues that science alone cannot resolve. In the midst of the U.S. debate over embryonic stem cell research in the summer and fall of 2001 it became evident that stem-cell research will move forward. Private industry was already involved and the British Parliament had already approved the research. Progress is hard to reverse, particularly if it produces popular products at competitive prices. There were once people who felt automobiles were evil and would never replace the horse and buggy. Future generations may look at GMOs in the same light.

Reports indicate there are so many GMOs in the global food supply as to render it virtually impossible to remove them. In the United States, surveys indicate public acceptance of GMOs is growing, and reports indicate over 50% of food products now contain some genetically modified components.

The secret to acceptance will be public understanding of the process and establishing trust in the scientific and regulatory communities. This will require transparency, education, and credible and responsible regulations.

In discussing GMOs and related issues, LHP-makers must seek to understand where the opposition is coming from. They should avoid arguments that cannot be won and resist the temptation to overreact and sound self-righteous when trading partners raise concerns about the safety of products derived through genetic manipulation.

Suggested strategies for dealing with this sensitive issue include making an effort to avoid propagandizing the merits of GMO products; explaining the process in terms comprehensible to average citizens; acknowledging the uncertainties regarding alleged risks from GMOs; continuing to explore the issues with the newest available scientific and epidemiological studies; confining biotechnological programs to problems not amenable to other approaches; and laying out reasonable expectations that biotechnology is not a panacea that will solve all the world's problems (Gerke 2001).

Challenges in Animal Welfare

Global sensitivity to the comfort and treatment of livestock continues to increase as the world becomes more civilized. In developed countries, the animal welfare movement is responsible for much of this progress and it continues to gain support. It has stimulated improvement in the care, feeding, handling, and movement of livestock and in the design of animal facilities. Many of these changes contribute positively to livestock health by reducing the stress, anxiety, and apprehension that contribute to disease and production shortfalls.

The animal rights movement, an extremist offshoot of animal welfare, is less effective because of its radical views and at times violent interventions. Animal rights advocates present a compelling vision of a more moral world, but this vision is ecologically foolhardy and based on a naive definition of animal happiness (Pollan 2000).

Dealing with issues of animal welfare will be a continuing challenge, but it will simultaneously present opportunities as LHP-makers strive to improve production efficiency, food safety, and public support.

Challenges in Deterring Terrorism

The new millennium and its age of terrorism bring increased attention to biosecurity in feedlots, farms, auction barns, slaughterhouses, and processing plants. Concerns about terrorist attacks on livestock facilities arise from the increasing emergence of eccentric individuals with erratic and extremist views and violent political or religious agendas.

LHP-makers and veterinarians will play key roles in the proactive reduction of the impact of terrorist attacks on livestock and of acts of extremism that utilize zoonotic pathogens against animals or people (Ashford et al. 2000).

The new millennium brought a need for increased **biosecurity** measures at every point in the food chain (Gillespie 2000). The entire livestock industry from the farm to the consumer will be developing precautions to address increasing threats of bioterrorism, added risks of exotic-disease incursions, and the potential of increasing violence from animal rights extremists. These challenges are compounded by societal changes, including increasing crime rates and a declining respect for private and public property. In combination, these developments challenge farmers, ranchers, feedlot operators, and meat and poultry processors to develop security measures and emergency management procedures in cooperation with national and local officials.

In nations that have traditionally supported individual freedom, these threats signal new relationships between individual rights and public welfare, food safety, and livestock health.

Challenges in Improving Management Practices

Rapidly changing and ever-improving livestock management practices designed to enhance animal comfort and increase profits are an ongoing component of LHPs. Evolving methods of rearing, feeding, managing, sorting, transporting, and slaughtering livestock offer constant challenges to the livestock health community. A change in livestock management practices can produce an environment conducive to disease reduction and improved animal comfort, or it can achieve the opposite result. Changes in management practices can also create environmental and food-safety concerns. The LHP-making community is faced with continually escalating challenges to balance production efficiency with these complex concerns and individual freedoms and the rights of farmers to make management decisions.

Challenges in Improving Monitoring, Surveillance, and Reporting (MS&R)

Information on the nature and global distribution of livestock diseases is essential for establishing and implementing livestock health, food-safety, and public health programs. These data are also needed for prioritizing and evaluating domestic disease-control programs and vaccination activities and for establishing credible **exotic disease** exclusion programs. Each member country is expected to participate transparently in the OIE global livestock health-reporting network.

Increasing demand for **transparency** by citizens of democratic societies and the international community requires that policy makers strive for improvements in livestock health monitoring, surveillance, and reporting (MS&R) systems. The achievement of these improvements requires participation by national and subnational governments, animal disease diagnostic laboratories, practicing veterinarians, and the entire livestock industry (Kahrs 1999).

Monitoring is defined as general oversight of the health of livestock populations, while surveillance focuses on specific disease testing and tracking. Surveillance can be active or passive. In **active surveillance**, disease-specific tracking programs are instituted. These involve testing, inspections, and other regularly conducted activities that seek evidence of a disease. In **passive surveillance** authorities react to suggestions that a disease may be present by following leads or performing tests to verify suspicions and maintain general livestock health oversight.

Monitoring and surveillance are inseparably tied to reporting. Both domestic stakeholders and the international community expect that transparent health data will be widely available through elaborate livestock health information chains. Complete and accurate disease reporting determines the credibility of **livestock health infrastructures** and defines each country's integrity and trustworthiness in the international community.

When countries apply disease-specific sanitary measures to exclude importations, their trading partners expect clear statements of the risks involved and documentation of the status of each referenced disease in the recipient country.

The domestic livestock health status of every nation has international significance. OIE member countries are required to complete annual, monthly, and special-situation reports documenting their animal health status. Merely filing required OIE reports does not fully address the expectations of domestic stakeholders or the international community. As soon as a country submits a report to the OIE it is available internationally and can be used by other countries to establish import requirements. The integrity of these reports is the basis of national credibility in international health and trade circles.

The OIE communicates with the **chief veterinary officers (CVOs)** of member countries. Requests for national disease data are sent only to CVOs and reports are accepted only from their offices. In many countries CVOs dispense information only to inner circles, or to those with a need to know. The "need to know" includes a far broader component of society than those traditionally receiving communications from national veterinary authorities.

In the absence of information from CVOs, informal non-governmental information sources emerge. Their information may be valid, but it can also be based on rumors, false reports on unedited web sites, erroneous media reports, or suspicious outbreaks ultimately determined to be false alarms.

Import measures to exclude exotic diseases are often questioned or challenged by exporting countries. In such cases satisfactory trade requires importing countries to document that their territory is free of the diseases against which sanitary measures are designed. In lieu of disease freedom there may be nationally sponsored control or eradication programs. Both of these situations require nationally operated MS&R systems for OIE-listed diseases.

There are wide variations in the MS&R systems among countries due to differing local conditions. Some nations try to respect the authority of subnational governments and the proprietary confidentiality of affected industries. This can result in haphazard MS&R systems and diminished national credibility. Most developed countries have effective MS&R systems. Developed countries should take the lead in MS&R activities and exhibit respect and understanding for the deficiencies of nations with less surveillance capacity.

Some countries are reluctant to report their animal health situations, because they can be used to their disadvantage (see Discussion Topic 8). Livestock health information systems are built on trust and credibility. Failure to report a disease is a more subtle violation of international trust than falsely claiming disease-free status.

In addition to submitting timely reports to the OIE, the ideal national MS&R system publishes an annual report. Such reports succinctly summarize progress in control or eradication programs, outline the national status regarding each OIE List A and List B disease, and indicate those diseases for which vaccination is permitted. These reports are distributed to livestock groups, personnel who interact with representatives of foreign governments, employees of the national agriculture and veterinary services, legislators and trading partners, and all participants in the national livestock health information chain. They are also available to the media and the general public. It helps to supplement annual reports with updates for each major livestock species.

Countries should clearly define the roles of national and subnational governments and of constituent and stakeholder organizations in their national animal health reporting systems (NAHRS).

There are three types of NAHRS: compulsory, voluntary, and cooperative. Compulsory requirements, as is the case with many bureaucratic exercises, often generate resistance and can be ineffective in many cultures. Voluntary programs are equally unsuccessful. Trading partners often refuse to recognize claims of disease freedom based on loosely administered voluntary reporting systems.

Cooperative animal disease reporting systems address the conflicting needs of governments, livestock producers, and their organizations. Cooperative industry-state-federal programs are frequently controversial during their development. They are most effective when all participants are involved from the outset and are represented at all levels in the decision-making process. It is desirable to have a cooperative NAHRS involving each industry and subnational unit needing assistance from the national veterinary services or requiring national governmental certification of animal products for export. This definition carries considerable force, because most countries require national officials of exporting countries to sign health certifications.

Livestock health information programs based on accurate information at every step in the MS&R chain should be developed cooperatively by all interested parties and implemented electronically. Participants in the information flow chain should include livestock producers, private and publicly employed veterinarians, inspectors at packing houses, regulatory officials, diagnostic laboratory personnel, veterinary drug and biological manufacturers, and the veterinary academic community. Successful disease-control and exclusion programs and MS&R systems require that these individuals gather all possible identification and point-of-origin data on every suspected exotic, emerging, or unusual disease. These data must be promptly reported to animal health officials so that timely epidemiologic investigation can be initiated. The final results of each investigation should be reported, preferably electronically, up and down the information chain. Transparency, prompt feedback, and active involvement are essential to retain the support of constituent groups and individuals.

As globalization and international trade expand NAHRS will become more critical. There is a growing tendency of countries to judge MS&R activities on the quality, not the quantity, of the NAHRSs of trading partners. Countries that are agricultural producers can have major problems in the global marketplace if they lack the resources for developing and implementing effective reporting systems.

LHP-makers must be strong advocates of cooperative NAHRS in their countries. They must understand the factors behind resistance to reporting. They must work to involve all essential constituents in the development and constant updating of systems that credibly represent the animal health status of the country (see chapter 10).

Challenges in Improving Animal Identification Systems

A system of permanent animal identification (ID) is important to national animal health infrastructures. National ID systems should be adequate to identify animals and trace them through the supply chain. This ability to trace has marketing value as it provides producers with real time information on the wholesomeness of their products and permits quality-incentive payments by slaughter facilities. Producer incentives to use ID systems would ensure continuous involvement in the program. A functional ID system also allows infected animals or contaminated products to be traced to the farm of origin. This capability is essential to national livestock health and food-safety programs.

It is challenging to develop a workable, consistently applied, and mutually acceptable ID system covering all livestock. Complications arise from species differences, costs, logistical difficulties, and resistance of producers and processors who fear being penalized for events and contaminants beyond their control.

Some European countries have led the way in effective national ID systems. These systems enhance public acceptance of products and help assure export markets. They use ear tags accompanied by electronic identification cards (passports) that indicate ownership, official tests, and vaccinations. This information is entered into a central computer and provides documentation for payment of EU subsidies to producers.

As diseases like **tuberculosis** and **brucellosis** approach eradication in the United States, ear tags inserted during routine tests and brucellosis vaccinations will gradually decline in numbers (Salmon 2000).

A variety of animal identification devices and electronic remote-reading equipment is available (see chapter 10). While understanding all the details is challenging to LHP-makers, they should be apprised of progress in animal ID programs in competing nations and be aware that acceptable animal ID systems may soon be required by importing countries. A credible animal ID system gives leverage in opening up export markets. Adequate identification and trace-back systems provide nations with the capacity to promptly localize disease problems and to regionalize to be able to continue exports from uninfected areas. Producer acceptance of national animal ID systems is expedited when governments supply identification equipment without charge.

Growing pressure for animal ID systems will continue to come from the international community and from fast-food and supermarket chains as they attempt to respond to increasing consumer demands for verifiable information on the environments in which source animals are raised (see Discussion Topic 2) and the humane conditions under which they are managed (see Discussion Topic 3).

LHP-makers will continually be asked to regulate the installation, monitoring, implementation, and ongoing improvement of animal ID systems.

Challenges in Overcoming Increased Disease Risk of Confinement Operations

The economic advantages of confinement livestock production systems result from mass production strategies. In some systems the feed production, feed mixing, animal housing, medication, slaughtering, processing, and packaging of products occur under single ownership. Sometimes all these operations occur on contiguous properties. This system standardizes procedures, produces quality uniform products, eliminates numerous middlemen, lowers transportation costs, and permits delivery of products at competitive prices. It can also provide opportunities for improving livestock health.

Large feedlots, dairy, laying-hen and broiler production facilities are sometimes called factory farms, concentrated livestock feeding operations, industrialized agriculture, or corporate farms. They have the potential to cause the demise of less competitive, small family-owned farms within a country. Where unrestricted free trade prevails, they can trigger the collapse of livestock industries in countries with less competitive agribusiness practices. They can often deliver quality animal products to foreign markets at costs significantly lower than can be produced in the importing country. This can occur in less developed countries or in those struggling in transition from controlled political systems to free-market economies.

Countries frequently invoke sanitary measures with borderline scientific validity in order to protect struggling domestic livestock industries, preserve rural ecosystems, and support family-farm cultures. Thoughtful diplomatic negotiations are required to establish and maintain markets in such countries without permanently damaging their economies or totally alienating their officials. This can sometimes be accomplished through technology transfer, scientific cooperation, or joint commercial ventures.

Proponents of ecosystem preservation, family-farm lifestyles, worker's rights, vegetarianism, animal welfare, and animal rights have significant political influence. They decry the evils of corporate agriculture and its stress-inducing discomforts and animal disease problems. There are significant health differences between livestock grazing contentedly in open pastures and those reared in close confinement. The free-ranging animals mature and grow more slowly even if shade, water, and feed are present. They are subject to less stress than confinement-reared livestock, which are often commingled from multiple sources and must compete for space, feed, water, and pecking-order status. This stress produces immunosuppression (Tizzard 2000), a key contributor to diseases like **bovine shipping fever**, **porcine reproductive and respiratory syndrome (PRRS),** and several viral infections of poultry.

In capitalistic societies confinement agriculture is apparently here to stay. Policy makers need an understanding of the contributions of integrated livestock industries to national economies and consumers.

In the United States, where **confinement livestock operations** are prevalent, consumers spend less than 12% of their disposable income on food. This bargain is largely unappreciated and must be placed in perspective with the environmental issues and animal health implications of confinement livestock rearing. Animal health officials must be sensitive to the unique potential of, and livestock health challenges presented by, corporate agriculture as they develop programs, regulations, and policies.

Gaining Support for Livestock Health Issues

There will be a continually increasing need for financial support for livestock health issues as a result of the growing impetus for new and expanding programs, for meeting increasing public expectations, and for keeping up with advancing technology. In the competition for limited federal funds, these items must be emphasized as issues of major national consequence. To date, this message has not been effectively delivered and needs to be raised to levels heretofore not achieved by livestock health interests.

Funding for national programs requires media attention and vocal public concern over significant issues including food safety and public health, availability of foods at reasonable prices, threats of bioterrorism, and balance of trade.

Positive support for these issues requires that citizens understand the need for critical programs like emergency preparedness and response, zoonoses surveillance, NAHRS, animal ID systems, MS&R systems, disease-control and eradication programs, diagnostic laboratories, and animal health research. This challenge must be addressed by LHP-makers.

Gaining Support for Diagnostic Laboratories

Diagnostic laboratories are critical to disease surveillance and exotic disease exclusion. They perform an unsung but valuable role in teaching veterinary students and in livestock extension programs. Diagnostic laboratories are a major contact point between the academic community and the real world of producers, consumers, and the media.

The increasing costs of diagnostic equipment and the reagents essential to remaining technologically contemporary are largely unappreciated by budgeting authorities.

The support of livestock disease diagnostic laboratories must be a high priority of LHP-makers. This is an ongoing challenge.

Gaining Support for Disease-Control and Eradication Programs

Like other aspects of LHPs, disease-control and eradication programs have languished with a lack of national attention. This situation must be changed by an invigorated partnership among the livestock health community, national officials, and the media.

The increased emphasis on food safety and added concerns about bioterrorism will increase public expectations for improved control of zoonotic diseases and upgraded biosecurity. These expectations will provide opportunities and challenges for LHP-makers to attain appropriate levels of support for livestock disease-control activities.

Gaining Support for Livestock Health Research

In many economies the declining political and economic importance of agriculture and the growing public interest in other issues has significantly influenced the livestock health-research agenda. In the wake of exciting new technologies, agricultural and veterinary academics, traditionally bastions for livestock health research, have diversified by adding new disciplines and specialties and focusing increasingly on fundamental life processes.

Some colleges of agriculture have shifted their attention from livestock production to explorations of environmental issues, natural resources, human nutrition, and food processing technology. They have emphasized research in the basic biological sciences and molecular biology. Despite a decreasing percentage of funding, as well as a major de-emphasis and lessened prestige in academic circles, agricultural research has produced major advances in livestock health, animal reproductive efficiency, and food production technology (see chapter 2). Hopefully this progress will continue.

In veterinary medicine the twentieth century focus on livestock health and food production has been drastically diluted by an emphasis on companion animal medicine and surgery and basic research. The emergence of specialties like anesthesiology, cardiology, dermatology, food safety, laboratory animal medicine, neurology, ophthalmology, pathology, radiology, and toxicology has moved the veterinary profession away from its early focus on food animals.

In agriculture and veterinary medicine few university employees have a farm background, and the mind-set of the academic community is far removed from livestock health problems. In the United States food is convenient, plentiful, and of high quality. This creates a lack of appreciation for the return on investment for agricultural research and development (R&D). The livestock health segment of the academic research community has found it progressively more difficult to secure advocates and bolster programs intended to increase productivity. Corporate investors, who preserve their findings for proprietary reasons, have faired better than the academics, who don't speak with one voice and have not utilized the power of the press to elevate their cause.

In the United States in the last few decades private funding has outpaced public funding in support of agricultural research and development (R&D). These changes in support have negatively impacted public funding for agricultural R&D, and the research agenda has shifted to more scientifically popular and socially acceptable programs.

Public supported U.S. agricultural research and related policies are now at a pivotal point. A long period of substantial growth appears to have ended, and an extended phase of general fiscal restraint is developing. There is an ongoing debate justifying R&D funds and the accountability for their use. The culture and operations of public research institutions are being called into question. Unlike funds for human health research, consumers are more skeptical and less supportive of agricultural R&D and the concept of its public good.

It will be a challenge to convince academic leadership or the public that active livestock health research programs are essential for agricultural prosperity and a safe and affordable food supply. Livestock health research is needed to address pressures from domestic interest groups and the expectations of trading partners in the international community.

There is always a need for aggressive and active pursuit of a continually expanding list of questions about livestock health and its relation to food safety, human health, international trade, domestic prosperity, and economic stability. Capturing the answers to these questions requires expensive facilities, sophisticated equipment, trained scientists with competitive salaries, and adequate operating funds. Appeals for livestock health research funding are frequently lost among other politically urgent priorities.

The future of livestock research is a major challenge for LHP-makers and their supporters. They must capitalize on emergencies or media-hyped issues like **bovine spongiform encephalopathy (BSE), foot-and-mouth disease (FMD)**, and bioterrorism to market the importance of essential livestock health research funding. They must also become more active in food-safety education and provide a continual flow of industry-supported news releases. The marketing effort should include clearly articulated, scientifically sound reports to convince the media, the public (including potentially contrary interest groups), and legislators of specific livestock health research needs in both basic and applied areas. Such efforts require careful coordination, prioritization, and cooperative strategic planning. They must involve veterinary practitioners, the academic community, industry, government, and private stakeholders and develop strategies permitting the livestock health community to maintain its record of productive research.

Assuring the Safety, Effectiveness, and Availability of Animal Health Products

LHP-makers are expected to develop policies, regulations and procedures to assure that animal health products are safe, effective, and without human health hazards. This includes assurances that quality therapeutic agents are available for minor livestock species and for uncommon applications. It requires up-to-date laboratories and personnel trained to address advancing product technology, such as genetically engineered pharmaceuticals and vaccines derived from plants, plant viruses, or bacteria.

There are four biosafety levels (BLs) for handling microbiologic agents without risk to humans and animals. These levels represent increasingly stringent systems for biocontainment, protective clothing for workers, and laboratory ventilation. BL-1 is a conventional microbiology laboratory. Higher BLs require more advanced containment facilities and procedures.

BL-4 laboratories have the highest security level. They have elaborate one-piece biosafety hoods in which microbes are manipulated and multiple filters in their ventilation systems. BL-4 laboratories are called shower-in-shower-out facilities, because workers must shower and put on laboratory clothing on entry and shower before leaving and donning civilian clothes.

Fulfilling the obligation for reliable livestock health products requires costly approval procedures. But these approval procedures reduce the financial incentives for companies to develop animal drugs with limited market potential. The unavailability of licensed products labeled for use on minor species presents a dilemma. It means that products licensed and labeled for use on major livestock species or humans cannot be used on minor species, largely because economic considerations have precluded needed testing. This dilemma leaves livestock producers and veterinarians with two options. One is not to use the best available therapies for treatment of minor animal species and uncommon diseases. The equally unacceptable alternative is to use products for purposes for which they have not been licensed or labeled.

In 2001, a coalition of U.S. animal health groups and concerned supporters introduced legislation, named the Minor Use and Minor Species Animal Health Act. If passed, this legislation will permit the Food and Drug Administration to authorize companies to produce drugs already approved for use on major species to fulfill the limited market potential associated with use on small ruminants, **cervids**, fish, zoo animals, pet birds, or reptiles.

Societies are tightening controls on animal drugs in an effort to decrease injection-site blemishes, reduce antibiotic and drug residues in foods, and slow the development of antimicrobial resistance in microorganisms. LHP-makers face major challenges in regulating products used in maintaining livestock health in a manner that assures safe, effective use without endangering health or overly restricting creativity.

Addressing the Challenge of Global Food Distribution

The operational details of delivering safe foods from surplus-producing regions to countries with starving populations present major challenges to the international community. Advancing production technology and improved transportation capabilities indicate the time is approaching when feeding the world is possible. But this achievement will require creative efforts to unselfishly overcome economic, political, cultural, and religious obstacles to integrated livestock operations and incentive-base capitalistic systems.

Maintaining Support of Livestock Producers and Industry Organizations

The strength of participatory governments and free societies is that the voices of the people, however irrational or overstated, must be heard and considered by policy makers as they invoke transparent procedures for the development of LHPs and regulations.

The people rarely speak with one voice. In issues of livestock health it is tempting to heed only the knowledgeable opinions of those closest to the situation, i.e., livestock producers and processors, practicing veterinarians, regulatory veterinarians, and biological and pharmaceutical manufacturers. Their vested interests can run counter to consumer concerns about food safety and environmental preservation. They also conflict with the goals of some animal rights activists who openly wish FMD would enter the United States. As with the general population, livestock interests rarely speak with one voice. In addition, the scientific community, which should provide the deciding information, is divided on many livestock health issues of national importance.

These divisions provide LHP-makers with dilemmas and challenges. They must listen carefully to all groups to determine their biases, agendas, and vested interests. They must separate fact from fiction and make thoughtful, balanced decisions that serve the best interests of the general population without crippling the livestock industry.

Addressing Concerns of Opposition Groups

Almost all LHPs encounter opposition. LHP-makers must resist the temptation to totally disregard aberrant or unclear positions. They may have merit. The principle of 10% wrong is often invoked in lieu of careful listening. This procedure completely discards ideas because they are 10% wrong and neglects the 90% of the argument that has merit. LHP-makers must resist the temptation to totally reject arguments of opposition groups and carefully analyze them to extract whatever wisdom is present. This challenge is ever present at organizational and governmental levels.

Balancing Legitimate Governmental Oversight With Excessive Central Control

Citizens of countries with participatory governments and free-enterprise systems cherish freedom and resent government intrusion into personal affairs and private-sector enterprises. Ironically, people most vocal in opposing government interference with the operation of businesses, farms, or ranches are sometimes the first to seek government programs to support their interests. They often criticize governments for not doing enough when emergencies arise and demand action from government agencies whose budgets they have fought to cut.

Policy makers must be aware that those who are the loudest opponents of proposed regulations are frequently most guilty with respect to violations of the public safety. Nonetheless, their objections frequently have valid components. LHP-makers must listen carefully to all comments and develop balanced policies that serve the best interests of the public at large.

Interacting Successfully With Varying Political and Cultural Viewpoints

LHP-makers are continually challenged to interact successfully with domestic stakeholders and trading partners. Spokespersons for these groups represent varying political, ethnic, cultural, educational, and religious backgrounds. They have differing agendas and often speak different languages.

On an international basis, the challenge of dealing with trading partners was amplified in the 1990s when health issues became key elements in the global movement of livestock products. This focus on livestock health followed establishment of the Agricultural Agreements of the General Agreement on Tariffs and Trade (GATT). These agreements were developed to reduce tariffs, increase international trade in agricultural products, and eliminate the use of sanitary measures as artificial trade barriers.

The GATT signatory nations established the WTO to oversee international trade, serve as the international dispute resolution body, and implement the SPS provisions of the treaty. The WTO formalized the SPS provisions of the GATT into the WTO SPS Agreement, which carries the force of international law. The WTO then named the OIE as the international standard-setting organization for animal health.

Efforts to fulfill commitments to the WTO SPS Agreement revolutionized global trade in animals and animal products (see chapter 5). They set the stage for endless bilateral and multilateral trade discussions aimed at developing mutually agreeable import and export conditions compatible with the agreement, the international standards established by the OIE, and the legitimate interests of individual countries.

Trade discussions involve negotiators from widely varying backgrounds with diverse agendas and prejudices. Discussions of sanitary issues require negotiators who are knowledgeable about animal health, tactfully diplomatic, culturally sensitive, and patient even when negotiations drag. Successful agreements for export of livestock products require understanding and a respect for the styles and viewpoints of the other side. This leads to gaining the trust of colleagues from other countries. Similar skills, perhaps to a lesser degree, are required for negotiation with fellow countrymen (see Skillful Negotiators in chapter 4).

Policy makers must insist that those representing their countries in international exchanges possess the interpersonal skills, patience, and animal health knowledge needed to be effective. Some people believe that multilingual skills are essential in trade negotiations and that translators, who may be unfamiliar with animal health jargon, should be replaced by multilingual negotiators. The presence of skilled translators helps overcome confusion that can occur when all participants are not fluent in the language of the host country and when arguments are presented rapidly in dialects with unfamiliar colloquialisms. Translations also offer a brief time for contemplation and note taking.

Although negotiations should be based on sound science, the negotiators themselves succeed because of interpersonal skills and trust. This trust is established by building long-term rapport with counterparts who have faith in their personal credibility and professional integrity. It is a challenge for LHP-makers to ensure that those who represent them are knowledgeable and diplomatic.

Bibliography

Ashford, D. A., T. M. Gomez, D. L. Noah et al. 2000. Biological Terrorism and Veterinary Medicine in the United States. *J. Am Vet Med Assoc.* 217:664-667.

Gerke, J. 2001. Putting GMOs in Perspective. Food Systems Insider. *Drovers Magazine* 1(3).

Gillespie, J. R. 2000. The Underlying Interrelated Issues of Biosecurity. *J. Am Vet Med Assoc.* 216:662-664.

Kahrs, R. F. 1999. The International Animal Health Communities Expectation's of the U.S. National Animal Health Reporting System (NAHRS). *Proc U.S. Animal Health Association* 103: 100-109.

Mohr, P. 2001. Portland General Electric Foots the Bill for Methane Production on Oregon Dairy Farm. *Dairy Today* (August):3.

Pollan, M. 2002. The Unnatural Idea of Animal Rights: An Animals Place. *The New York Times Magazine* (November 14):58-66.

Salmon, M. D. 2000. Surveillance Methodologies for Diseases Approaching Zero Prevalence in a Country/Region. *Proc. U.S. Animal Health Association* 104:289-290.

Tizzard, I. R. 2000. *Veterinary Immunology.* 6th ed. Philadelphia: W. B. Saunders Company.

Tweeden, L. G. et al. 2001. *Vertical Coordination of Agriculture in Farming-dependent Areas.* Ames, IA: Council for Agricultural Science and Technology Report 137:1-40.

Chapter 8

A Look at the Future

INTRODUCTION

The future of global **livestock health policies (LHPs)** will be shaped by predictable trends and complicated by unforeseeable events and unexpected issues. Upcoming decades will bring scientific and technologic achievements and further modernization of livestock production and processing practices. This will be accompanied by political, social, and cultural dynamics; alterations in governing styles; continued resistance to globalization and international governance; elevated concern about new or emerging diseases; bioterrorist attacks against livestock; and the use of **zoonotic** agents against people. These trends will increase the pressures on livestock agriculture to conform to social, environmental, food-safety, and animal welfare expectations.

Driving forces and events will call for a new generation of LHP leaders. They will need both scientific and political savvy to address new obligations and challenges. Leaders with foresight will look to livestock health as a springboard for addressing global starvation and world peace.

The challenges facing animal agriculture and LHPs in the twenty-first century will be increasingly complex. They will require global outlooks and a skillful balancing of public perceptions, scientific uncertainty, and positive and equitable policy-making actions.

Predictable Twenty-First Century Trends

Advancing science and technology are inevitable results of the passage of time. If historic trends prevail, new techniques to increase production and processing efficiency will come with increasing frequency and rapidity. They will impact both livestock and human health. In developed countries, some advances will become common practice and will be in daily use before policy makers, government officials, and public interest groups suspect their existence.

New developments in livestock technology will face continuing opposition despite their value to society. This opposition will come from individuals and organizations opposing change and fighting progress to protect firmly ensconced beliefs, long-standing traditions, or vested interests. LHP-makers will confront many dilemmas. They must sort out legitimate technological advances from profit-motivated activities that infringe on food safety, the environment, animal welfare, and other public concerns.

The future will probably bring a deluge of new vaccines, medicinal implants, feed additives, therapeutics, disinfectants, and other disease-control products. They will be developed using technology that is so new that it will be unfamiliar to regulators and much of the scientific community. It will become commonplace to employ genetic manipulation to increase disease resistance and to alter infectious agents to reduce their pathogenicity. The controversy over microbial resistance to antibiotics will probably be resolved by efforts on multiple fronts.

Unexpected Events and New Issues

The triggering events of future LHP issues will arise from unimaginable scientific progress, adaptations of diseases to changing ecological niches, political turnarounds, and slowly moving cultural accommodation to a rapidly changing world. Acts of agroterrorism or bioterrorism will alter public thinking about livestock health, food safety, and zoonotic diseases and generate support for the livestock industry.

The future will bring major scientific progress including the discovery of new pieces of the disease puzzle: new and previously unimagined classes of infectious and non-infectious pathogens; new chapters in the role of the immune system; new understanding of the multifaceted nature of human and animal disease; and revolutionary mechanisms for detecting invisible infectious materials, toxins, and residues in live animals, food, and the environment.

Some findings will be shocking. They will cause a collapse of long-standing dogmas about the causes, prevention, and cure of disease and may refute the disease-free claims of some countries. This progress may create an increased willingness to invest public moneys in research. The cost of sophisticated scientific inquiry will continue to outstrip available resources. People allocating research moneys will need the capacity to distinguish between projects with the potential for progress and those designed to garnish the coffers of research institutions.

The gap will continue to expand between accelerating science and a human reluctance to change. This will produce conflicts in and among the livestock and food industries, regulatory agencies, and consumers. LHP-makers will need to adjudicate increasing differences between the scientific community and profit-driven industries. Vocal interests representing consumers, the environment, human rights, and animal welfare may damage their causes by becoming increasingly antiscience and antigovernment. These behaviors may end up alienating the very people most able to help them.

LHP conflicts will be complicated by firmly established cultural and religious attitudes that change more slowly than LHPs or global food preferences. Resolving these conflicts will set the stage for livestock health to address global starvation and influence world peace.

Advancing Technology and LHPs

While the future is unpredictable, the lessons of past decades and the potential for increasing scientific and technological progress suggest events that will shape LHPs. These will include:

- Emergence of new human and animal diseases
- New discoveries about disease causation that clarify the roles of environmental, genetic, infectious, immunological, parasitic, and metabolic disease agents
- Therapeutic agents for conditions formerly considered untreatable
- Advances in immunology providing highly effective vaccines and more rapid diagnostic tests
- Rapid electronic **monitoring, surveillance, and reporting (MS&R) systems**
- Electronic identification for tracking animals and animal products

These changes will impose new obligations and present challenging opportunities for the leadership of nations. Leaders will be called upon to resolve cultural conflicts and infrastructural disparities in order to establish animal health as a springboard to world peace. This will give tomorrow's LHP leadership the potential to change the world.

Twentieth century dogma suggests a certain amount of animal disease is inevitable, some diseases are uncontrollable and without successful treatments, and there will never be enough animal protein to satisfy the nutritional needs of the world's expanding population. The next century will see technology to debunk these assumptions.

Livestock production will benefit from crop production efficiencies and the increased yields possible with genetically engineered plants resistant to plant pests and requiring fewer applications of pesticides and herbicides. Soon animals will be genetically engineered to grow faster; produce larger amounts of higher quality meat, milk, and eggs; and resist diseases.

Every discovery raises new questions. Nonetheless, science is paving the way for previously unimaginable success in raising disease-free livestock. This progress results from a mix of advances in genetics, immunology, management, nutrition, vaccinology, treatments, preventative therapy, and diagnosis. It will result in less expensive, more nutritious, and safer foods.

Intensive Modernization of Livestock Production Practices

Production efficiencies should produce increased supplies of animal protein. Worldwide availability of animal products will ease global tensions if appropriately distributed, accepted as dietary components by protein-starved cultures, and encouraged by opponents of modern livestock production. Firmly ensconced cultural beliefs can conflict with science and with the goal of feeding the world's starving people.

Political, economic, societal, and cultural dynamics and **globalization** issues reach beyond livestock health to pressure agricultural policies. They cannot be ignored and must be factored into forecasts. These combined dynamics have the potential to:

- Heighten conflicts between have and have-not countries
- Increase rural-urban tensions within countries
- Stimulate a movement toward international egalitarianism
- Increase public involvement in governments
- Increase tensions among livestock producers, environmentalists, and animal welfare advocates
- Create added pressure for global resource sharing
- Set the stage for food-surplus-endowed nations to be the arbiters of world peace

Changing Political and Cultural Dynamics

Changing political, cultural, and social dynamics will shape the future direction of LHPs. The idealistic notion of science-based LHPs that are transparent and non-discriminatory will eventually prevail globally. It will overcome many political and cultural forces that sometimes tend to countermand science, logic, and common sense.

Political Dynamics

Frequent governmental changes in the nations of the world, the attitudes of their leaders, and the persuasiveness of their challengers will determine the directions of global LHPs in upcoming decades.

If the movement toward democracy continues, transparent participatory processes will govern the development and implementation of LHPs in most of the world. This will permit policies to be discussed and debated at length before enactment so they can address the concerns of non-agricultural interests.

If there is a reemergence of monarchies this input will be lacking and policies will be narrower in scope and more rigidly enforced. Should there be a reemergence of communism or other socialist regimes, affected countries will likely regress to non-competitive livestock industries that rely largely on sanitary measures to protect struggling industries, rather than increasing their competitiveness by incentive-based efficiency or shifting to industries more adapted to their ecosystems.

Cultural Dynamics

Culture is a summation of the regional, behavioral, technological, esthetic, and intellectual achievements of a civilization. It impacts livestock management practices and processing, transportation, and refrigeration methods. Firmly ensconced cultural beliefs preserve proud traditions and support cherished lifestyles. They correctly assume that change does not necessarily represent progress, particularly when it involves personal and societal values. These values can conflict with science, foresight, and the idealistic goal of feeding the starving people of the world.

The impact of culture on LHPs is less volatile and energetic than political reactions. But it exerts steady pressure that resists inevitable changes. Barring momentous and earthshaking unforeseen events, LHPs of the twenty-first century will be faced with the same cultural divides present at the turn of the century. The cultural differences among the continents will combine with differences between developed and less developed countries, industrialized and non-industrial nations, and those with subsistence versus industrialized livestock production, to heavily impact LHPs. Racial and religious differences between countries will persist and perhaps intensify.

These developments will create controversy over LHPs. There will be continued public dissatisfaction with LHPs throughout the world and continued rural-urban conflicts in developed countries. There will probably be greater recognition and concern about new and **emerging diseases**, higher expectations to reconcile public perceptions of risk with scientific uncertainty, and increasing pressure on livestock agriculture to conform to social and environmental expectations.

Cultural differences will impact LHPs in different ways. They will require talented and understanding leadership to resolve differences so all cultures can benefit from advancing livestock production and health.

Inevitable cultural conflicts will continue to magnify global tensions within and between countries. Deeply ingrained religious beliefs accompanying cultural leanings will underlay many international conflicts.

Changing Governmental Styles

The dynamics of governmental style will, to some extent, dictate the LHPs of every country. Even in countries with elected government officials, swings of popular opinion produce a cycling of liberal and conservative, business and worker, and industrial and environmental influences. All of these are affected by firmly entrenched cultural and religious institutions such as prohibitions on pork or beef consumption, and climatic and geographic influences on work ethics that are crucial to agricultural success. Less-developed nations, unless enriched by natural resources, have difficulty with high expectations for livestock health infrastructures. Unless there are large-scale food aid undertakings, major political upheavals, or wars followed by massive repatriation projects, there will be an inevitably widening gap between rich and poor nations. Exceptions for increasing production may exist for those poor nations with climate and geography supportive to livestock production. Thus, there will be a continuing worldwide need to exclude exotic diseases, improve livestock health, increase production of animal protein, and preserve environments supportive of livestock production.

Continued Resistance to Globalization

Worldwide, the forces opposing globalization include isolationist interests in all nations, labor unions, and industries that are non-competitive in free-market economies. These interests have yet to accept the realities of increased movement of populations within and between countries, expedited global transportation of goods and services, and improving communication technology that flashes news of events around the world.

Despite these realities, leaders of all nations will continually be pressed to withdraw from worldly involvement and to exclude imports, though not exports. They will be urged to withdraw by those who emphasize the inequities and opportunities for abuse presented by the global free-market economy. The **World Trade Organization (WTO) Sanitary and Phytosanitary (SPS) Principles** and international standards promulgated democratically by the OIE are the best evidence of global influence on LHPs. Despite their shortcomings, they offer positive programs for world peace.

It will require remarkable foresight and wisdom for LHP-makers and national officials to respond positively to anti-globalization interests in their countries and to act in the best interests of the citizens of their nations and the world.

Concern With Emerging Diseases

The timing and nature of new and emerging diseases is unpredictable. Nonetheless, the future will bring continuing bacterial and viral mutation as organisms adjust to environmental changes, livestock management activities, new drugs and **antimicrobials**, and human and animal immune responses. These pressures and random mutations will result in new strains and previously unknown infectious agents. These will be revealed in increasing numbers and more rapidly by advancing diagnostic methods. Keeping up with the development of new threats to food safety and newly recognized insect-transmitted zoonoses will be a challenge that will leave the health communities one step behind nature regardless of how fast technology advances. The diagnostic and public health communities will continually be appealing for additional funding.

Bioterrorism and Agroterrorism

Economic and cultural differences and terrorist groups obsessed by jealousy and hatred of other cultures or religions will undoubtedly continue cowardly sneak attacks on innocent civilians in an effort to deliver vaguely defined messages. They will include both biological warfare against the livestock populations of developed countries and zoonotic agents against human populations. Preventive counter-terrorism measures are essential to avoid Monday morning quarterbacking and unjust criticism of the leaders of attacked countries. Livestock populations are vulnerable to bioterrorism (Ashford et al. 2000) and veterinarians and livestock producers will play a key role in its prevention and recognition. The measures necessary to prevent terrorist acts involving zoonotic agents and attacks on livestock will without doubt cause inconvenience, encroach on civil liberties, and limit traditional freedom of access to farms and government facilities. These changes will be resisted by some interest groups.

Preventive activities will be costly but imperfect. They will impact the entire food chain and will require increased border security, immigration checks, and disease surveillance activities. There will be increased security and controls over research facilities, vaccine and drug-manufacturing operations, and stringent security measures at farms, ranches, feedlots and food-processing plants.

Social and Environmental Expectations

In spite of intensive efforts to reconnect the public and agriculture, vocal critics of the consumption of animal products and of the discharging of animal wastes into the environment will continue to block production practices that offer hope of relieving global starvation. The affected industries can respond with cost-effective improvements but will strenuously object to regulations that have the potential to bankrupt them. LHP-makers must attempt to successfully adjudicate these differences with tactful, scientifically sound recommendations.

Obligations and Challenges of National Leadership

LHP-makers will be among the few in leadership roles who see the big picture, have the capacity to evaluate risks and make science-based decisions that serve the interests of the general population rather than serving the interests of the multiple special-interest groups involved in animal health and food safety. Upcoming decades will bring unimaginable challenges and new responsibilities to the livestock industry and the agencies that regulate it.

Livestock Health: A Springboard to World Peace

It can be convincingly argued that starvation is one of the many causes of wars and terrorism. Starvation is not easily overcome. To say "drop food instead of bombs" is a gross oversimplification. Nonetheless, a fat and fully fed society is likely to seek diversions other than slaughtering the groups deemed responsible for their plight.

Delivery systems must be devised that can distribute inexpensive food to all countries and cultures of the world. Delivering food and getting people, however hungry, to eat the food, are different tasks. Cultural barriers to consumption of readily available foodstuffs are not easy to overcome but it can be done.

International Egalitarianism and Resource Sharing

International egalitarianism, the belief that all people are created equal and deserve similar opportunities for survival and happiness, is a goal toward which LHP-makers can strive.

Some of the world's peoples have their opportunities squelched by economic deprivation and suppression by governmental styles that diminish ambition and initiative. The global movement toward transparent, participatory governments that permit election of leaders willing to address the people's needs for food, clothing, and shelter is spreading slowly but surely. Many people will die of starvation, genocide, and terrorist acts spawned by starvation and oppression before egalitarianism prevails. Advancing livestock production technology, underpinned by solid livestock operations providing meat, poultry, milk, and cheese in supplies adequate to feed all the world's people, is one approach to turning the tide of starvation and hatred. It can introduce global resource sharing and eventually yield world peace and tolerance.

Public Perceptions and Scientific Uncertainty

As technology advances, the public will increasingly distrust the scientific and regulatory communities in some societies. Interest groups will emerge that criticize governments for excessive spending and intervention in private affairs. They will simultaneously chastise them for dealing inadequately with their favored causes. These clashing expectations present a challenge for policy makers. They must deal with consumers who repudiate reasonable scientific evidence in favor of demands that hypothetical risks be proven not to exist, rather than accepting lack of evidence that they do exist. They seek negative proofs, which is comparable to saying there is no needle in the haystack. This skepticism prevails instead of an acceptance that there is no evidence of risk.

This **precautionary principle** philosophy fails to recognize the concept of scientific uncertainty and demands that products be banned unless there is indisputable proof that they are risk-free. Supporters of this approach frequently object to the experimentation needed to properly render evaluations. Societies dominated by supporters of the precautionary principle present challenges to their domestic leadership and are even more challenging to exporting countries who must fulfill one set of regulations at home and another set to meet export requirements.

As technology advances, new and more sensitive detection methods for residues or contaminants are evolving. Adherence by some societies to a zero-risk mentality seems incongruent in a world where there are so many starving people. The zero-risk mentality opposes science-based risk assessments and instead favors precautionary principles and labeling to identify each product's country of origin, food safety, environmental, and animal welfare details.

Summary

The future will bring ever-increasing challenges in LHP-making and will require creative and thoughtful leadership and broad understanding. The future holds widespread potential for both conflict and positive action. The national controversies over work ethics, incentives for productivity, government intervention, confidence in government programs, precautionary principles, and protection of the interests of all peoples can be overcome. This will require positive actions toward egalitarianism and the establishment of national and international harmony and trust based on a worldwide effort to overcome global starvation by nations capable of producing food in excess of global requirements and by overcoming the multiple obstacles to its distribution.

Bibliography

Ashford, D. A., T. M. Gomez, D. L. Noah et al. 2000. Biological Terrorism and Veterinary Medicine in the United States. *Jour Am Vet Med Assoc.* 217:664-667.

Chapter 9

Who Will Be the Leaders?

Introduction

There is a shortage of effective leaders in **livestock health policy (LHP)**. Opportunities exist for interested people with a wide variety of backgrounds, training, and experience. A person with leadership potential should have a positive attitude, certain personality traits, and special skills. These rarely come naturally. They must be learned and cultivated. Regardless of life stage, intensive self-study is essential to identify and hone the skills that can increase leadership potential and effectiveness.

The character traits of good leaders include knowledge, experience, wisdom, realistic optimism, dedication, persistence, drive, accountability, a sense of closure, professional credibility, personal integrity, and interpersonal and communication skills supportive of colleagues and subordinates. Each is a valuable asset in policy-making leadership. Successful leaders may not have all these qualities, but they need a generous mixture of them. Those who seek to make a difference should exert leadership and this can be done by working on the skills identified in this chapter.

Background of Leaders in Livestock Health

People who rise to leadership positions and policy-making roles in livestock health have varied backgrounds, education, training, and life experiences. A background in farming, ranching, or other business dealing in livestock production, processing, or distribution provides a logical pathway to involvement in LHP leadership. Education in colleges of agriculture or veterinary medicine provides a direct entree. However, leaders in LHP can have training in economics, biology, food science, food processing, business administration, international studies, transportation, law, and other seemingly unrelated fields.

People of various backgrounds who follow career paths in government, academics, business, or industry become involved with livestock-oriented organizations, institutions, or corporations. Eventually they address the challenges of LHPs. Whether they are effective and eventually attain leadership roles depends on their ambitions, goals, skills, abilities, knowledge, and experience, and on the success of their interactions with others.

Leadership Skills and Abilities

During the 1950s, society appeared to be mired in a leadership crisis characterized by mediocrity, irresponsibility, and a lack of clear standards for assessing successful leaders (Burns 1978). The rapid technological advances that introduced the new millennium have dramatized the need for leaders who can develop and maintain enthusiasm and maximize the potential of the people around them (Manz and Sims 2001).

In most organizations, their colleagues and superiors recognize those demonstrating leadership qualities and a talent for energizing others. They gradually move upward. Leaders possess qualities that emerge from their work in organizations, grow with effective networking, and result in speaking invitations and nominations for offices. Some people with unhealthy personal ambition also achieve leadership roles, but their insincerity and pursuit of self-gratification are soon evident.

Some people initially lack interest in leadership roles. They feel that family priorities, hobbies, and other activities are more important. However, priorities shift over the years. When leadership inadequacies in their organizations become evident many people eventually realize that if promoted they could outperform present supervisors, increase their income, and improve their job satisfaction.

Some realize they must begin thinking, listening, talking, and dressing like leaders in order to be considered for leadership roles. Those who vigorously push their own careers may rise to leadership positions. However, if they lack most of the essentials described below their shortcomings will soon be recognized and will halt their progress and effectiveness.

Walters (1987) describes true leadership as supportive but not dictatorial; working with people and not over them; regarding people as more important than things; requiring continual efforts to learn; applying sensitivity; and differing significantly from position or title. His book, *The Art of Leadership* (Walters 1987), indicates that individuals who fail in leadership roles emphasize the contrasting side of the above definition, glory in their own positions, and lose the support of their team members. By contrast, true leaders:

- Work to temper their arrogance
- Focus on the job without seeking praise or self-aggrandizement
- Have a serious sense of responsibility
- Are willing to accept responsibility, though sometimes undeserved, for failures
- Put their personal wishes last, not first
- Ask for what is needed, not what they would like
- Sacrifice their own feelings to those of subordinates
- Remain impersonally attuned to the flow of events
- Possess humility
- Are loyal to staff
- Possess intuition but exercise it cautiously

This idealistic view of leadership qualities is borne out over time. History records that the efforts of organizations reflect the attitudes of their leadership. The essential skills for LHP-making and leadership are similar to those needed for success in business, industry, government, or academia.

Knowledge

No one can know everything about livestock health but a broad knowledge of the area is essential. It can be acquired through study or by experience with animals or poultry. Education or training in the fields of livestock husbandry, animal nutrition, livestock management, animal reproduction, agricultural economics, or veterinary medicine enhances one's ability to function effectively in livestock health matters. This training is helpful but not absolutely essential.

Experience

Experience is a great source of confidence and knowledge. Those with practical experience can be effective teachers, speakers, and leaders. People who have studied animal science and worked with farm animals have considerable advantages in LHP-making. Veterinarians with a few years of food-animal or poultry practice are valuable additions to policy-making teams.

Wisdom

Knowledge, skills, experience, and even brilliance are sometimes inadequate to confer the discretion and common sense that comprise wisdom. Wisdom is that immeasurable power acquired over the years that permits some people to instinctively discern what needs to be done and to act accordingly. Wisdom implies appropriate application of knowledge, an understanding of when to talk and when to listen, a sense of when to proceed and when to wait, and sensitivity to the concerns of others. An essential component of wisdom involves resisting the temptation to partake in corruption or graft. Wisdom has more to do with understanding human nature and the operational aspects of real issues than with intellectual capacity. In fact, intelligent people often make dumb mistakes.

Freeman and DeWolf (1992) propose techniques to avoid pitfalls that trap intelligent people. These include tendencies to overreact and get worked up over relatively insignificant matters, to assume they know what people are thinking and that others can read their minds, and to take things too personally. They tend to be overconfident, overly sensitive to criticism, stifled by perfectionist tendencies, over competitive, overcautious, and reluctant to take risks. Intelligent people tend to be burdened by guilt, and to be nitpickers who say "yes-but" more frequently than simply "yes."

These tendencies are not the sole dominion of smart people. They are uniformly present and are obstacles to understanding. They can be overcome by carefully focused self-discipline. Wisdom to function effectively in LHP issues is best acquired through years of involvement.

An important component of wisdom involves capitalizing on experience gained over the years. Old sages have wisdom but must overcome losses accompanying the aging process. Feeling old comes from slowing down physically and mentally, and most dangerously, relaxing intellectually.

Wisdom acquired over time is useful if accompanied by physical conditioning, regular exercise, and mental conditioning that permits one to capitalize on life's experience and knowledge. LHP needs the valuable contributions of those with applicable work experience and wisdom. The wisdom of LHP-makers can be expanded if they:

- Try to learn something new every day
- Believe in themselves and are assured that they can make a difference
- Attend courses and continually learn
- Reduce stress by ignoring matters that are out of their control
- Write about their opinions and experiences

Personal improvement can be achieved proactively and positively by identifying habits and mannerisms that increase interpersonal skills. In his book *The Seven Habits of Highly Effective People*, Covey (1989) describes principles for persons who wish to take charge of their lives with a positive attitude. He recommends

- Being proactive by beginning each undertaking with a goal in mind
- Putting first things first
- Developing interdependence with people you trust by treating human relationships as bank accounts that require more deposits than withdrawals

- Using a win-win thought mode
- Striving first to understand and then to be understood
- Practicing cooperative synergism
- Practicing balanced and creative self-renewal

Numerous self-study programs can reap life-changing benefits if pursued with conscious, continuous effort.

Realistic Optimism

Realistically optimistic individuals have positive attitudes about what must be done to achieve goals. They know this often involves hard work and organizational sacrifice. The naive optimist is unaware of the realities that need to be overcome and assumes good things will just happen. Effective leaders need realistic optimism balanced with an understanding of the effort, time, and compromises required to accomplish worthy, clearly defined, and prioritized goals.

Dedication

Those seeking LHP leadership roles must continually demonstrate dedication to some aspect of animal health. This dedication must be evident in thoughts, words, and deeds. It requires a sense of commitment that is evident to coworkers, colleagues, subordinates, supervisors, and competitors. Dedication is evidenced by positive attitudes and contributions. Its recognition by colleagues surfaces when truly dedicated individuals are selected to receive increasingly challenging assignments and are chosen to represent their organizations in sensitive situations.

Dedication is often missing among employees of governments and academic institutions. Though bureaucratic structure is needed to achieve noble goals, bureaucracies can be impersonal and rigid. In such environments, individuals can be swallowed up in organizational machinery and power struggles and become alienated from their work. They can be inundated with paperwork that is designed to enhance communication and efficiency but ends up blocking and distorting these objectives. Complex bureaucracies can lose sight of their organizational goals in the rush to perfect methodologies. The result is that the method becomes more important than the accomplishment of the goal (Burns 1978).

When dedication is missing, career government and academic personnel can gradually fall into an anti-establishment demeanor characterized by negative attitudes toward their employing institutions and their people. This gradually becomes evident in speech and actions. In its advanced form, the professional entrapment syndrome is detrimental not only to the organization but to the careers and personal lives of victims. Without fully realizing it, entrapped employees feel put upon by the system and its management. Often unconsciously, they grumble and become increasingly critical of supervisors. After years on the job, without ever demonstrating leadership abilities, interest, or thought they gradually conclude, correctly or not, that they are more qualified than their supervisors, particularly those with less tenure in the organization. This can lead to further bitterness.

Victims of the professional entrapment syndrome feed on each other's gripes. Their discontent can be contagious. Eventually victims become counterproductive, unmarketable, and are gradually excluded from challenging assignments or opportunities. They can't represent their companies, nations, or agencies publicly because they unconsciously express contempt for organizational policies. They are often considered loose cannons. Such individuals usually cannot be fired due to tenure guidelines, seniority policies, or fear of costly and demeaning anti-discrimination actions. They are often promoted sideways into irrelevant positions with limited responsibility. This unhappy scenario plays out in lieu of enthusiastic participation, creative activities, cooperative attitudes, and commitment to the mission.

Avoiding the professional entrapment syndrome does not require unthinking agreement with every utterance of superiors. It allows for diplomatically expressed disagreements accompanied by positive alternatives and backing off when the decision is to go another way. Many victims are unaware that the professional entrapment syndrome exists. They slip into it gradually and are unaware that demeaning the organization and boss-bashing in lunchrooms, rest rooms, and hallways is a disease. The best prevention is to recognize it, walk away, and be very cautious about associating with afflicted individuals because it tends to spread to unsuspecting colleagues.

Leaders in organizations with professional entrapment syndrome must accept partial responsibility for the situation. This pattern arises where leaders lack true dedication to organizational goals and vigorously pursue their personal ambitions. It rarely develops in supportive environments where organizational goals are clearly articulated and employees are encouraged, thanked for their contributions, and listened to.

Reversal of entrenched entrapment syndromes requires changes in the attitude and *modus operandi* of existing leadership or the gradual introduction of new leaders who work to subtly change the organizational culture. This is a long-term task of monumental proportions. It requires thoughtful listening, careful analysis, and cautious decision making.

Leaders attempting to alter organizational cultures must avoid being judgmental and use caution in accepting the views of outspoken individuals attempting to influence actions in ways beneficial to their personal agendas. They must carefully seek to learn both sides of every story and sort out the power struggles involved. The cure requires rare leadership ability. In some cultures it is challenging to remain dedicated and even more challenging to establish a sense of dedication to organizational goals among individuals who are convinced the organization has mistreated them or failed to recognize their contributions. Bridging entrenched cultural gaps between employees and management requires time-consuming efforts and sensitive diplomacy to establish mutual trust and broad-based cooperation.

With persistence and patience, leaders who are liked and trusted by their colleagues can turn these situations around and ultimately, perhaps years later, be recognized for their accomplishments.

Persistence

Effective and potential leaders who are truly dedicated tenaciously and diplomatically pursue worthy goals of their organizations and their countries. They persist in courses of action despite discouragement, opposition, and temporary failures. Persistence must be accompanied by flexibility, with a willingness to shift direction when the need becomes evident or circumstances warrant.

Drive

Successful leaders have a strong desire for accomplishment of program goals. This drive overcomes aspirations for personal gain. They work hard to develop their interpersonal skills and encourage employees to regard organizational objectives as their personal accomplishments. They go the extra mile to make essential programs work. This requires immense drive, a careful sense of priorities, and a willingness to be accountable for organizational shortfalls.

Accountability

A big part of gaining trust is accepting responsibility for tasks, sharing the responsibilities of successes, and personally accepting blame for failures. A prompt apology for a failed effort or bungled enterprise is respected far more than evasive denials, multiple excuses, or efforts to divert responsibility to others.

Accountability involves actions, attitudes, and words. Truly accountable leaders acknowledge when they don't know an answer and readily admit when they have been wrong or when changing situations require a shift of previously endorsed positions. Accountable leaders neither say nor do anything they wouldn't want to read about in the next day's newspaper. They advise their employees to do the same.

Closure

Closure is a vital characteristic of effective leaders. It is the ability to complete tasks and assignments in a reasonable timeframe and close the door on them even if they are not perfect. This ability does not come easily to smart, thorough, or perfectionist people.

Closure can be achieved by assigning a reasonable amount of time to each task or decision and wrapping it up on deadline. If the outcome falls short of expectations, or the decision later proves incorrect, so be it. Accept the responsibly and move on.

One component of closure is delegation of authority and responsibility to others, expecting them to meet deadlines, and accepting their results even if you know you could have done better yourself. Remember you didn't have time.

Lack of closure can cause frustration and loss of self-esteem. Closure can be assured by analyzing the reasons for the problem such as inefficient use of time, excessive distractions, unreasonable expectations for perfection, or inability to prioritize tasks. All are correctable. Lack of closure is a common symptom of writer's block and can be an obstacle to leadership ambitions.

Essential Communication Abilities and Skills

Many of the skills essential to successful leadership involve communication. In this changing world, communication is the key to survival (Kroeger and Thuesen 1992). Disciplined thinking and clear communication of thoughts, both keys to successful leadership, require attentive listening, clear speaking, effective writing, and a variety of interpersonal skills. These abilities rarely come naturally.

Concentration and practice are required to overcome pre-existing habits and prejudices. With hard work shy people can become excellent speakers, most people can become excellent writers, and people who are always interrupting can become good listeners. When these skills are practiced faithfully they eventually become second nature but they must be practiced constantly and consciously to become permanent personal assets. If developed and then neglected, essential skills, such as good listening, slip away in favor of old ingrained habits.

Listening Skills

Listening skills may be the most important characteristic of effective people. Good listening does not come naturally (Brusaw et al. 1993). Thoughtful listening requires concerted effort to overcome poor habits that develop over the years. Listening during private conversations requires concentration and avoiding the temptation to interrupt.

One key to good listening involves saving questions until after speakers finish making their points. Questions seeking elaboration are usually received more favorably than arguments. Brusaw et al. (1993) and Toropav (1997) present guidelines for good listening:

- Try conscientiously to listen carefully without letting your mind wander
- When your mind is ahead of a conversation or speech, review what you have heard, try to list the points already made and anticipate the conclusion

- Work hard to avoid being distracted by the speaker's mannerisms, personality, or dress
- Do some advanced homework so you have some background on the topic of upcoming appointments, discussions, and meetings
- When listening, make eye contact and signal attention by nodding
- Before responding, rephrase the speaker's points in your own words, seek verification, and immediately yield the floor
- Ask open-ended questions such as "what do you think?" or "how would stakeholders respond to this?"
- Ask for clarification before assuming statements are incorrect
- In tense situations avoid asking questions, because they often are perceived as attacks. Instead, rephrase proposed questions as presumptions. Instead of saying "Who created this mess?" try saying "Let's all pull together to straighten this out"
- When asked a question, rephrase it before answering
- Take notes; this encourages speakers or others in a conversation and improves your attention

Respectful listening is a valuable leadership skill and one of the most difficult to master. It requires constant effort and patience but pays high dividends in effectiveness.

Speaking Skills

Most people are instinctively fearful of speaking. Polls indicate that people fear public speaking more than they fear dying (Wilder 1999).

Speaking is a skill that can be easily acquired through practice and participation in programs such as Toastmasters Clubs, which are active in many communities, or the Dale Carnegie Course (Carnegie 1998). These and other speech-training programs provide practice before critical, but supportive, audiences. They reinforce positive steps for improving preparation, organization, and presentation of speeches and for overcoming mannerisms that detract from speaking effectively.

Most libraries have an array of books on public speaking, such as *The Seven Steps to Fearless Speaking* (Wilder 1999). This book guides the reader through a seven-step do-it-yourself program that proposes techniques for improving speaking skills, practicing speeches in daily conversation, and using voice exercises. The book presents procedures for increasing verbal effectiveness including:

- Learning proper pronunciation
- Relaxing and breathing properly
- Getting an immediate audience response by asking questions
- Describing shared experiences

- Providing updates on issues of common interest or seeking audience participation
- Structuring your thoughts with an introduction, body, and conclusion
- Establishing a dialogue by posing questions
- Relating an anecdote
- Observing and commenting on audience reactions or reviewing a brief handout
- Tapping your creativity by seeking new ways to express old ideas and using exciting examples
- Learning to persuade by exploring how things can be done in down-to-earth terms
- Achieving higher objectives for your agency or country by pursuing what should be done and why it matters
- Giving the gift of your convictions

Effective and persuasive speaking, before audiences and in conversation, is a valuable asset for LHP-makers.

The Process of Writing Effectively

Writing skills are valuable skills for leaders. Many opportunities will arise for individuals with a reputation for preparing reports and issue analyses that are brief, clearly written, easily understandable, and flow logically from start to finish. Unfortunately such writing is not common.

Much of the cynicism about government and academia stems from the ponderous language commonly found in regulations, research reports, and textbooks. Many arguments within the scientific community focus on differing definitions of words or descriptions of processes, organisms, or structures. Some of these disagreements arise directly from misunderstandings attributable to awkward writing.

Aspiring leaders must choose between a focused effort to achieve writing excellence and a lifetime of ponderous manuscripts laden with confusing jargon, bureaucratese, and legalese. Many scientists, professionals, government officials, and politicians lack writing skills. Like athletic and artistic excellence and speaking proficiency, writing excellence is achieved through hard work, practice, and determination.

The steps to successful writing are preparation, research, organization, drafting, and revision (Brusaw et al. 1993). These are followed by submission of the manuscript to a publisher and proofreading, the final pre-printing reading and marking of manuscripts for corrections.

In getting ready to write, authors must clarify their objectives and target audiences and decide on the content, emphasis, and appropriate technical level of each document. Long before starting, it helps to make notes of spontaneous thoughts, relevant articles, books, and meetings. Schedule dates for completion of drafts, final revisions, and submission.

Little effective writing occurs in busy offices. Thus, it is essential to establish a writing hideaway, preferably at home, and schedule a daily writing time in very early or very late hours that won't interfere with other obligations.

Organization is crucial. Writing must follow a logical sequence. An outline helps to improve the flow, expedite smooth transitions from topic to topic, and determine where charts, diagrams, and side-bars are to be placed.

Writing begins with organization and a rough draft consisting of an introductory paragraph, details supporting each point in the introduction, and a clear statement of conclusions. Each paragraph needs an introductory sentence, clarifying sentences, and a closing sentence that introduces the next paragraph.

The first draft is always a challenge. Successful writers have favorite approaches. Many get right at it and move quickly with little attention to grammar, spelling, or details. The temptation to polish and revise should be resisted until a first draft is completed. Many experts prepare abstracts or summaries after the draft is finished. Others prefer to draft a summary initially as a guide to content and order. The summary should briefly mention each main point to be covered.

After a work is drafted, writers are urged to read it aloud several times (Brohaugh 1983). Then the following questions should be answered from the reader's perspective:

- Is it easy to understand?
- Does it get to the point?
- Does it stick to the point?
- Is it logically organized?
- Are there unnecessary words?
- Is it complete?
- Is it positive?
- Is it accurate?
- Does it flow smoothly?

After these questions are answered multiple revisions may be required to achieve the desired effect. Both the summary and the entire draft are repeatedly revised to make the work more readable. Careful editing and multiple revisions to improve organization, spelling, grammar, word usage, clarity, succinctness, and check for the use of the active rather than the passive voice will produce clear and effective writing (Williams 1985).

Proofreading, the final reading and marking of manuscripts for corrections, is an art of its own. Often done by professionals, proofreading identifies typographical errors and errors in grammar, spelling, capitalization, punctuation, and word usage. Proofreaders' marks are symbols that identify corrections to be made in manuscripts before final printing.

Elements of Effective Writing

The essentials of good writing are correct spelling, grammar, clarity, organization, and succinctness. These are achieved by repeated revising and editing.

Correct spelling reflects on the author's credibility and ensures the desired interpretation. The spell-checker on the computer is helpful but imperfect. Hastily spell-checked manuscripts often contain obvious errors. Authors must personally check spelling.

Grammar is a system of rules for language usage (Shertzer 1986). The word grammar carries a negative connotation because it is usually taught in terms of what is wrong. Good grammar expedites communication by the selection of appropriate words or phrases and makes for easy reading. Because grammar governs the choice and placement of words and phrases, the search for writing excellence eventually turns to grammar. Most writers keep a grammar book handy.

Punctuation is the appropriate use of standard marks to convey intended meanings to readers in the same fashion that spoken pauses and changes in tone transmit emphasis to listeners in conversation or speeches. When used correctly with short direct sentences, correct punctuation is the key to clarity (Alward and Alward 1997).

Clarity, one of the most challenging aspects of good writing, requires clearly stated points tied together logically, and it is best achieved by carefully planning the ideas and connecting them with smooth transitions.

Major obstacles to clarity include ambiguity, clichés, wordiness, gobbledygook, jargon, pretentious words, and vagueness (Steinmann and Keller 1999). Excessive use of the passive voice also defeats clarity. Clarity is best achieved by putting carefully selected simple words in the best possible order to emphasize points without being pretentious. Words should be chosen to express thoughts, not to impress readers.

Increased effectiveness, personal satisfaction, and a reputation for professional competence will reward LHP-makers who aggressively seek to improve their writing. This usually leads to challenging assignments. In the academic world, faculty members need a record of successful professional publication to receive tenure.

Interpersonal Skills

Interpersonal skills are a major factor in leadership ability and a principal criterion for choosing leaders. If people like you they are likely to cooperate with you. If they hate or distrust you your effectiveness and tenure as a successful leader is limited.

Successful leadership attributes are evident upon meeting someone with modest self-confidence, a cheerful greeting, a smile, and a firm non-aggressive handshake. Potential leaders are usually upbeat, have positive attitudes, show consideration for the rights and concerns of others, habitually ask people about themselves, listen attentively without interrupting, and provide encouragement rather than criticism. Successful leadership also requires an understanding of your own personality style and that of the people you deal with (Kroeger and Thuesen 1992).

Appearance is often regarded as a superficial attribute, but it is one determinant of leadership effectiveness. Experts say if you want to lead you must look and act the part. An appearance of being bright, alert, and intelligent, walking with a positive brisk carriage and good posture, and dressing in a professional manner adds to the image of leadership. It builds self-confidence and the esteem of those who seek your guidance.

On the contrary, sloppily dressed individuals and those inconsiderate of established styles in their cultures have a leadership disadvantage because their dress suggests a lack of self-confidence and disregard for tradition. A trim physical appearance suggests stamina and the capacity to address numerous challenges. Though not necessarily true, many people feel that obesity suggests poor self-discipline, physical shortfalls, slow movement, and a potential for inaction.

The principles in *How to Win Friends and Influence People,* written by Dale Carnegie in 1937, remain a gold standard for the development of interpersonal skills (Carnegie 1998). Although they require some modification as technology and society have evolved, Carnegie's ground rules for success have held up through years of social and technologic turmoil. His fundamental techniques for handling people are

- When considering changing or improving someone, start with yourself
- Avoid criticism
- Speak ill of no one
- Tell all the good you know about everyone
- Endeavor to understand people

Many people correctly insist that effective leadership is not a popularity contest. Nonetheless, leaders have more opportunities for success if their subordinates, peers, and superiors like them than if they dislike or detest them. In fact, leaders who have antagonized their associates have one strike against their success. Carnegie's six big secrets for getting people to like you have relevance in LHP-making:

- Become genuinely interested in people
- Smile
- Remember, a person's name is the sweetest and most important sound in any language
- Be a good listener

- Encourage others to talk about themselves
- Talk in terms of the interests of others
- Make others feel important, and do it sincerely

Carnegie's strategies for effective leadership, for winning people to your way of thinking, and for changing people without giving offense or arousing resentment include:

- The only way to get the best of an argument is to avoid it
- Show respect for the opinions of others, and never tell anyone they are wrong
- When wrong, admit it quickly and emphatically
- Begin in a friendly way
- Get others saying "yes, yes" immediately
- Let others do a great deal of the talking
- Let others feel it was their idea
- Try honestly to see things from the other person's point of view
- Be sympathetic to the ideas and desires of others
- Appeal to nobler motives
- Dramatize your ideas
- Throw down a challenge
- Begin with praise and honest appreciation
- Call attention to the mistakes of others only indirectly
- Talk about your own mistakes before criticizing other people
- Ask questions instead of giving direct orders
- Let others save face
- Praise the slightest improvement and praise every improvement. Be hearty in your approbation and lavish in your praise
- Give others a fine reputation to live up to
- Use encouragement
- Make faults easy to correct
- Make the others happy about doing the things you suggest

These pointers are all applicable to the discussion and negotiation of LHP issues. They have particular relevance to those seeking leadership roles. Despite its age, Dale Carnegie's book (Carnegie 1998) should be required reading for anyone aspiring to leadership in animal agriculture, trade policy, or human health. The classic work of Norman Vincent Peale, *The Power of Positive Thinking* (Peale 1996), has also stood the test of time.

Recent theory calls for personality-type recognition (Kroeger and Thuesen 1992). Knowing your personality type, or brain type, and the personality types of colleagues can provide a foundation for solid interpersonal relationships and successful interactions. Understanding your personality type and preferred way of doing things and relating to people is key to the success of personal and professional relationships.

The Meyers-Briggs Type Instrument (MBTI) is a test designed to determine individual style preferences (Kroeger and Thuesen 1992). It asks questions about choices and uses the answers to identify the relative strengths of people on the basis of four pairs of contrasting preferences. Groups who take the MBTI test in team-building exercises can gain valuable insights about workplace dynamics. If applied conscientiously, this knowledge can help attain organizational goals.

Torapov (1997) describes personality types in terms of four mind-sets, namely: the lone ranger, the sharpshooter, the professor, and the cheerleader. The ability of workers to recognize and understand the mind-sets and personality types of others is a valuable organizational asset.

Professional Credibility and Personal Integrity

Professional credibility implies knowledge and expertise in a chosen area and the ability to discuss technical issues in a believable manner. It is characterized by a reputation for professional knowledge and scientific clarity adequate to engender the trust of colleagues and adversaries. Professional credibility demands adherence to current knowledge even if it fails to support a personal cause; ready admission when the facts are unclear or unknown; and a willingness to defer to someone more experienced or qualified. The trust engendered by a reputation for professional credibility is a valuable asset of leaders and negotiators.

Personal integrity is essential for leaders. It implies that a person can be trusted to consistently tell the truth, to maintain confidentiality when appropriate, and to be a dead-end host for gossip and unfounded speculation.

In the long run, professional credibility and personal integrity are among the most cherished and most fragile of leadership skills. Leaders possessing both attributes can be counted upon to avoid talking when they should be listening; to mean what they say and say diplomatically what they mean; and to admit when they are wrong or responsible for unfortunate incidents. Rather than covering up, they adhere to the adage that one prompt apology is worth a hundred denials. They strongly subscribe to the rule of thumb that if you lie now you will pay later in triplicate. Establishment of trust is the first step in setting the stage for effective leadership.

Running Effective Meetings

Well-run meetings can be effective, enjoyable, and a productive use of time. Studies indicate that about half of the time spent at meetings is wasted. There are strategies for increasing the productivity of meetings. The chairperson is the key to seeing that meetings:

- Start on time to avoid penalizing those arriving promptly
- End on time

- Are kept short and last less than one hour
- Have a pre-circulated agenda with strict preprinted times for reports and discussions
- Are accompanied by pre-circulated essential information and report summaries
- Are attended by no more than five to eight people. If numbers exceed this limit consider two meetings of essential people
- Are run so as to encourage diplomatic disagreement
- Are verbally summarized at the end
- Are promptly reported in writing

Meetings should be announced well in advance with a call for agenda topics. They should have a clear purpose. Attendees should leave the meeting with clear assignments for action within assigned time intervals.

Who Will Be the Leaders?

The future leaders in global LHP will come from a wide variety of backgrounds. The effectiveness and professional credibility of each country's LHPs in the national and international community will depend upon its leadership.

The leadership characteristics outlined above can be acquired and cultivated through reading, training programs, and continual practice. Their regular application will further the goals of organizations and nations and increase the probability of the survival of national livestock industries in the expanding global free-market economy.

Individuals who actively seek to expand their leadership skills will increasingly represent their organizations, agencies, or nations in challenging situations and will receive constant inquiries about sensitive assignments and new job opportunities.

Bibliography

Alward, E. C. and J. A. Alward.1997. *Punctuation: Plain and Simple.* New York: Barnes and Noble.

Brohaugh, W. 1993. *Write Tight: How to Keep Your Prose Sharp, Focused and Concise*. Cincinnati, OH: Writers Digest Books.

Brusaw, C. I., G. J. Alred and W. E. Olin. 1993. *Handbook of Technical Writing*. 4th ed. New York: St. Martins Press.

Burns, J. M. 1978. *Leadership*. New York: Harper and Row Publishers, Inc.

Carnegie, D. 1998. *Dale Carnegie's Lifetime Plan for Success: How to Win Friends and Influence People* and *How to Stop Worrying and Start Living.* New York: Galahad Books.

Covey, S. R. 1989. *The Seven Habits of Highly Effective People*. New York: Fireside Books, Simon and Schuster.

Freeman, A. and R. DeWolf. 1992. *The Ten Dumbest Mistakes Smart People Make and How to Avoid Them*. New York: Harper Collins Publishers, Inc.

Kroeger, O. and J. M. Thuesen. 1992. *Type Talk at Work*. New York: Bantam Doubleday Dell Publishing.

Manz, C. C. and H. P. Sims. 2001. *The New Super Leadership*. San Francisco: Berret Koehler Publishers, Inc.

Peale, N. V. 1996. *The Power of Positive Thinking*. New York: Fawell Columbine.

Shertzer, M. 1986. *The Elements of Grammar: The Essential Guide to Refining and Improving Grammar*. New York: Barnes and Noble.

Steinmann, M. and M. Keller. 1999. *Good Grammar Made Easy*. New York: Gramercy Books, Random House Value Publishing.

Torapov, B. 1997. *The Art and Skill of Dealing with People*. New York: MJF Books.

Walters, J. D. 1987. *The Art of Leadership: A Practical Guide for People in Positions of Responsibility*. New York: MJF Books Fine Communications.

Wilder, L. 1999. *Seven Steps to Fearless Speaking*. New York: John Wiley and Sons Inc.

Williams, J. M. 1985. *Style: Ten Lessons in Clarity and Grace*. 2nd ed. Glenview, IL: Foresman and Company.

Chapter 10

Strategies for Effective LHP Action

INTRODUCTION

Strategies are tactics, plans, methods, and procedures for deploying resources and personnel to achieve goals. Each **livestock health policy (LHP)** strategy has multiple components.

LHPs require carefully crafted building blocks and a firm foundation of public support and scientific knowledge. The building blocks, such as laws and regulations, are constantly shifting and require continuous repositioning to avoid collapse. This chapter examines LHP foundation stones and building blocks, and it lays out strategies for effective action.

As outlined in chapter 6, the goals and objectives of LHPs are to protect the health and welfare of consumers, to improve the health of livestock, to advance the prosperity of livestock producers and associated industries, and to maintain and expand domestic and foreign markets. Achieving these goals involves a seven-stage process that traverses a five-tiered hierarchy. Success depends on consensus, trust, and cooperation among individuals in each tier of the hierarchy at each stage in the process.

LHPs that address these goals include laws, regulations, and guidelines for controlling specific diseases of livestock, enhancing food safety, excluding **exotic diseases**, addressing new and emerging diseases, and establishing transparent and equitable import and export measures.

Strategies for national policy makers boil down to:

- Establishing clear goals and objectives
- Selecting program-evaluation criteria
- Developing stakeholder involvement
- Gaining public support
- Involving academic and diagnostic communities
- Building communication networks
- Developing action-oriented skilled leadership
- Building **livestock health infrastructures**
- Creating mechanisms to enhance international credibility and understanding
- Employing transparent policy-development processes

Some secrets to success include working in the abstract, anticipating unforeseen challenges, incorporating flexibility, using analogies to improve clarity, and constantly reviewing policies by stakeholders and interest groups so results are workable for affected industries.

Foundation Stones of LHPs

LHPs do not appear spontaneously. Neither do they fall smoothly into place like poured concrete walls. Instead, they are fabricated like an endless mortarless stone wall by an ever-changing team of workers whose expertise varies and who sometimes pursue separate agendas. Like walls, LHPs require a solid foundation and carefully placed building blocks.

Previous chapters outlined the foundation and building blocks of effective LHPs. The foundation stones consist of public trust and support, knowledge of the livestock health dynamics of the past century, and an appreciation of the critical events of the last three decades. Successful LHPs must be built on this foundation.

The building blocks are biotechnology, communication technology, livestock health infrastructures, national animal disease-control programs, the **World Trade Organization (WTO) Sanitary and Phytosanitary (SPS) Agreement**, and international standards established by the **Office International des Epzooties (OIE).** These blocks must be carefully set upon their foundation stones.

Foundation Stone Number One: Public Support

The most difficult challenge facing LHP-makers is gaining broad-based public support and trust. Thoughtful concerns revolve around the controversial issues of livestock rearing, slaughter practices, and food safety. It is essential that the people of each country and the leaders of the global community trust the policy makers, particularly those at the national level. This trust must be continually cultivated and evident in words and deeds.

Foundation Stone Number Two: Understanding the Past Century

LHP-makers who know about twentieth century progress can capitalize on its lessons and predict future needs. In the face of population explosions and political, economic, and technological change, the twentieth century yielded livestock health progress (see chapter 2). These advances include improvements in animal reproduction, feeding, and management practices, advances in diagnosis and control of infectious diseases, modernization of processing procedures, and improvements in the transportation of perishable products. The implementation of these advances calls for new disease-control programs; innovative food-safety initiatives; and assurances that animal feeds, pharmaceuticals, and **biologicals** are safe, effective, and not hazardous to human health. This implementation must involve thoughtful strategies at each step in the LHP hierarchy.

Foundation Stone Number Three: Appreciation of Critical Events of the Last Three Decades

The last three decades of the 1900s brought changes that permanently altered LHPs and demanded new strategies. The framers and managers of LHPs in the new millennium must understand these events and respond to them. These changes expanded the venue of livestock health beyond the interests of farmers, ranchers, and processors to capture the attention of consumers, the general public, and global leaders.

These critical events are addressed in chapter 3. They include outbreaks of **foot-and-mouth disease (FMD)** and **bovine spongiform encephalopathy (BSE)**, recognition of the **transmissible spongiform encephalopathies (TSEs)**, increased emphasis on emerging diseases, onset of the age of biotechnology, advances in communication technology, the ratification of the WTO SPS Agreement, the establishment of international standards for trade, and the inclusion of **risk analysis** in livestock health issues.

These events coincided with the emergence of newly independent nations, a global movement toward democracy and free-market economies, the formation of multinational trading blocs, and the establishment of international trade agreements. They ushered in the new millennium with a need for new perspectives on LHPs. They added a new dimension to LHPs and complicated trade agreements, health certifications, and international trade in livestock and poultry products.

Collectively, the events that closed the twentieth century opened a new era in LHPs for the next century.

Outbreaks of FMD

FMD has been known for centuries. Extensive and costly outbreaks in the 1980s and 1990s brought new attention to the disease and to the environmental and humane aspects of its control that involved the slaughter and disposal of millions of infected and exposed animals. Outbreaks in Taiwan, Great Britain, the Netherlands, and elsewhere brought extensive criticism to the LHP-makers and caused public misgivings about the methods used by the livestock health community. These concerns revived U.S. fears about potential FMD introductions and caused a reevaluation of FMD policies worldwide (see Discussion Topic 10).

BSE and the TSEs

Appreciation of the risk of TSEs to livestock and human health began in England in 1984 with recognition of BSE, also known as mad cow disease. BSE is a slowly progressive condition manifested by behavioral, postural, and locomotor disorders. Its discovery ushered in a period of disillusionment with agricultural and veterinary officials in Europe. People felt the public health had been neglected in order to protect beef markets by supporting a later disproved thesis that BSE presented no risk to humans. These events reactivated consumer support of the **precautionary principle**, which holds that hypothesized risks to human or animal health can be considered real until there is positive proof that they are not (see Discussion Topic 6).

The controversy surrounding the outbreaks of BSE has resulted in international concern, distrust, politically and economically motivated trade barriers, uncertainty within the veterinary profession, and dissension within the European Community. Despite efforts of the OIE to develop BSE standards for international movement of livestock products and criteria for countries to be recognized as free of BSE, this distrust has not been completely alleviated.

The TSEs were originally called "slow virus" infections due to their long incubation periods and progressive clinical courses. They are now known to be caused by agents called prions, which produce several similar but unrelated diseases.

Human **Creutzfeldt-Jacob disease (CJD)** was known long before BSE. It occurs worldwide. For years it was regarded as a genetic defect. In 1993 a slightly different disease called **variant Creutzfeldt-Jacob disease (VCJD)** was recognized in England. It is a fatal psychiatric locomotor disorder with an earlier age of onset and slightly different symptoms than classic CJD. VCJD is rare. The causative agent is indistinguishable from the **prion** that causes BSE. VCJD probably results from human consumption of meat from cattle with BSE. Milk, milk products, gelatin, and properly rendered tallow are considered safe, but cosmetics, pharmaceuticals, and other products using animal-derived materials or glands are now considered to be potential causes of VCJD.

The other TSEs of animals are **scrapie**, feline spongiform encephalopathy, **chronic wasting disease (CWD)** of deer and elk, and **transmissible mink encephalopathy (TME).**

Scrapie is considered a prototype spongiform encephalopathy. It occurs in sheep and rarely in goats. It has been present in Great Britain for several centuries and was first diagnosed in the United States in 1947. Scrapie was presumably introduced into the United States by Suffolk sheep imported from the United Kingdom. Following an incubation period of one to two years or more, affected sheep develop locomotor incoordination and behavioral changes including rubbing against objects, staggering, tremors, and walking in circles. They experience progressive weight loss and ultimately die. Scrapie is seen mostly in black-faced sheep from two to eight years old. It has received new attention due to the relationship of BSE to VCJD.

CWD of deer and elk is a fatal progressive condition first identified in the United States in 1977. It is characterized by weight loss and emaciation. It has been seen in elk, mule deer, and black-tailed deer in the western United States and Canada. Affected animals drink more than usual and salivate and urinate excessively. They may have blank stares in both eyes and develop life-threatening pneumonia, which is frequently the cause of death. CWD victims have spongiform brain lesions but rarely exhibit behavioral or nervous signs. The causative agent is probably distinct from both scrapie and BSE. Knowledge of CWD and the other TSEs will probably expand with further surveillance and advancing technology.

The TSEs opened a new era in disease diagnosis and control. They cannot be detected by classical methods, are not amenable to standard live-animal testing, do not stimulate classic immune responses, and are resistant to all known therapies and disinfectants. Prions survive conventional sterilization methods including most rendering and incineration procedures. These diseases have created skepticism about the scientific and regulatory communities in Europe.

The Age of Biotechnology

In the closing years of the twentieth century, applied molecular biology and genetic engineering produced new understanding of fundamental life processes and added working technologies to LHPs.

The significance of **deoxyribonucleic acid (DNA)** had been known since the 1950s. The day-to-day use of DNA technology in animal health research and diagnostic laboratories was seriously adopted several decades later. It yielded advances in diagnosis, prevention, and treatment of livestock diseases and methods for manipulating the genetic makeup of plants, animals, and people.

The introduction of DNA technology to animal disease study provided the **polymerase chain reaction (PCR).** Application of the PCR has increased the rapidity and specificity of procedures for isolating and identifying infectious agents, improved the measurement of disease-specific **antibodies** in **serum**, and helped define the components of the immune system.

Molecular technology introduced controversial new techniques for manipulating animal, plant, and human genes and for altering the activities of pathogenic microorganisms. With these techniques came new hopes for overcoming livestock diseases, human pestilence, and global starvation.

The new technology increased the speed, accuracy, and specificity of isolating and identifying infectious agents. Prior to the age of molecular biology, infectious agents were extracted from samples collected from live animals or post-mortem specimens by cultivation in selective media. These were determined by previous trial-and-error exercises to support the growth of pathogenic agents. Nutrient broths or gelatin-like agars were used to grow out bacteria, which could then be identified microscopically using various staining techniques.

Viruses, however, multiply only in living animals or cells. They require painstaking cultivation in laboratory hosts before they induce recognizable changes in the host. Their specific identity can be determined by neutralizing the changes with hyperimmune sera.

The new technology permits identification of DNAs specific for each microorganism. DNA technology offered improvements in the detection and measurement of antibodies. Antibody detection permits retrospective disease diagnosis and helps estimate the prevalence and geographic distribution of infectious agents. Molecular technology has defined the components of the immune system, permitting improved diagnostic and preventative measures.

The production of **genetically modified organisms (GMOs)** can result from cloning of animals, insertion and deletion of genes from organisms or animals, transplantation of genes from one species to another, and the introduction of stem-cell technology. These advances raise thoughtful, and often divisive, moral, ethical, and ecological questions (Holdredge and Talbot 2001) and give rise to controversies that cannot be ignored.

Cloning is the production of multiple identical copies of desirable animals. It has the potential for replicating rare individuals and preserving endangered breeds or species. It can be used to produce cows and goats genetically engineered to produce milk proteins of medicinal value. Cloning has been accomplished with varying degrees of success in sheep and other small ruminants, cattle, and horses.

In its developmental stages, animal cloning was a costly and risky process. It is conducted in research institutions and on a limited commercial basis. Once perfected, it has the potential for developing highly productive disease-resistant herds and flocks capable of making foods of animal origin available to a hungry world.

Cloning of cattle has produced calves with oversized bodies and undersized organs and a variety of neonatal abnormalities. Some cloned calves required expensive veterinary support in intensive care facilities. These complications suggest potential problems in other species, including humans.

Cloning is controversial. It raises moral, ethical, and religious issues. Nonetheless, the possible beneficial effects of this technology will be explored, because future work holds promise and its potential benefits appear worth pursuing.

The cloning process involves harvesting unfertilized eggs from females, removing all nuclear (genetic) materials, and replacing them with the nuclear material from the animal to be duplicated. The resulting fertile eggs are briefly nurtured in the laboratory. They are then implanted in surrogate females who give birth to offspring identical to the selected parent. The application of cloning and other genetic procedures to human reproduction raises controversial moral, ethical, and religious issues. These controversies could spill over into livestock applications.

The decisions facing LHP-makers is whether animal cloning should be regulated and if so how. This decision is likely to differ between countries. It will depend partly on the question of the safety of foods produced by cloned animals (National Academy of Science 2002) and their potential dangers to the environment. Similar discussions will be required to address the issues of the insertion and deletion of genes in animals and microorganisms and the questions surrounding **stem-cell technology**.

Communication Technology

The emergence and application of computer and wireless communication revolutionized LHPs of all nations. By the turn of the century there was instantaneous dissemination of national and international information. The world now has immediate access to information on livestock disease outbreaks, new research findings, newly available diagnostic results, and proposed regulations. Details of these matters, some reliable and some not, are available on web sites sponsored by individuals, organizations, corporations, and government agencies.

Livestock health officials and stakeholders can access information prior to its publication. This permits rapid spread of both accurate information and rumors. Its accentuates the need for credibility in **monitoring, surveillance, and reporting (MS&R)** activities and equitable application of sanitary measures.

Animal identification (ID) technology is expanding globally. Some countries are planning import measures requiring exporting countries to have identification systems capable of tracing any carcass or animal product with bacterial contamination or excessive residues to the farm of origin.

WTO SPS Agreement

The WTO SPS Agreement grants importing countries the right to establish appropriate levels of protection and to impose risk-mitigating measures necessary, but not more than necessary, to achieve them. It indicates that import measures must be science-based, transparent, non-discriminatory, and based on **regionalization** and **risk assessment**. The WTO imposed a new code of ethics on the international livestock health community. This created the need for disease-specific international standards.

International Standards for Trade

The WTO SPS Agreement and the OIE international standards are principal building blocks of LHPs. It is essential that everyone in the field of livestock health understand them. They are discussed in detail in chapter 5.

Emergence of Risk Analysis as a Livestock Health Mechanism

Risk analysis was introduced into LHPs in the 1990s. The WTO SPS Agreement states import measures must be in accord with international standards or based on scientifically sound risk analyses.

The application of risk analysis to biological problems from its origins in engineering is described in chapter 3. Engineering applications of risk analysis involve mathematical calculations of strengths and quantities of construction materials necessary to resist predictable maximum stresses. These concepts were transferred to estimating the risk of acquiring livestock diseases via importations. Application of risk analysis to livestock products is subject to less quantification and greater variation than its engineering uses.

Despite the vagaries of its application to trade, the concept of risk analysis is sound. Using transparent estimates of the likelihood of untoward consequences as a basis for imposing tests or other risk-mitigating measures adds new dimensions to international trade in livestock products. This is a change for countries that previously tried to achieve the unattainable goal of zero risk.

Some risk assessments are no better than intuitive decisions by knowledgeable and experienced officials. They are, however, superior to those developed by inexperienced workers and have the distinct advantage of expecting a documented basis for requirements that exceed international standards.

The risk-assessment process forces countries to define acceptable levels of risk. The expectation for stated acceptable risk represents a step toward equitable and effective global trade measures. Risk assessment is described in detail in chapter 5. It will continue to be used in international trade and will help focus discussions about import requirements and market access.

Building Blocks of LHPs

The most visible and most fragile portion of the LHP structure are the building blocks, rocks of various sizes and shapes needing careful placement and timely repositioning to stand firmly and resist collapse. The building blocks of LHPs have rigid outlines. They must be chipped and shaped to fit specific niches. The skills and agendas of LHP-makers and their willingness to work as a team in laying these blocks will determine the validity and utility of their efforts.

These building blocks are

- Livestock health infrastructures
- Competitive and equitable national LHPs
- International livestock health standards

- Addressing ever-changing challenges
- Understanding the complex forces driving the global free-market economy
- Policy makers who look to the future
- The critical need for competent leadership

These building blocks resemble items previously discussed. The descriptions presented earlier set the stage for strategic action.

Building Block Number One: Livestock Health Infrastructures

Livestock health infrastructures are the basis and cohesive guiding force for livestock health, food-safety, and international marketing programs (see chapter 4). Livestock health programs, usually overseen by national governments, require support from subnational agencies, livestock and veterinary organizations, the academic and diagnostic communities, and individual stakeholders.

Food-safety programs involve the inspection of food-processing facilities and testing of foods for contaminating organisms or residues. They are often administered by the same branches of government that oversee livestock health programs and must be integrated with livestock health activities.

Brokers, food processors, representatives of national and subnational governments, and animal health officials who establish import and export requirements share international marketing activities.

The quality of livestock health infrastructures is basic to sanitary measures imposed on livestock products. To be functional, they must follow strategies that:

- Gain the support of owners and veterinarians who comprise a first line of defense against livestock diseases
- Provide a network of diagnostic laboratories with personnel and facilities capable of determining the exact cause of disease outbreaks
- Maintain national control programs for carefully selected domestic diseases
- Establish a disease MS&R system at farms and ranches and in slaughtering and processing plants
- Maintain national animal ID systems
- Include border security, emergency disease management, information management systems, regulatory oversight of animal drugs and biologicals, and a network of subnational livestock health programs that cooperate in the national endeavor
- Cooperate closely with livestock producers and processors, the academic and diagnostic communities, the nation's veterinary profession, and numerous governmental agencies and sustaining industries

- Establish working partnerships with the media

Livestock health infrastructures establish the credibility of national governments within domestic and international animal health communities. They determine the success of each nation's livestock health and food-safety programs. The strength and integrity of each country's infrastructure are primary criteria for decision making by importers of livestock products.

It is the responsibility of LHP-makers to develop strategies that secure resources and authority that permit the successful implementation of livestock health programs and their management by knowledgeable professionals with communication skills and leadership abilities. Periodic external reviews of national livestock health infrastructures are highly recommended.

Building Block Number Two: Competitive and Equitable National LHPs

Policy makers of all nations must address the establishment of competitive and equitable LHPs for the twenty-first century. State, national, regional, and international governing bodies play a role in these activities.

LHP development processes can be masterpieces of intergovernmental cooperation. However the process is sometimes flawed by divisiveness and tensions as stakeholders and special interest groups struggle to advance their own agendas. In dealing with LHPs, it is sometimes difficult to sort out the scope and authority of supporting legislation, regulations, and guidelines. The policy development and oversight roles of executive and legislative branches of national governments are sometimes difficult to separate from those of local, state, and national government agencies.

Satisfactory outcomes of LHP-development processes can emerge after extensive positioning by groups with conflicting interests and eventually produce compromise and cooperation. The LHP-building process appears to be increasing in complexity due to advances in livestock health, demographic and economic changes, and ever-increasing global demands.

LHPs should be equitable. They should be capable of being applied in an impartial manner to domestic industries, consumers, and international interests. Equitable application also implies recognition of differences between situations and countries. For example, regulations imposed upon countries affected with FMD can be equitable but different from those applied to FMD-free nations. The distinction is that equitable application applies to situations where similar conditions prevail. Efforts to maintain equitable conditions in policy-making are challenging when country differences are subtle.

The strategies for building competitive and equitable LHPs will vary among nations. All will require the input of multiple stakeholders, the cooperation of national, subnational, and local agencies, and extensive informational meetings and consultations with various groups with conflicting agendas.

Strategically, it is ideal if the industry to be regulated recognizes the need for government oversight and initiates voluntary **quality assurance programs** before there are outcries from consumers, environmentalists, animal welfare agencies, or other interested groups. This sometimes occurs.

Industry groups and livestock health organizations like the **U.S. Animal Health Association (USAHA)** are often the first to recognize program needs. They can serve as intermediaries between producers and governments and expedite strategic approaches.

Building Block Number Three: International Livestock Health Standards

Changing global dynamics dictate that LHPs must be consistent with international standards. Knowledge of international standards and of the organizations that promulgate them is essential for maintaining markets in an era of expanding international trade.

Establishing credibility in the international community is more challenging than dealing with domestic stakeholders because of physical separations, language barriers, and political and cultural differences. A constant turnover of personnel within nations makes long-lasting international relationships problematic.

A significant measure of international credibility is the integrity of a country's national MS&R system. Nothing damages a nation's image more than officially claiming freedom from a disease when veterinary textbooks, published articles, product advertisements, or diagnostic laboratory reports indicate the disease exists within its territory. It is important that trade officials lacking a background in animal health be cautioned against ill advised statements about national livestock health status.

Credibility must be a national goal at all levels in the national livestock community. It should be constantly reinvigorated by precept and example and by forceful reminders from top officials who themselves demonstrate a willingness to admit when they don't know something. Officials can openly state that comments must wait until further information is available, as long as they follow up and don't use insufficient information as a dodge.

There is no place for corruption or graft in credible livestock health infrastructures. Temptations for unsavory behaviors are best combated by the appointment of officials with personal and professional integrity. Careful appointment policies can be supplemented with internal communication and supervisory oversight that reinforces the importance of honesty. **Multijurisdictional authority**, where several governmental agencies share oversight of critical areas, helps deter sloppy or dishonest practices.

In maintaining a credible national livestock health infrastructures, areas of particular sensitivity are food safety, residue monitoring, livestock disease control, and the issuing of import permits and export certificates.

Building Block Number Four: Addressing New Challenges

Complex and continually changing challenges face LHP-makers in the twenty-first century. Some are issues of broad public and consumer concern and others address matters directly affecting the livestock industries.

The issues of concern to the general public are food safety, ecosystem preservation, animal well being, potential loss of the cherished small-farm lifestyle, and questions about genetically modified organisms (GMOs) and other products of biotechnology.

Challenges of more direct concern to the livestock industries include overcoming the disease risks associated with confinement livestock rearing through biosecurity measures and managerial improvements, improving animal disease MS&R systems, and upgrading animal ID systems (see chapter 4). LHP-makers will be key players in deterring terrorist activities involving animal diseases or zoonoses.

Livestock health strategies must include provisions for necessary changes in direction in the attitudes of the general public or the livestock industry.

Building Block Number Five: Understanding the Complex Global Free-Market Economy

The emergence of the global free-market economy dictates new strategies for LHP-makers. These strategies must maximize food production and distribution efficiency, minimize human food-borne illness, and reduce restrictions to the movement of animal products from production to consumption points.

These goals can best be accomplished by policies that support internationally competitive livestock industries. This will require checking policies, domestic regulations, and international standards for clarity as well as recognizing the realities of a global free economy. For many countries this will involve an analysis of the missions of national livestock health infrastructures and veterinary programs for compliance with the WTO SPS Agreement, OIE standards, and the principles of contemporary science.

Global relationships can be strengthened by active membership in international organizations and consistency with international standards. To comprehend the forces of free-market economies LHP-makers must

- Examine the strengths and weaknesses of their regulatory culture
- Scrutinize domestic and international regulations for **transparency**

- Review the relationship of national governments to livestock producers and other **stakeholders**
- Upgrade livestock health personnel with regard to intra- and inter-agency communications, interpersonal skills, cultural sensitivities, negotiating capabilities, and knowledge of animal husbandry and livestock health

Understanding the free market and its complex driving forces is a key strategy for the development and implementation of sound LHPs.

Building Block Number Six: Policy Makers Who Look to the Future

Predictable trends, unexpected events, and unforeseeable issues will shape the future of global LHPs. LHP-makers need to be forward looking, anticipatory, and proactive. There is an ever-decreasing lag period between the discovery of new technologies and their actual application. Policy action should begin when the scientific community is first aware of potential breakthroughs. It cannot wait until advances are in regular use to initiate reactive policy discussions.

The future will bring new scientific and technologic achievements. Intensified modernization of livestock production and processing practices will require proactive policies. There will be changing political, societal, and cultural dynamics and continued resistance to **globalization** and international governance of trade in livestock products.

Throughout the world, understanding and public appreciation of livestock industries will rise and fall with producer-consumer and rural-urban conflicts. There will be greater recognition and concern about new and emerging diseases and increasing pressure on livestock industries and regulatory agencies to conform to social and environmental expectations.

The future will bring ever-increasing challenges in LHP-making. This will require creative, thoughtful, and proactive leadership.

Building Block Number Seven: The Critical Need for Competent Leadership

The success of a country's LHPs will depend largely on the strength and professional credibility of its leadership. The leadership characteristics outlined in chapter 9 can be acquired and cultivated through reading, training programs, and continual practice. In this way the goals of aspiring leaders and their organizations can be met and their national livestock industries strengthened in the expanding global free market economy. The LHPs of each nation should include clear strategies that recruit and continually upgrade the effectiveness of its livestock health leadership.

Goals and Objectives of LHPs

LHPs must address a broad range of industry and public concerns. Each national or subnational unit should list the areas they categorize as LHPs, delineate organizations responsible for their development and implementation, and commission appropriate officials to succinctly document the range of authority and responsibility and the goals and objectives of each policy category. This sounds basic, but most LHPs have developed piecemeal over the years with minimal attention to the big picture. They can contain anachronistic and redundant measures that are inapplicable to current conditions.

There are several approaches to this task. Eventually, goals and objectives must be prioritized. Public prioritization is bound to offend supporters of vested interests. People will assume any list of goals and objectives is presented in order of importance. Alphabetizing lists helps neutralize arguments over priorities. Start with a list that contains general areas such as:

- Protecting consumers
- Improving livestock health
- Producing profits for livestock industries
- Developing domestic and foreign markets

Specific programs are then added under each goal. These goals and programs will vary widely among countries.

The achievement of goals will be expedited if each law or regulation is crafted via a seven-stage process that traverses a five-tiered hierarchy. The success of this task depends on consensus, trust, and cooperation among individuals in each tier in the hierarchy, at each stage in the process.

Protection of consumers is a deviation from traditional goals of livestock health interests. It must head most lists. In this age of food production by ever-decreasing, highly industrialized segments of society, serving the larger public interest ultimately determines the fate of industries. Blatant disregard for public concern generates distrust and regulatory action.

Improvement of livestock health has three components. Each is crucial to consumer welfare. First, livestock health underlies food-safety programs, which flounder in the absence of a sound livestock health infrastructure. Second, healthy livestock populations are crucial to minimizing transmission of zoonotic infections from animals to humans. Third, healthy livestock populations are the keys to the availability of affordable quality food.

The goal of producing profits for the national livestock industry is crucial. In incentive-driven capitalistic free-market economies, industries must produce adequate income to pay their employees and obtain return on investments. Otherwise, they succumb to competitive pressures. Competitive success requires achieving those goals. It demands attention to the economic, scientific, political, and cultural characteristics of domestic and international marketplaces.

These complexities emphasize the need to clearly outline the goals and objectives of national LHPs and regularly review existing policies, procedures, regulations, and strategies to accommodate rapidly changing domestic and global conditions.

Seven Stages of LHP Development

There are seven stages of LHP development: need identification, methodology selection, policy drafting, discussion of proposals, revisions, final publication, and ongoing communication. These stages should be addressed at each tier in the hierarchy. Livestock health officials must interact positively throughout this process.

Need Identification

The recognition and identification of need for new or amended LHPs can arise from any level in the LHP hierarchy. Need for regulation is recognized when disturbing trends are observed by public interest groups, government officials, professionals, or academicians. Trading partners often indicate reluctance to import products without evidence of control programs or MS&R systems. This can trigger regulatory actions that industries have previously resisted. Attention to issues of public or industry concern can emerge from media coverage, journal articles, or public officials who have been lobbied by concerned citizens. Broad-based or vaguely articulated issues require definition and focus so they can be referred to organizations or agencies with the practical and technical skills to evaluate their merit and their economic and public health impact. Once an issue is recognized, identified, defined, focused, and clarified in succinct written proposals, it is assigned to the most appropriate arm of the national government for consideration and review by scientific experts, affected industries, and public advocacy groups.

Methodology Selection

Regardless of the legitimacy of an issue, potential methods of handling apparent livestock health or food-safety needs can emerge early in the process. They are sometimes discussed concomitantly with identification of issues. This is productive because the need for action is inseparable from the nature of the needed response. Discussion of appropriate measures to decrease risks advances from the "something has to be done" stage to the "what can be done" stage. Determining what needs to be done requires study of available diagnostic and preventive procedures and their scientific, economic, and political ramifications for the general public and affected industries. Such discussions eventually focus on methodology and should proactively address emerging technologies, international standards, existing policies, and the costs of implementation within existing livestock health infrastructures.

Policy Drafting

The scientific community and principal stakeholders often remain aloof to impending legislation or regulatory action hoping that if is ignored it will go away. Once a regulatory agency proposes a rule the climate changes. At this stage, the proposed policy receives serious scrutiny and intense evaluation.

Strategies for policy drafting must be seriously crafted so that regulations are clearly written by individuals who understand the issues.

Discussion of Proposed Regulations

Drafts of policies, laws, regulations, or voluntary pilot programs are described and discussed in newsletters and at organization meetings. They sometimes appear in the media.

At this point there is a surge of activity, and proposals are seriously studied, analyzed, and criticized by widely divergent interests. Opposition groups and supporters become vocal, and the true merits and disadvantages of proposals are aired. Thoughtful input then emerges.

Revision

Revision of policies, regulations, or standards attempts to include scientifically sound, workable, and economically feasible suggestions. The final version of a proposed measure may differ considerably from what was originally proposed or intended.

In the United States, proposed rules are prepared after input is considered, viable suggestions are included, and extensive revision is completed. Revision involves careful editing to assure the proposal is clearly worded and transparent in its intentions. The proposed rule is then published in the **Federal Register** with a request for comments. Each written comment is reviewed and either included or rejected. The author receives a written acknowledgment of receipt of the comment and an explanation as to why it was included or rejected.

Final Publication

In the United States, final versions of regulations are published in the Federal Register and incorporated into the **U.S. Code of Federal Regulations** as they become effective.

Ongoing Communication

Each issue or potential policy should be clearly articulated and opened for discussion and debate by the sponsoring agency at each stage in the development process. This dialogue must reach out to include all five levels of the policy-development hierarchy, persist through each step in the process, and continue after the policy is in effect.

Five-Tiered Hierarchy of LHP Development

LHP-development processes are most likely to succeed and produce lasting and effective laws, regulations, guidelines, and educational programs if they are debated and shaped by thoughtful people at each level of the five-tiered hierarchy. Wisdom, biases, and political and cultural influences of individuals must emerge as early as possible in the discussion in order to receive maximum consideration. After review, discussion, and modification, individual opinions are merged into organizational positions. They appear again at subnational, national, and global levels. While not all positions survive the consensus-building process, these contributions refine and strengthen the public appeal of a policy. They also dilute the strength, specificity, and effectiveness. Ideally these inputs and changes leave adequate oversight to deter violative activities and penalize offenders.

Effective Personal Strategies

Everyone involved in LHPs must initially address issues on a personal level and apply their background knowledge, skills, abilities, and biases to each issue. They must first determine what, if anything, they would personally propose. Personal opinions expand and dilute as issues emerge and are discussed with colleagues and at meetings.

Regardless of background and previous involvement with animals, LHP-makers must continually expand their knowledge and adapt to changing conditions. This will permit their contributions to have an impact beyond their personal preferences. There are times in the process when individuals with private agendas must adapt to broader goals of employers, organizations, or industry groups.

There are limits that one can't exceed and lines that cannot be crossed. The boundaries that cannot be crossed include distorting scientific facts, sacrificing professional credibility, or forsaking personal integrity. The pressures and temptations to abandon personal standards, renounce professional ethics, or reject science-based reasoning escalate as the stakes increase. As the chain of command broadens, personal or organizational views are challenged at the national or international level.

When confronted with challenges to personal and professional ethics, policy makers must move carefully, be sure of their facts, speak softly, behave diplomatically, and stand firmly. Confidence to assume this positive posture requires a scientifically based understanding of issues and an appreciation of the complex interactions of science, economics, politics, and culture. It also requires the identification of fundamental concepts that deserve support and of those that are unacceptable and should be repudiated. Those involved in LHP-making must be prepared for career-long struggles to espouse goals and discard non-scientific, unethical, or otherwise unacceptable alternatives. A diplomatic but firm and non-condescending posture in opposition to questionable proposals earns the trust of colleagues and adversaries and can significantly advance personal achievement.

Effective Strategies for Professional or Industry Groups

Professional or industry groups are non-governmental and have volunteer members, most of whom are not organizational employees. The priorities, goals, and strategies of professional or industry groups must represent the best interests of their membership. Organizational strategies must also address the greater needs of society and the country. This is where some overly self-serving interest groups go astray.

When organizations oppose the best interests of their countries, they are at risk, and their priorities may need reevaluation. They must carefully evaluate their positions with respect to the best interests of society and their nation. Where there is divergence or direct conflict between organizational goals and the public interest, courageous individuals must speak up and urge organizations to reconsider.

Effective Strategies for Subnational Governments

Subnational governments represent towns, cities, counties, provinces, parishes, states, and territories. Their needs and contributions in LHPs are often lost in the scramble to address the concerns of professional or industry groups and national governments. In every country, subnational contributions play thoughtful and often moderating roles in LHP development.

The cooperation of subnational officials is essential in national livestock disease-control and border-security programs (see Discussion Topic 7). Their concerns about propriety and confidentiality in MS&R activities make them key players in national matters. Their support of educational institutions and diagnostic services is indispensable to national LHPs.

Subnational governments are close to the action. They usually have clear, science-based policies that incorporate the best interests of local governments, organizations, and industries.

Eventually these must be reviewed with respect to what is best from the national or global outlook. This broad perspective can be difficult for subnational governments and is a challenging component of the LHP strategies.

Effective Strategies for National Governments

By the time an issue or potential sanitary measure has traversed the hierarchical tiers needed to reach serious consideration at the national level, it may contain compromises, dilutions, and some loss of focus.

Like those of industry groups and subnational governments, national priorities, goals, and strategies must represent the best interests of the citizens. National policies are complex. They are difficult to solidify and don't always represent the majority of interested citizens. They are more difficult to express clearly than those of subnational interest groups. They are also at greater risk of deviating from sound science and professional credibility. To prevent these deviations, national livestock health and food-safety policies must be monitored carefully by courageous technical experts who speak out in a non-confrontational, non-public manner. In extreme cases, honest experts will blow the whistle. Whistle blowers must have documented facts, clear arguments, and positive ethical stances. They must repeatedly present written recommendations or arguments to several higher levels of authority before going public.

National officials assume a unique role in LHP management. They have to play a leadership role that respects the various political, industrial, and special interest groups that come to bear on the issues. National officials need to respect the sovereign rights of subnational jurisdictions. They must understand the needs of different geographic and ecological entities within their nation. They must represent their countries with credibility and integrity in the international community and negotiate international issues in the best interests of multiple stakeholders. All involved parties are not always happy with the activities of national LHP-makers.

The demands of LHP-making require the understanding of chief livestock and agricultural officials. LHP needs are often too demanding for direct involvement by high officials because of time limitations and other diversions.

High-ranking nationals should appoint a competent director of LHP who has time and vision to anticipate needs for domestic disease-control activities, food-safety oversight, and exotic-disease exclusion. This leader should consult with wise people from various constituencies, review issues with internal groups and national organizations, prepare issue analyses, consult with leaders of other agencies, and attempt to stay in touch with the media by scheduling regular press conferences. This leader should also prepare reviews and regular updates of the entire national LHP program, agency goals and missions, and organizational effectiveness.

Effective Global Strategies

International, or global, LHPs are developed by representatives of national governments in forums such as the OIE and the WTO. They are brought forward by representatives of countries, trading blocs, regional commissions, or scientific panels. These bodies rely heavily on developed nations for financial support.

Before reaching international tribunals, LHPs are usually filtered by national or multinational organizations and may lose some of their originally intended virility.

Representatives at international LHP-making meetings have usually worked their way through the personal, organizational, and national battles. They sometimes still push for wording favorable to individual or national agendas. They may be so far removed from reality that they have lost track of the scientific and practical merits of issues.

Ideally, at this level there is enough concern for global welfare that parochial interests are set aside. The interests of underdeveloped, developing, and developed nations are recognized, and the needs of the various regions of the world are addressed. Still, agendas of individuals, organizations, and nations can resurface. Caution is needed so interventions are presented diplomatically in an air of cross-cultural understanding. They should be based on good science, sound logic, and professional integrity. This requires a realization that the building blocks of global policies are extensions of personal, organizational, and national positions and that they emerge from broader perspectives that expand and slightly subvert individual and national objectives.

Policy-Development Strategies

Strategies for the development of effective LHPs require the establishment of broad goals. These can include protecting consumer health through food-safety programs, improving livestock health and profitability, or enhancing international trade.

Within each broad category, a series of specific objectives can then be outlined. For example, within the goal of improving livestock health, specific program objectives for excluding exotic diseases can be identified. For each specific objective, a sequential plan is outlined. Such a plan can include

- Selecting program-evaluation criteria and schedules
- Encouraging stakeholder involvement
- Gaining public support
- Involving the academic and diagnostic communities
- Building a communication network
- Developing action-oriented skilled leadership
- Building a livestock health infrastructure

- Creating mechanisms to enhance international credibility and understanding
- Employing highly transparent policy development processes

Within each component of the plan, program-specific descriptions and activities must be documented.

Establishment of Clear Goals and Objectives

Goals and objectives for livestock health and food-safety programs spell out specific livestock or human diseases that need exclusion, reduction, or eradication. A challenging aspect of goal setting is identifying the most logical point in the food chain to focus the attack. The point of attack may be during production, as is the case with most livestock diseases. Human diseases of animal origin are traditionally addressed during food processing. There are increasing calls for farm-to-fork food-safety efforts that address each link in the food chain.

Key components of goal setting are the identification of **risk**, the recognition that zero risk is unattainable, and the outlining of realistic, workable procedures to reduce risk to acceptable levels.

This exercise, while seemingly self-evident, is sometimes overlooked in newly proposed programs. Reevaluation of the goals of existing programs, particularly those that have been in effect for many years, is an essential process.

Selecting Program Evaluation Criteria

One of the most enlightening and often neglected aspects of program development strategies is the categorizing of criteria according to which activities are being evaluated. Development of program evaluation criteria requires focus on methodological details like the surveillance and testing procedures needed to accurately diagnose a disease and estimate its prevalence and geographic distribution. Each livestock health program should have a list of evaluation criteria and a time scheduled for regular evaluations employing outside review committees.

Developing Stakeholder Support

In transparent participatory societies the probability of success of LHPs is directly proportional to the level of support by stakeholders, that is those with a direct financial interest. The support of stakeholders will vary depending on the proposed program and its likely effects on their *modus operandi* and profits. It is essential to demonstrate to stakeholders that in the long run proposed policies or regulations enhance the credibility of the industry and do not reduce profits.

Policies should not create unnecessary burdens and should ward off later, more drastic, prohibitions. Often, convincing stakeholders is a monumental task. It requires long-term understanding, trust, and communication among livestock health officials and producers and processors. It also requires painstaking discussions at all levels and within all segments of the industry far in advance of proposed regulations.

Involving the Academic and Diagnostic Communities

LHP-makers and regulatory agencies traditionally neglect cultivating the agricultural and veterinary academic communities. These groups appear to be happy to be ignored by regulatory and government officials unless there is grant money involved. Then they can be very cooperative. Academics also cherish the prestige of serving on national committees or advisory boards. The commingling of these two worlds is as inevitable as the commingling of nations in the globalization movement. Both encounter resistance.

The mutual benefits of academic-regulatory interactions are numerous. Benefits for universities include government funding for their research, diagnostic and public health programs, and the introduction of an element of reality into teaching programs often isolated from worldly affairs.

The potential benefits of academic interactions to LHPs include injection of scientific credibility into regulatory programs and access to respected authorities.

Extension outreach programs, long a feature of the **land-grant system**, have traditionally provided information to consumers and farmers. Modernized livestock operations have moved toward the use of private consultants. These technical experts focus on specific needs rather than on general information offered by university extension personnel.

Extension specialists have somewhat shifted focus from livestock production to consumer programs. They still provide valuable livestock services by delivering information at public meetings and in informational bulletins. National livestock health and regulatory agencies, however, have a unique, and as yet unfulfilled, opportunity to capitalize on federally financed extension programs to engage in public dialogue. Most state extension directors would gladly discuss LHPs as potential program components.

Diagnostic laboratories, particularly those associated with land-grant universities, have traditionally bridged the gap and provided the major academic-regulatory communication network. This contribution has not been fully utilized by the regulatory community. Increasing this interaction should be a major component of the strategies of LHP-makers. It can involve diagnostic laboratory workers in MS&R activities and advisory committees.

Gaining Public Support

Public support can be more easily gained than stakeholder support. Gaining public support requires transparent and continual communication that is best accomplished through good media relations. Successful media management requires sustained, conscientious efforts by articulate spokespersons who gain public respect through continued interactions and openly providing information.

This can be achieved by regular distribution of brief and well-written activity updates. These must be succinct and fully suitable for reproduction in newspapers and magazines. Because media moguls are always pressed by deadlines and looking for factual and well-written stories, these items may begin appearing almost word for word, and the message of the livestock health community will be disseminated. When such materials are distributed, officials at all levels of the livestock health hierarchy must also receive them and be prepared to elaborate when queried. Regular press conferences help.

The down side of this strategy is that, in seeking public attention, the party line can be distorted. This policy confusion opens further healthy debate and is far better than keeping positions, policies, and plans veiled in secrecy. Furthermore, such openness often raises hitherto unconsidered issues that are vital to the national interest.

Building a Communication Network

Clear and forthright communication underlies success in LHPs. Conversely, ineffective information transmission undermines messages and outcomes.

Government agencies are constantly under fire from regulated industries, the public, and the media. There is a tendency to withhold information for fear of exposing program deficiencies, being offensive to stakeholders or the public, or being misinterpreted or proven wrong. This is particularly challenging to leaders who lack self-confidence or tend toward introversion. It is also true among extroverts, who can be labeled "loose cannons" and banned from important assignments and promotions because of their tendencies to talk when they should be listening. The potential for encouraging and rewarding verbal and written communicators at each tier in the LHP hierarchy is unlimited. It should be the basis of LHP activity.

Developing Action-Oriented Skilled Leadership

The potential for implementing strategies is contingent on the presence of action-oriented and skilled leadership at all levels of the LHP-hierarchy. As detailed in chapter 9, leadership ability is a complex function of heritable and learned traits. Fortunately, positive and productive leadership characteristics can be learned, cultivated, and nurtured within organizations. With conscientious efforts, positive examples, and an upbeat rewards system, secure and confident leadership can gradually emerge. This can occur even in organizations with cultures in which non-communication and face-saving have been driving forces.

Building Livestock Health Infrastructures

The importance of infrastructure to livestock health and food safety cannot be overestimated. Both the general public and the livestock industries stand to benefit from every improvement in livestock health programs. Countries must analyze and prioritize each infrastructural component to adapt to changing global expectations and domestic issues (see chapter 4).

Infrastructure development requires financial support, which will be forthcoming in direct proportion to the communication skills of leaders and their ability to gain the support of stakeholders, the general public, the media, and the national and subnational officials who control the purse strings.

Creating Mechanisms to Enhance International Credibility and Understanding

The credibility of national livestock health infrastructure and leadership in the international community will determine the success of each country's efforts to maintain export markets and its influence in developing international standards and policies supportive of its interests. The selection of individuals to represent national interests in international forums is crucial. These representatives must be knowledgeable of animal health and disease issues, politically alert, and culturally sensitive. They should be good listeners, non-interrupting, and open to suggestions from colleagues from all over the world. The credibility of a nation in the international community is enhanced if its negotiating officials have **fast track authority**.

Employing Highly Transparent Policy-Development Processes

The process of policy development is far more effective if conducted in the open and in an environment that welcomes input from diverse interests. Policies, regulations, and proposals for livestock health matters must be transparent in order to meet the expectations of both domestic and international communities.

Policy-Development Strategies Must Seek Workable Solutions

LHP-makers and regulatory officials should see to it that sanitary requirements are understandable and can be implemented by the industries upon which they are imposed. This is best accomplished by concerned and knowledgeable veterinary officials. LHPs should be free of indecipherable details, legalese, scientific jargon, and unworkable details.

The key to workable strategies is that policies, laws, or regulations must be clearly written and amenable to practical application. This strategy can be subverted by legal staff who evaluate proposals for conflict with existing codes and then clarify them by rewording in legal jargon that can be incomprehensible to readers. Legalese and jargon are particularly frustrating to individuals with limited formal education and to trading partners who speak other languages.

The best strategy to keeping LHPs workable is, at all stages in the policy-development process, consultation with those who are being regulated.

Policy-Development Strategies Must Address Broad Goals and Specific Objectives

Both broad goals and disease-specific objectives have a place in LHP-making. It is essential to initially identify whether a policy effort is directed toward broad goals or disease-specific objectives. Each requires development at a different level.

General goals are often met by enabling legislation generated by lawmakers who are unfamiliar with livestock health details.

Disease-specific regulations are usually generated by livestock health officials who are familiar with diseases and their ramifications and qualified to answer questions and communicate with stakeholders and interest groups. Specific regulations should always be a part of a broader comprehensive program.

Effective Policy-Development Strategies

To achieve maximum effectiveness at each step, strategies should be developed in the abstract and be anticipatory, flexible, and transparent. The process should seek constructive analogies, involve review by stakeholders and special interest groups, strive for policies that are practical and workable for the affected industries, and address both general and specific issues.

Abstract Policy Development

The strategy development process should be undertaken in an abstract environment free from conflict surrounding specific issues that can distract from the big picture and bias discussions. It is difficult to identify broad-based program goals and clear objectives when facing the pressures of specific issues, a desk full of requests for projects or exceptions, and a phone overloaded with calls from politicians and friends extolling the virtues of specific ideas. Abstract policy development requires separating the country's best interests from the wishes of individuals and interest groups.

Some criteria for potential policies are scientific soundness, capacity for administration in a non-discriminatory manner, consistency with existing laws and regulations, harmony with international standards, compatibility with agency authority and mission, transparency, practicality, and amenability to oversight and enforcement.

Anticipatory Policy Development

The recommendation for an abstract policy development process should not prevent policy makers from anticipating needs to handle challenges. Such challenges could be accusations that disease-control programs discriminate against small or large farmers, that import policies are non-scientific and overly restrictive, or that one industry is being treated differently than another. Anticipation of these and similar arguments enable leaders to do their homework and better consider the ramifications and validity of potential positions.

Flexible Policy Development

A strategic goal for those developing LHPs should be to seek program policies and regulations that are flexible enough to be easily amended, adaptable to multiple circumstances or changing technology, and amenable to translation into other languages.

Policy-Development Strategies that Use Analogies

The use of carefully selected analogies in verbal or written arguments regarding potential LHPs can make points more easily understandable. Hopefully, the complexity of LHP-making was illustrated by comparing the policy-development process to a constantly changing team of stone masons with differing styles and agendas, building a never-ending mortar-less wall of variously shaped stones.

Another effective analogy is to compare disease-surveillance tactics to trying to catch fireflies in the dark. They are virtually invisible until they light up and become visible just as previously hidden diseases suddenly become visible in epidemics. Animal-health risk analysis and risk mitigation become understandable when compared to traffic controls and safety education programs. Both reduce, but don't totally eliminate, accidents.

Developing Equitable Transparent Regulations in Cooperation with Stakeholders

The early and frequent involvement of all interested or affected parties is the key to successful policy development. It permits the airing of different views. When conducted in open forums this strategy encourages supporters and opponents to become acquainted, recognize valid concerns of interest groups, and translate them into larger issues. Ideally this can lead to cooperative team approaches, increased understanding, and compromise.

Open discussions documented in clear articulate language, and readily available to interested parties, are the best means of developing transparent policies.

In an ideal world LHPs would be proposed by regulated industries to protect the best interests of the public. This bottom-up development process for laws and regulations is virtually nonexistent. It is sometimes replaced by top down processes in which officials develop LHPs without input from regulated industries and stakeholders. Understandably, livestock producers, processors, and transporters don't want to be regulated by governments unsympathetic to their needs and financial aspirations.

The solution to these extremes lies in a middle ground called "cooperative" or "participatory" regulatory approaches. In cooperative approaches initiatives are discussed jointly among industry and government officials. This process is time consuming and can involve lengthy and sometimes contentious discussions. The outcome is often significantly different from the one initially envisioned by policy makers and may result in the abandonment or postponement of an idea or its initiation as a voluntary pilot program.

Barring emergencies, threats to export markets, or media publicity, the successful launching of disease-control programs, mandatory animal ID, or MS&R systems usually requires lengthy discussions and compromise among the livestock industries, interested stakeholders, and government officials.

In such discussions, industries are represented by commodity groups. These include cattlemen's associations, dairy producers' associations, organizations representing the interests of poultry and egg producers and processors, pork producer groups, associations of meat and food-processing organizations, and representatives of the rendering industry.

It is helpful if other groups are available to broaden perspectives. In the United States, organizations such as the **National Institute for Animal Agriculture (NIAA)**, the **U.S. Animal Health Association (USAHA)**, and the **Coalition for Animal Agriculture** help policy makers hear the concerns of commodity groups and subnational livestock health officials and modulate extreme positions to achieve a consensus acceptable to national officials.

The process of developing equitable and transparent regulations requires that LHP-makers must be excellent listeners. The strategies outlined above require that LHP-makers and regulatory officials communicate directly and honestly with the livestock health communities, national and subnational officials, legislators, and interest groups that support and oppose their efforts. Direct communication with the national and local news media is essential for transparent LHPs.

Major Categories of LHPs

Variable strategies are needed to cover the broad range of activities addressed by LHPs. The techniques described above can be customized to suit the personal and organizational preferences of LHP-makers and adjusted to accommodate the specific issues in question. At a minimum the issues addressed using these strategies should include development of laws, regulations, and guidelines for:

- Controlling specific diseases of livestock
- Enhancing food safety
- Excluding exotic diseases
- Addressing new and emerging diseases of animals and people
- Developing national animal health reporting systems
- Assuring animal ID
- Establishing transparent and equitable import and export measures

Controlling Specific Diseases of Livestock

Strategies for developing disease-specific control programs are largely the responsibility of national governments. Involving livestock producers from the start is advisable. Control strategies must consider the financial and public health implications of the disease and the level of support by the livestock industry and the general public.

Livestock diseases are considered for control or eradication when they cause serious economic losses, are transmissible to people, or impact trade. Some pathogenic organisms are more easily controlled and eradicated than others. The biological characteristics of diseases amenable to control efforts are manageable incubation periods, readily recognizable symptoms, availability of diagnostic tests to identify the causative agents, and the absence of persistent infections in individual animals.

Before committing to eradication or control programs, policy makers and national veterinary services must carefully explore the criteria for controllable or eradicable diseases listed in chapter 4 and address each in their proposed strategy.

Enhancing Food Safety

Strategies for food-safety policies must initially address the farm-to-fork dimensions of the issue, identify links in the food chain most amenable to intervention, and narrow the programs to those that are scientifically sound, economically feasible, and practical.

Selected strategies must recognize the complexity of the issue. Strategists must address public tendencies to take risks in spite of warnings, ignore simple preventive measures unless major catastrophes occur, and blame the government for the problem.

Food-safety measures must also address the ubiquity of constantly changing microorganisms in the excrement of all species and the small likelihood of major successes.

Food-safety programs require close cooperation among multiple agencies to avoid duplications or counterproductive resource expenditures.

Excluding Exotic Diseases

For the last sixty years, U.S. experts have contended that the major exotic-disease issue in the United States is FMD. The question has always been when, not if, FMD will appear. Exotic- disease exclusion measures have been less successful in Europe.

Strategies for disease exclusion in the new millennium face increasing challenges (National Association of State Departments of Agriculture Research Foundation 2001). Exotic-disease exclusion includes measures easily amenable to regulation. It also involves issues less easily controlled, like border security, farm security, and bioterrorism.

The most effective exclusion policy is to expand and improve current programs and to develop creative policies that exploit new technologies.

Addressing New and Emerging Diseases of Animals and People

The topic of new and emerging diseases raised public concern at the close of the twentieth century and the beginning of the new millennium. This was largely due to the presence of AIDS, BSE and other TSEs, **West Nile fever**, **Nipah virus**, and others. Advances in diagnostic technology have expedited the recognition of emerging diseases. Most are zoonoses, and many have insect vectors and mammalian host reservoirs. Most fall within the purview of LHPs.

The U.S. **National Center for Disease Control and Prevention (CDC)** has prepared a document entitled *Preventing Emerging Infectious Diseases: A Strategy for the 21st Century* (CDC 1998). The strategy includes improvement of disease surveillance and response to outbreaks, supporting research on emergent infectious-disease threats, preventing infectious diseases through control programs, communicating public health information, and strengthening the infectious disease-control portions of the public health infrastructure.

LHPs can expand on these goals by addressing border controls and security on livestock-producing premises. With human infections, security is virtually impossible due to travel, civil liberties concerns, and human rights considerations. With respect to research, scientists can conduct experimental studies on animals that would be impossible with human subjects. Veterinary medical diagnostic laboratories will play key roles in emerging-disease surveillance and control.

Developing National Livestock Health Reporting Systems (NAHRS)

An NAHRS must be part of the national strategy of countries seeking healthy domestic livestock populations and a competitive position in global markets. This is an urgent reality that does not allow time for decades of discussion, analysis, and debate.

Each country's NAHRS needs a proactive steering committee comprised of industry organizations, veterinary medical associations, national and subnational animal health officials, diagnostic organizations, national and subnational food-safety officials, and the country's **chief veterinary officer (CVO).** The group needs an executive board comprised of action-oriented leaders.

The NAHRS mission should be the development of a cooperative, transparent disease reporting system that involves every industry and state needing federal assistance in livestock disease control or requiring export certifications to be endorsed by officials of the national government. The NAHRS should provide data for the nation's livestock-disease reports to the OIE and produce an annual report on the national livestock health status for general distribution. Specifics of the NAHRS are described in chapter 4.

The NAHRS should be a major component of larger national livestock health trade strategies that address changing global trade paradigms and national market objectives. This strategy should include, at a minimum, the following components:

- Credible animal disease data
- A nationally coordinated livestock identification system capable of tracing to the farm of origin any animal, carcass, or product with signs of reportable diseases, potentially harmful residues, or contamination with pathogens
- An industry-driven disease-by-disease, species-by-species, commodity-by-commodity review of the OIE Code to identify inconsistencies, scientific deficiencies, and national noncompliance
- A review of existing national import and export regulations to determine scientific accuracy and harmony with the OIE Code
- A non-political, first-come-first-serve basis for prioritizing and addressing foreign requests for importations or regionalization
- Development of a list of questions to be answered before national **veterinary services (VS)** or industry spokespersons suggest that foreign import requirements are unscientific or overly restrictive
- Endorsement by veterinary associations of an overhaul of national LHP
- A nationally coordinated livestock disease MS&R system participated in by all industries and subnational agencies desiring federal financial support for disease-control efforts or endorsement of export certificates
- A "one-animal-per-needle" policy when testing and vaccinating livestock
- Provision of adequate resources and personnel to assure national agencies can develop and implement these measures

If the livestock industries of a country are to remain competitive, national authorities must meet domestic and international expectations in regard to commitments to international trade agreements, consistency with international standards, credible disease reporting, and conformance with legitimate import requirements.

These obligations are basic to establishing and preserving foreign markets. They are essential to the survival of the livestock industries in a competitive global economy. Meeting these obligations requires compliance with provisions of the WTO SPS Agreement; conformity with OIE disease reporting, testing, and trade standards; and meeting livestock disease MS&R and health certification requirements of trading partners.

If they are to fulfill these obligations, countries need a nationally coordinated alliance of producers, regulatory and practicing veterinarians, processors, transporters, brokers, industry organizations, the academic and diagnostic communities, and subnational regulatory officials. Input from these groups is essential to assure the participation of all parties who ask that health certificates be endorsed by national governments. Cooperation and input from stakeholders are also essential for establishing a credible MS&R system so that each country's certifications accurately reflect their animal-disease situation.

International organizations and trading partners deal exclusively with representatives of national governments. Policy makers should pressure national livestock health officials to take the lead and speak out for cooperative national MS&R enterprises.

Assuring Animal ID

LHPs must include strategies for assuring animal ID systems adequate to meet domestic quality-control standards, to conduct rapid disease trace-back, and to fulfill the requirements of importing nations.The animal ID technologies applicable to each livestock species must be analyzed. National officials must decide on required formats for compulsory ID of each species.

Establishing Transparent and Equitable Import-Export Measures

The strategy of developing import-export measures that are both equitable and transparent will be a major determinant of each country's success in the global free-market economy.

Transparent import-export measures are developed with an openness that permits domestic stakeholders and trading partners to be involved at all stages in the process.

Transparency complicates the process by engendering comments, controversy, and contentiousness, which adds unpleasantness early on in the policy development process but provides early recognition of potential stumbling blocks. Early recognition of obstacles helps to address them in the initial stages of policy making.

Policy-development strategies should strive for equitable LHPs. This requires a built-in assurance that they can be justly and fairly administered.

This expectation applies to domestic and international issues and reaches beyond trade and is consistent with the equivalency requirements of the WTO SPS agreement. LHPs will be equitable to the extent that diverse domestic and international interests are involved in each step of the LHP-development process and that equal treatment is applied to equal conditions in policy administration.

Import-export measures are inexorably linked. Measures imposed on each nation's livestock-related exports often emulate the requirements the nation imposes on imports into the country.

Strategies for Success in the New Global Economy

The LHP goals of most countries are to protect the health of the people and the domestic livestock and to expand export markets. Protection of domestic animal populations is contingent on exclusion of exotic diseases, a goal that requires stringent import measures. The United States has rigid import requirements and little need to import animal products. This combination hinders efforts to expand exports, because it leaves very little to offer in give-and-take trade discussions upon which foreign marketing agreements are based.

International movement of livestock commodities involves complex intentions, goals, viewpoints, and agendas of livestock producers and processors, veterinarians, regulators, bureaucrats, politicians, and scientists.

Spokespersons for these interests represent several generations, many nations, and various religious, cultural, and linguistic backgrounds. They should be carefully chosen and well trained.

Development of a Cooperative Participatory Livestock Health Infrastructure

A cooperative participatory animal health infrastructure is the backbone of livestock disease-control and eradication programs and is essential for expanding foreign markets. Sound livestock health infrastructures require partnerships that maintain healthy livestock programs with diagnostic capacity, border security, MS&R activities, and a myriad of other activities outlined in chapter 4.

Establishing Credibility among Domestic Stakeholders and Foreign Counterparts

Credibility is a cherished and fragile possession of livestock health officials and regulatory agencies. Credibility is essential in domestic and international communities. It develops from forthright and honest representation of the country's animal health status, programs, and policies. It requires open and direct communication with the press, domestic stakeholders, and representatives of foreign governments. Measures of credibility within domestic communities are

- The levels of transparency and non-discrimination with which national livestock health officials develop and enforce regulations
- The openness with which they deal with subnational livestock and public health officials and the public
- The willingness to admit mistakes and program deficiencies
- The extent to which they willingly cooperate with other, sometimes competing, governmental agencies on issues of common interest
- Their willingness to cooperate on non-livestock issues of broad national interest
- The directness and honesty with which they deal with interest groups opposing their programs and criticizing their policies
- The openness with which they respond to media questioning

Establishing international credibility is challenging because of physical distances, language barriers, political and cultural differences, and a constant turnover of personnel that makes long-lasting relationships problematic. Nonetheless, international credibility is measured by the same standards as national credibility.

A major measure of international livestock health credibility is the integrity of each country's national MS&R system. Claims of disease-freedom must correspond with information in veterinary textbooks, published articles, product advertisements, or diagnostic laboratory reports that are available worldwide electronically. It is important that trade officials be cautioned against ill advised statements about national animal health status.

Livestock health credibility must be a strategic component of each country's LHPs and official behaviors.

Developing Equitable Transparent Regulations in Cooperation with Stakeholders

Strategies for gaining the cooperation of stakeholders must involve cooperative or participatory regulatory programs and initiatives discussed jointly among industry and government officials. This approach is time consuming and requires lengthy and sometimes contentious discussions. Outcomes often differ significantly from regulator's ideas and may result in postponement of the plan or in its initiation as a voluntary pilot program. Except in emergencies, successful launching of domestic livestock disease programs requires lengthy discussions and compromise among the livestock industry, interested stakeholders, and government officials. The process of the development of equitable and transparent regulations requires that LHP-makers be excellent listeners.

SUMMARY

The strategies outlined above will be achieved to the extent that LHP-makers and regulatory officials make extraordinary efforts to communicate directly and honestly with all segments of the livestock health communities, national and subnational officials, legislators, and interest groups that support and oppose their efforts. Throughout the entire laborious process, direct communication with the national and local news media is essential.

Effective, clear, and workable LHPs can be generated and implemented by a seven-stage strategy that works its way through the five-tier hierarchy and involves developing policies in the abstract, anticipating unforeseen challenges, using analogies, offering constant review by stakeholders and interest groups to assure workability, and including both general concepts and specific issues. Communication is the key to the development and implementation of effective livestock strategies.

BIBLIOGRAPHY

CDC. 1998. *Preventing Emerging Infectious Diseases: A Strategy for the Twenty-first Century*. Atlanta, GA: Centers for Disease Control and Prevention.

Holdredge, C. and S. Talbot. 2001. Sewing Technology: The Ecologic Argument against Genetic Engineering Down on the Farm. *Sierra*. July-August 2001.

National Association of State Departments of Agriculture Research Foundation. 2001. *The Animal Health Safeguarding Review: Results and Recommendations*. Washington, D.C.

National Academy of Science. 2002. *Report of the Panel on the Risks of Genetic Manipulation of Animals to the Environment and Potentially to Human Health*. Washington, D.C.: National Academy Press.

Chapter 11

Discussion Topics

Introduction

These topics provide information on hypothetical situations for group discussions. They mix fiction and fact and should not be quoted as historical truths. They are designed to stimulate thought and discussion of **livestock health policy (LHP)** issues that could potentially arise.

Perusing this chapter will acquaint readers with the complexities of LHP-making. Group discussions of these topics will provide participants with unique insights into the realities of livestock health issues in the public domain.

Use of the Discussion Topics

These topics can be used in seminars, short courses, committee meetings, at symposia, or in formal course work. In group settings, their application will depend on available time, number of participants, goals of the program, and preferences of discussion leaders. They are largely fictitious and can be modified at will.

These discussions divide attendees into groups with differing opinions and direct them to develop and present opposing positions. Everyone benefits from the varied perspectives that emerge. Participants will benefit most from discussions if they prepare, listen carefully, and participate actively.

Attention and involvement will improve if attendees know at the outset that groups will elect spokespersons, advisors, reporters for news articles, and speakers to deliver summaries to special interest groups. Participants can also be told that non-contributing individuals may be asked to present spontaneous summaries or analyses at any point.

If participants have the book, they can be asked to read the selected topic in advance. Discussion leaders should assign groups randomly to maintain numerical balance.

If participants don't have the book, discussion leaders can prepare color-coded handouts for each group. The handouts can outline general information for all participants and include separate position information for each group. Handouts can be distributed before the session or as participants enter the room. The initial confusion resulting from surprise assignments will mimic the real-life bewilderment that arises from hidden agendas, language difficulties, and political and cultural differences between people gathering to discuss policy issues.

Program goals and available time will determine the discussion strategy. Ancillary assignments or groups can be deleted, or new ones can be added.

Discussion Strategies

Discussion leaders should introduce the issue and explain the ground rules and time restrictions. Participants should be divided into groups as indicated. Initially, each group meets separately. They should spend about one quarter of their allotted time discussing the issue and preparing a case. Then they pause to elect a spokesperson and advisor to present their arguments at upcoming meetings. They reassemble to coach their group representatives and help them prepare their presentation.

After a break, each group presents its case to a decision-making body, which usually includes all participants.

After the presentations and the question sessions, all attendees can complete a secret multiple-choice ballot to select the arguments that have been most clearly and convincingly presented, most scientifically sound, are in the best national interest, and are most likely to be selected by the decision-making body.

Use of Ancillary Assignments in Discussion Topics

Assignments to prepare summaries, deliver speeches, or write newspaper articles help emphasize the importance of communication and listening skills.

Speeches are most effective if limited to fifteen to twenty minutes and presented to an assembly of all participants representing a decision-making body or special interest group. Time should be allowed for hostile questions after the speeches. This scenario emphasizes the importance of tailoring talks to audiences without compromising accuracy.

The assignment of newspaper articles with short deadlines offers participants an opportunity to see issues from a media perspective. Reporting assignments are most effective if the articles are limited to 200–300 words and are distributed to the group for comment. The reporting and speaking assignments will illustrate that people hearing the same discussion can gain different impressions and that it is challenging to summarize discussions succinctly and correctly under the pressure of deadlines.

In several topics specific audiences are selected for speeches, and specific newspapers are suggested for stories. Discussion leaders can adjust these to suit the situation.

Discussion leaders wishing to illustrate certain concepts may modify a topic with creative handouts. Groups should be encouraged to modify or expand the positions initially assigned. As time passes, new issues will emerge. These strategies can be adapted to almost any issue.

If these topics are not utilized in a group setting, reading them can provide LHP-makers with provocative insights into some aspects of LHPs.

Discussion Topic 1: The **European Union (EU)** Beef Hormone Ban

The Issue

Since the late 1980s, the EU has refused to buy U.S. beef because it may contain residues of hormonal growth promotants. The hormones estrogen and testosterone are approved by the U.S. **Food and Drug Administration (FDA)** for use in the United States. They increase growth rates from 5 to 10%, increase feed conversion rates, and reduce fat-to-lean ratios. Most are implanted in the ear because it is one of the few parts discarded at slaughter. These compounds are rapidly metabolized, and beef from treated cattle often has hormone levels similar to beef from untreated animals.

The EU invoked the ban as a precautionary measure fearing unknown, possibly harmful, effects on humans eating beef from treated cattle. They claim the issue is surrounded by scientific uncertainty. European pressures for precautionary measures come from a public that feels the scientific community and agricultural officials withheld information on the dangers of eating beef from cattle with **bovine spongiform encephalopathy (BSE)**.

U.S. cattlemen feel the Europeans are using the ban to exclude U.S. beef because the European beef is non-competitive in price and quality. This noncompetitiveness lies largely in the differences in production systems and the availability of affordable grain supplies, which are in short supply in Europe and must be imported. In the United States, the fertile U.S. corn and grain belts provide abundant supplies of corn, wheat, oats, barley, and soybeans. Beef prices also reflect the comparative efficiencies of large integrated U.S.

feedlots versus the small family farms, which Europeans cherish as a way of life and for ecosystem preservation.

The demise of small farms, family values, and work ethics is also evident in the United States. The decrease in family farms in the United States is believed to be a result of advancing technology, changing lifestyles, and integrated livestock operations.

U.S. trade officials have insisted that the hormone ban is a protectionist measure. They say it violates the requirements for **transparency**, non-discrimination, scientifically based risk assessment, and equal national treatment of the **World Trade Organization (WTO) Sanitary and Phytosanitary (SPS) Agreement**. After years of frustrating discussion, they took the issue to the WTO dispute resolution board.

Countries generally work to avoid advancing issues to the WTO dispute resolution process, which is expensive, time consuming, and unpredictable. The United States negotiated with the EU to change the policy before seeking WTO dispute resolution.

In 1999 the WTO ruled in favor of the United States and awarded them $117 million in trade sanctions. Beef industry leaders urged the office of the **U.S. Trade Representative (USTR)** to impose the sanctions hoping it would cause European exporters to pressure their governments to back down.

The EU refused to discontinue the ban even though their technical review committees found it to be without basis. They literally dared the United States to invoke the WTO-endorsed sanctions because they were holding in abeyance about $4 billion in WTO-awarded sanctions from their successful dispute with the United States on U.S. taxation of foreign sales corporations.

This discussion topic involves beef industry leaders. They have run out of patience because the United States hasn't invoked the WTO-decreed retributions on the EU. Calling themselves the Beef Industry Coalition (Group 1), they have been joined by the American Meat Institute, the American Farm Bureau, the National Cattlemen's Beef Association, and several purebred breed associations. Group 1 has requested a meeting with U.S. trade officials to present their case. The request has been granted.

The meeting will bring together the Beef Industry Coalition and officials from the **United States Department of Agriculture (USDA)**, the office of the USTR, and the Joint Congressional Committee on Agriculture.

Discussion Strategy

The discussion participants should be divided into four groups as follows:

Group 1 represents the Beef Industry Coalition. It will chair the meeting. It supports invoking the sanctions on the EU.

Group 2 is the USTR. It operates out of the office of the President and is the lead organization on all U.S. international trade issues. It supports a watch and wait approach that avoids confrontation with the EU, a U.S. ally on other issues, partly because it has not yet invoked the $4 billion in WTO-decreed sanctions on the United States.

Group 3 represents the USDA. It is caught between the USTR and the Beef Industry Coalition, whose members cooperate in their disease-control efforts and programs to expand international trade. The USDA would have to prepare and endorse health certifications for exported beef if the EU decides to accept it.

Group 4 represents a delegation from the Joint Congressional Committee on Agriculture. Several of the members are from beef states and are up for reelection. This group must weigh the merits of the discussions and prepare a recommendation for the Joint Congressional Committee on Agriculture.

Each group should meet, choose a spokesperson and an advisor to present their arguments, outline their case, and prepare a fifteen-minute presentation for a meeting of all groups. The spokespersons and advisors from the four groups will assemble for the upcoming meeting before an audience comprised of the remainder of attendees.

Before the meeting begins, two participants should be designated reporters. One is from the *Washington Post* and the other is from the *Des Moines Register*. They must meet a six-hour deadline for written stories about the meeting.

The discussion leaders will look on at the group meetings and insist on timely closure. They will also force a timely conclusion to each presentation at the joint meeting.

At the next session, the representatives from the Joint Congressional Committee on Agriculture (Group 4) will present their report and recommendation to the Congress. Then the newspaper reporters will read their stories.

At the conclusion, forty-five minutes will be allowed for instructor critiques and closing discussions.

Discussion Topic 2: Food-Safety Concerns in Integrated Agriculture

The Issue

Increasing public concern about the safety of the U.S. food supply has caused special interest groups and the media to declare a food-safety crisis. They claim the breakdown is due to intensive livestock production systems, confinement operations, and automation of slaughtering processes.

Proponents of the breakdown argument have formed an organization (Group 1) called Citizens for Food Safety Advocacy (CFSA). Along with animal welfare groups and environmental groups, they contend that large livestock operations mistreat animals, destroy the environment, and contaminate the food supply. They are lobbying the House Committee on Agriculture to develop national legislation that limits animal concentrations, both the numbers of animals per farm and the number of farms per square mile. They insist such legislation is essential to preserve rural ecosystems, reestablish small farm lifestyles, and save the lives of the approximately five thousand citizens who succumb to food poisoning each year.

CFSA says industrialization and mass production in livestock production and processing has caused an epidemic of food-poisoning outbreaks. They quote data that says each year 76 million people experience vomiting and diarrhea and 325,000 patients require hospitalization for food-borne illnesses that cost the nation $34 billion in medical costs.

They say that since the 1980s ***E. coli*** **O157:H7** and ***Listeria monocytogenes*** have been added to the existing list of food-borne infections. They argue that veterinary and animal science textbooks report that animals raised in confinement experience stress-induced infectious diseases far in excess of livestock grazing on pastures. They insist that legislation is the only means to restore sanity to U.S. agriculture, increase food safety by reducing livestock infections, and preserve the work ethic and family values associated with small farms.

Not surprisingly, this proposal has encountered considerable resistance from corporate agriculture represented by the Association for Integrated Agricultural Interests (AIAI) (Group 2). They contend that the proposed legislation would triple the cost of food, damage U.S. export markets, and have minimal effects on food-borne illnesses. Food industry spokespersons say the alleged increase in food poisoning results from advancing diagnostic technology, increased disease reporting, and media hype. They contend that most food-borne disease is preventable by proper cooking and food handling. They say that human gastrointestinal tracts carry levels of pathogenic organisms comparable to those of animals. They insist the key to food safety is the personal hygiene of food handlers and kitchen workers and thorough cooking of foods. Group 2 alleges that increased incidence is an artifact of increasing surveillance and reporting.

Other agricultural groups, like the National Farm Bureau (Group 3), say their membership is divided in their views on the subject. They say that combining animal welfare, the environment, and food safety into a single issue adds unnecessary complexity. They would like the issue to be narrowed to food safety and to be reviewed by expert committees before any legislation is considered.

The **U.S. Department of Agriculture (USDA)** (Group 4) contends that the issue would be better resolved by increasing the budget of the Department of Agriculture to provide more inspectors at U.S. packing plants and ports through which tons of contaminated fruits and vegetables, fertilized abroad with human waste, enter the country annually.

Many state and federal legislators feel there is inadequate scientific evidence to support the CFSA claims and wish to postpone action until the subject can be researched by academic and government scientists.

A 1997 report entitled *Food Safety from Farm to Table*, a joint report of the **Food and Drug Administration (FDA)**, the USDA, the **Environmental Protection Agency (EPA)**, and the **National Center for Disease Control (CDC)**, outlined the complexity of the issue. It concluded there was a need for enhanced surveillance and inspections, better compliance with existing regulations, improved response capacity, additional **risk assessments**, more public education, and further research. The report stated that some food-borne diseases have been reduced by pasteurization of milk, and **botulism** has been virtually eliminated by advances in canning technology. As detection technology has advanced, other diseases, such as food-borne ***E. coli* O157:H7** that can cause fatal renal failure in some patients, ***Listeria***, and strains of ***Salmonella*** and ***Staphylococci*** that are resistant to multiple antimicrobial agents, have been detected and reported with increasing frequency.

The 1997 report concluded that in the animal health arena, newer diagnostic procedures and laboratory expertise, active surveillance, prompt epidemiological investigations, and close partnerships among academia, industry, and regulatory agencies are all necessary to aid in the prevention of food-borne illnesses. It also concluded that basic education, communication of risks, and prevention strategies for the general public are critical to food safety.

Many concerns about food-safety hazards associated with integrated livestock enterprises surfaced in preliminary discussions. Some experts say the problem is not on the farm or in the packing plants but in kitchens, where unsanitary food-handling practices and improper cooking procedures prevail. Others assert the most practical solution is to require the irradiation of meat, poultry, and dairy products following the example of the highly successful and initially resisted practice of pasteurizing milk.

Discussion Strategy

The participants should be divided into five groups as follows:

Group 1 represents the CFSA. They support the proposal and urge immediate legislative action.

Group 2 represents the Association for Integrated Agricultural Interests (AIAI). They represent the interests of livestock producers and processors and support further study of the matter.

Group 3 represents the National Farm Bureau. They are relatively ambivalent about the issue and do not place it among their legislative priorities.

Group 4 represents the USDA's **Food Safety and Inspection Service (FSIS)**. They say budget increases are the solution.

Group 5 represents the Joint Congressional Committee on Agriculture. Several of their members are from states with integrated beef, dairy, poultry, or swine industries. Some are up for reelection. This group must weigh the merits of the discussions and prepare a recommendation for a presentation to the next meeting of the Joint Committee.

Each group should meet, choose a spokesperson and an advisor to present their arguments, and prepare their case and a fifteen-minute presentation at the meeting of all groups.

The spokespersons and advisors from the five groups will assemble for the meeting before an audience comprised of all attendees. Two attendees should be designated reporters from the *Denver Post* who must meet a six-hour deadline for a 300-word story on the meeting.

The discussion leaders will observe each group's preparatory meetings and insist on timely conclusions. They will also force timely conclusions of each group's presentation at the joint meeting. After the CFSA, the AIAI, the National Farm Bureau, and the FSIS have made their presentations the instructors will allow twenty minutes for audience questions.

At the next session, the representatives from the Joint Congressional Committee on Agriculture will present their recommendations to Congress. Then the *Denver Post* reporters will read their stories.

At the conclusion, forty-five minutes will be allowed for critiques by discussion leaders, final comments, and a discussion of national policies that could address the issue.

Discussion Topic 3: Animal Welfare Policies as Exclusionary Factors

The Issue

Country A is an exporter of livestock products. They have been told by a large trading bloc (Trading Bloc B) that consumers in the bloc's member countries are upset about abuse of animals in Country A. The countries of Trading Bloc B are major importers of livestock products from Country A.

The alleged practices were reported by animal rights groups from Trading Bloc B. Their members had traveled in Country A. The complaints include confinement of laying hens in individual small cages; crowding of chickens in broiler houses; confinement of sows in farrowing pens; crowding of feeder pigs; housing of cows in tiny stalls and crowding them in pens and walkways awaiting milking; herding beef cattle through chutes with electric stock prods; and crowding feedlot cattle in manure-littered pens.

The chairman of the Standing Veterinary Committee of Trading Bloc B sent a letter to the **Chief Veterinary Officer (CVO)** of Country A. The letter says officials of Trading Bloc B are sensitive to the concerns of consumers and feel they must respond to these animal-rights issues which also affect food safety. The letter says Bloc B countries make every effort to adhere to the principles of the **World Trade Organization (WTO) Sanitary and Phytosanitary (SPS) Agreement** and to abide by international standards. Accordingly, they expect Country A to do the same.

The letter indicates that unless Country A takes responsible corrective action and passes appropriate legislation within two years, the countries of Trading Bloc B may be forced to discontinue importing milk, cheese, poultry, eggs, beef, and pork from County A.

The letter requests a meeting, within six months, of veterinary officials of Trading Bloc B with Country A's CVO and staff to discuss their plans for addressing the issue.

Discussion Strategy

The participants should be divided into four groups as follows:

Group 1 represents food-safety regulators from Country A and national food-safety organizations. They are charged with preparing a response to the food-safety comment. They must decide if their response should indicate that no legitimate food-safety issues are involved; if they can present scientific findings to show there is no such relationship; if they want to develop recommendations for proposed quality-assurance and quality-management guidelines to address the complaint; or if they should outline legislative initiatives they deem necessary.

Group 2 represents Country A's CVO and staff. They will develop strategies and positions for the proposed meeting. They must decide which livestock producers and processor groups they will ask to present position statements and attend the meeting. They must decide which parts of the letter require action or if they should say there is no legitimate basis to the allegations.

Group 3 represents the high-level officials of Country A's department of agriculture. They have seen the letter and believe that they, and not the CVO and staff, should oversee the issue, respond to the correspondence, and meet with officials of Trading Bloc B. They feel they should represent Country A, because the delegation from Trading Bloc B will undoubtedly include the secretaries of agriculture from some member countries. Protocol indicates they should have discussions with officials of comparable level. They will prepare a letter to the CVO of Country A, which will be copied to the chairman of the Standing Veterinary Committee of Trading Bloc B.

Group 4 represents the National Trade Office, a unit within the administrative branch of Country A's national government. They have also heard of the letter, and they will meet to decide if possibly neither the department of agriculture nor the CVO are of high enough level in the national government to address this diplomatically sensitive international issue. Some National

Trade Office officials believe they should prepare a response for presentation at the proposed meeting. They would, however, need extensive briefing from agricultural and veterinary officials.

Each group should choose a spokesperson and advisor. They should meet for an hour to prepare their cases or draft their letters then present them in fifteen minutes to a meeting of all attendees. The discussion leader(s) will time each group's presentation and allow twenty minutes for questions after the four groups have reported.

Then the spokespersons and advisors from all four groups will meet collectively at a twenty-minute session chaired by a "Secretary of State" elected by the participants. Everyone will watch as the Secretary of State hears the arguments of each group and takes notes in preparation for an administrative decision. The Secretary must consider Country A's representation with the delegation from Trading Bloc B and issue assignments to appropriate agencies to prepare briefing papers in preparation for the initial meeting. The Secretary of State's report can be presented at the next session.

Finally, forty-five minutes will be allowed for critiques and closing questions.

Discussion Topic 4: Russian Importations of U.S. Poultry

The Issue

The United States exports approximately 700,000 tons of poultry meat to Russia each year. From time to time, Russia threatens to discontinue importations.

In October 2001, Russia temporarily shut off imports of poultry meat from Florida ports because human **anthrax** was reported near Miami. This produced an uproar among exporters who indicated that products shipped from Florida ports are raised and processed in other states. The Russians backed off when U.S. officials convinced them that poultry meat posed negligible risk of carrying anthrax and transmitting it to people.

Shortly thereafter, Russia again shut off U.S. poultry exports for other reasons. Exports were resumed in late 2002 but the details of the agreement were unknown, and additional Russian restrictions on U.S. and European meat products loomed on the horizon.

The 2001-2002 issues caused academicians, poultry scientists, and diagnostic workers to examine the Russian sanitary requirements on U.S. poultry meat. They found that veterinary inspectors, employed by the **U.S. Food Safety and Inspection Service (FSIS)** in packing plants, were signing certificates containing considerable amounts of questionable and irrelevant information.

The certificates included statements that the United States is free from **foot-and-mouth disease (FMD)** and **African swine fever** and that the poultry meat originates from counties that are free of six avian diseases. Several of these diseases are considered globally ubiquitous and widespread in the United States, where vaccination is practiced. The avian diseases involved are **psittacosis, Newcastle disease, highly pathogenic avian influenza (HPAI), paramyxovirus infection, avian encephalomyelitis, and infectious laryngotracheitis (ILT)**.

The topic arose during discussions at a combined meeting of the **U.S. Animal Health Association (USAHA)** and the **American Association of Veterinary Laboratory Diagnosticians (AAVLD)**.

A self-appointed committee, calling themselves the Conscience of American Animal Health Reporting Systems (CAAHRS), decided to examine the poultry certifications and hold a half-day session on the subject. They received permission to hold a symposium at the meeting of the Committee on Animal Health Information Systems at the next USAHA meeting.

Members of CAAHRS volunteered to pursue various portions of the issue. They volunteered to prepare position statements from involved organizations and present them as proposed USAHA resolutions.

Discussion Strategy

The participants should be divided into four groups. Each group will prepare a presentation for the session at the USAHA-AAVLD Meeting.

Group 1, the history group, agreed to review the history of the Russian poultry export certificate. They found differences of opinion about its background. They located a detailed anonymous report written in 1996, called the *Russian Poultry Embargoes* (see below). They mailed it to all CAAHRS members and agreed to prepare a background statement and possibly a resolution that the USDA should convene a committee to review the process by which U.S. export certificates for livestock commodities are developed.

Group 2 agreed to outline the position of the American Association of Federal Veterinarians (AAFV), whose membership includes employees of the Food Safety and Inspection Service (FSIS) working as **Inspectors in Charge (IIC)** in poultry packing plants and signing the certificates. They found that the AAFV was unable to discuss the issue, due to a pending settlement of a lawsuit claiming their members had been forced to sign certifications without knowledge of the health status of flocks supplying poultry for export. They found individual food inspectors who had been ordered to sign the certificates despite minimal information. Group 2 tentatively decided to resolve that no further export certificates be endorsed until a valid national animal health reporting system is developed.

Group 3, the FSIS group, agreed to present the official position of that agency. Along with representatives of the USDA **Foreign Agricultural Service (FAS)**, the FSIS had negotiated the conditions in the certificate. However, the FSIS also refused to supply information due to a court order not to discuss it. In light of the agency's inability to comment, they agreed to study the paper provided by the history group and develop an unofficial position for presentation. Group 3 has tentatively decided to resolve that all export certificates for livestock commodities be reviewed within 18 months.

Group 4, the industry group, was charged to consult with the poultry industry to determine their feelings on the issue. Industry spokespersons told them poultry was currently being exported and to let a sleeping dog lie. In light of the industry's unwillingness to comment, Group 4 also studied the history group's paper. They developed a fictional position for discussion purposes only. They decided to represent industries' position of no action. They suggest addressing each request for export certificates on their individual merits and on the estimated value of the potential market.

The members of CAAHRS were frustrated by the lack of cooperation and the apparent secrecy surrounding the issue but decided to proceed with the symposium.

After studying the attached report and talking informally with many people, each group developed a position statement in the form of a resolution for presentation at the meeting of the USAHA Committee on Animal Health Information Systems. As the time for the meeting approached, they recommended each group have a final discussion to refine their positions.

To accomplish this, the groups should meet separately to develop positions. After thirty minutes, each should choose a spokesperson and advisor to present their position to the attendees, which will represent the Committee on Animal Health Information Systems.

After the group meetings, the participants should elect two representatives who will prepare fifteen-minute invited speeches. One speaker will address the AAFV. The other will talk to a combined meeting of the American Association of Avian Pathologists and the poultry producer organizations. Both speeches must be presented to the next session. Participants should also elect an Assistant Secretary of Agriculture who will attend the committee meeting, evaluate the presentations, and prepare a fifteen-minute USDA recommendation for the Senate Committee on Agriculture.

Participants will then attend the meeting of the USAHA Committee on Animal Health Information Systems. The discussion leaders will limit groups' presentations to twenty minutes and allow twenty minutes for audience questions after the four groups have reported to the Committee on Animal Health Information Systems.

After all resolutions have been presented and the assistant secretary has made a recommendation, participants will vote yes or no on each proposed resolution.

Immediately following the speeches, there will be a twenty-minute question and answer session for all participants. Then forty-five minutes will be allowed for critiques and closing questions.

Attachment: Russian Poultry Embargoes

In 1993, Russian officials indicated unhappiness with U.S. poultry certification procedures, temporarily discontinued importing poultry, and resumed when U.S. officials agreed to certify that exported poultry came from states free of certain diseases.

In 1995, a threatened embargo was based on the contention that U.S. products did not fulfill Russian sanitary measures outlined in the *1993 Veterinary Certificate for Poultry Exported into the Russian Federation*. Some U.S. officials felt the embargo was intended to protect Russia's poultry industry from U.S. competition.

In the Russian view, U.S. plants were not fulfilling their import requirements, poor-quality shipments were being received, and requests to rectify the situation were ignored. In 1995 and 1996, the Russians indicated that U.S. certifications did not accurately reflect the health status of source flocks or adequately certify product freedom from contamination with ***Salmonella*** bacteria or residues of hormones, antibiotics, pesticides, and heavy metals. The Russian position emanated from their tradition of strict controls and a continuous paper trail documenting required tests and inspections by full-time employees of national governments. Conversely, U.S. procedures included:

- Federally supervised and company-implemented quality-control programs
- Private laboratories for product testing and residue analyses
- Certifications by private or company veterinarians
- A national residue program based on statistical sampling

The Russians were concerned about apparent conflicts of interest in the U.S. system and were reluctant to recognize privatized regulatory oversight or quality control.

Throughout the 1990s, declining Russian poultry production was supplemented by U.S. imports of legs, thighs, and pulverized mechanically de-boned meat (MDM). U.S. legs and thighs were of higher quality and priced 40% lower than domestic products. The MDM is scraped from backs and frames after white meat is removed and can contain *Salmonella*. In Russia, it was sold at outdoor markets without admonitions that cooking is required and was sometimes eaten raw.

In April 1993, USDA and Russian veterinary officials agreed upon the health certificate. It contained language uncomfortable to U.S. officials. Russian negotiators offered verbal assurances that standard U.S. procedures fulfilled the spirit of the agreement.

The certificate stated that the meat was derived from clinically healthy birds grown in states free during the past six months from **psittacosis, Newcastle disease**, influenza, **paramxyovirus infection**, **avian encephalomyelitis**, and **infectious laryngotracheitis (ILT)**, and that the exporting country is free from **African swine fever** and **foot-and-mouth disease (FMD).** It stated that the meat is fit for human consumption and shows no evidence of infection with *Salmonella* or other bacterial infection and does not contain residues of hormonal substances, antibiotics, or **insectoacaricides.**

For several years, these certificates were signed by FSIS IICs and were accepted by Russian officials as evidence of product soundness with respect to animal and human health. Some IICs refused to sign them because they lacked personal knowledge or written certifications that the states of origin were free of the six diseases. Because of this, some certificates were signed in Washington, D.C.

The FSIS relied on the **Animal and Plant Health Inspection Service (APHIS)** to report national or state changes in poultry health status regarding the six diseases. However, APHIS had no formal surveillance program and had to base its assumptions on lack of reports from state authorities who relied on industry officials or diagnostic laboratories.

In the spring of 1995, Georgia and South Carolina reported ILT outbreaks. When APHIS reported this, the FSIS instructed IICs not to sign export certificates for poultry from those states. Their industry and animal health officials responded angrily. They said

- ILT was widespread in the United States
- Vaccination with **modified-live-virus (MLV)** vaccines was common
- MLV-induced disease could not be routinely differentiated from naturally acquired clinical infections with pathogenic ILT strains
- The reported outbreaks were caused by vaccine
- The USDA was penalizing them for honestly reporting disease that was widespread in the United States and unequally reported by other states

At a meeting in Paris in May 1995, APHIS officials convinced the Russians that the reported ILT was of vaccine origin. By mutual consent the certificate was changed to read that counties, rather than states, are free of **virulent** field strains of ILT.

In 1995, the revised certificate read "the meat originates from premises in a county free from, and not adjacent to, a county infected with ILT during the last six months." Shipments were resumed. These events revived the feeling that the Russian poultry meat-import requirements lacked a scientific basis.

In early 1996, the Russians suddenly discontinued importations of U.S. poultry meat. After several days of discussions, on February 22, 1996, U.S. and Russian veterinary officials agreed in principle on a poultry health-monitoring system proposed by a U.S. state-federal industry group. The plan included individual flock health inspection certificates on flocks slaughtered each week in plants exporting to Russia. These reports, endorsed by federally **accredited veterinarians**, certified that the flock is clinically healthy. They were submitted to IICs at federally inspected processing plants. States exporting poultry to Russia were to require that the six diseases become reportable. Upon receipt of reports of their diagnosis, the FSIS was to direct IICs to discontinue endorsing certificates for poultry from that state.

The notifiable diseases are **psittacosis**, exotic **Newcastle disease**, **highly pathogenic avian influenza (HPAI)**, **paramyxovirus infections** other than Newcastle disease, **infectious encephalomyelitis (avian encephalomyelitis)**, and non-vaccine-induced **infectious laryngotracheitis (ILT)**.

Annual comprehensive epidemiologic reports were to be prepared by state veterinarians and submitted through USDA **Area Veterinarians in Charge (AVICs)** to APHIS for compilation and forwarding to Russian officials. These reports would list, by species, all avian diseases diagnosed in each state in the past calendar year. Chief State Veterinarians, in consultation with AVICs, were to conduct quarterly reviews of each poultry company within their jurisdiction supplying Russia. This would ensure that individual flock health certificates are signed by accredited veterinarians and that appropriate documentation procedures are followed.

After agreeing on poultry health reporting, the 1996 discussions turned to human health issues. They were farthest apart on Russian requests to certify absence of all types of ***Salmonella***. Trade resumed after high-level negotiations. The certificate that resulted, however, left technical experts on both sides feeling uncomfortable. They raised legitimate questions about the reporting, processing, and inspection methods employed to assure recipient countries that poultry exports meet their sanitary requirements.

Russia held the upper hand in these negotiations because the United States wanted to sell chicken, and Russia was unbound by the constraints of the WTO SPS Agreement. If Russia had been signatory to that agreement, the scientific basis of their measures could have been challenged and risk assessments required.

After somewhat contentious negotiations in 1996, trade was resumed using the certificate described above. But in 2001 Russia again shut off U.S. poultry exports for similar reasons. Exports were resumed in late 2002, but the details of the agreement were not widely publicized.

Discussion Topic 5: **The World Trade Organization (WTO)** and National Sovereignty

The Issue

Within many countries there are interests opposed to the concept of **globalization** and the involvement of those countries in the WTO and foreign trading blocs. This discussion topic addresses a potential scenario.

A group of U.S. livestock-exporting states are initiating a movement to develop a bloc of U.S. WTO-Independent States (USWTOIS). The group is led by state departments of agriculture under pressure from livestock producer groups objecting to compulsory animal identification (ID) and the proposed **national animal health reporting system (NAHRS)**. They also object to the disease reporting requirements of the **Office International des Epizooties (OIE)**, which they feel foster questionable claims of disease-free status by some countries.

USWTOIS says the United States has subverted its national sovereignty to the WTO and international politics. They feel the WTO supports trade measures of a lowest common denominator that are unfair to developed countries and set the stage for incursions by **exotic diseases**.

USWTOIS plans to work in cooperation with milk, poultry, and meat processors to conduct independent trade negotiations to export livestock and foods without bureaucratic impediments imposed by the **United States Department of Agriculture (USDA)** and other government agencies. They also hope to develop interstate regulations and policies that protect the livestock populations of their states from exotic diseases that could enter the country under USDA policies.

Discussion Strategy

Participants should be divided into four groups as follows:

Group 1 represents the directors of agriculture of the USWTOIS member states. They will meet to prepare strategies for import-export policies and legislative initiatives to break the shackles of the federal bureaucracy. They have received permission to present their proposals at the annual meeting of the **U.S. Animal Health Association (USAHA)**. Many commissioners of agriculture who support the proposal say they will stand firm only if the USAHA approves a resolution urging them to proceed.

The USAHA has announced a two-hour session at its meeting for proponents and opponents to present arguments that will be considered by association directors if any standing committee of the association presents a resolution.

Group 2 represents members of a labor union that has always opposed globalization and the free-trade movement because it causes loss of U.S. jobs due to competition from countries where salaries are low. They oppose importations from countries that utilize child labor and the movement of U.S. corporations to countries where labor is cheap. This group has sponsored protests at several WTO meetings.

Group 3 represents **Chief Veterinary Officers (CVOs)** of states supporting the USWTOIS proposal. While reluctant to argue with commissioners of agriculture who are their supervisors, these CVOs feel the initiative is divisive and ill advised. They say it will lead to chaos in U.S. livestock health and export programs and cause loss of foreign markets. They will meet to develop strategies to convince the secessionist states of the impracticality of the proposal.

Group 4 represents officials of the USDA's **Animal and Plant Health Inspection Service (APHIS) and Food Safety and Inspection Service (FSIS).** They want to convince supporters of USWTOIS that their federal agencies have legal authority for international trade.

Group 4 says the USDA alone can develop sanitary measures for imports and exports and negotiate the content of health certificates that their employees sign. They believe the USWTOIS proposal is impractical and perhaps unconstitutional. The USDA has cautiously supported compulsory animal ID and an NAHRS. Group 4 has the support of the National Trade Office, which is a branch of the federal government that feels the idea is possibly illegal and counterproductive to the national image and the country's international credibility. They have consulted with government attorneys who state the constitution grants the federal government full authority over international commerce and laws delegate this authority to the USDA, the **Food and Drug Administration (FDA)**, and other federal agencies. But the lawyers say authority for commerce within and between states is relegated to the states. They hedge this interpretation by saying the USDA usually permits states rights to prevail in health matters. They hesitate to challenge states appearing to overstep their authority because of flexible interpretation of constitutional verbiage.

Each group should choose a spokesperson and advisor to present their arguments, meet to prepare their case, and present their case in fifteen minutes to the group that will represent USAHA members attending the special session. The group as a whole should elect five silent adjudicators who are not already spokespersons or advisors for groups 1–4, but who represent the USAHA Executive Board, which has veto authority over proposed resolutions.

The discussion leader(s) will time each presentation and allow twenty minutes for audience questions after the four groups have reported.

The discussion leader will then announce that of thirty-two USAHA standing committees, one has submitted a resolution recommending support of the USWTOIS movement and one has submitted a resolution requesting that the organization oppose it. The remaining thirty committees were silent on the issue.

During a fifteen-minute break, the adjudicators from the USAHA Executive Board will prepare their decision. The attendees should select two official spokespersons who will witness all proceedings and prepare fifteen-minute speeches. Speaker #1's talk is for the annual meeting of the labor union, and Speaker #2's speech is for the **American Veterinary Medical Association (AVMA)**. They should also select two reporters who will attend all sessions and prepare, without mutual consultation and on deadline, 200-word news articles. The two newspaper articles should be distributed at the next session after the speeches have been delivered.

Both speeches will be presented at the next session. Following the two fifteen minute talks, there will be a twenty-minute question and answer session for all. Then, twenty minutes will be allowed for instructor critiques and closing questions.

Discussion Topic 6: **Bovine Spongiform Encephalopathy (BSE)** and the **Precautionary Principle**

The Issue

The precautionary principle permits regulatory actions where scientific knowledge is uncertain or debatable if officials believe that human or livestock health will be protected by preventive actions based on suspicions of risk.

The uncertainty surrounding the manner of spread of BSE has caused apparent violations of the **World Trade Organization (WTO) Sanitary and Phytosanitary (SPS) Principles** regarding the need for a scientific basis for import measures. This rekindled debates that have plagued the **General Agreement on Tariffs and Trade (GATT)** and the WTO for years.

Discussion Strategy

The attendees should be divided into two groups that represent strongly opposing views on the precautionary principle as follows:

Group 1 represents several food-safety, environmental, labor, and consumer groups. They espouse the position that the interests of the United States would best be served by abandoning support of the WTO provision that **sanitary measures** be based upon sound science. They suggest adopting a policy of restricting imports based on suspicion of risk. This contrasts with the prevailing U.S. position that widespread application of precautionary principles permits uncontrolled use of sanitary measures as artificial trade barriers, abuses the concept of free trade, and violates the principles of the WTO SPS Agreement.

Members of Group 1 say their position has widespread bipartisan support on Capitol Hill and among the people. They hold that U.S. insistence that import measures be based on sound science is an error because of:

- Rapid advances in science
- Constant conflict and turf wars within the scientific and academic communities
- Incomplete understanding of many long-studied diseases
- Traditions in the science community of continually saying further work is needed before conclusions can be drawn

- Conflicts of interest resulting from big business sponsorship of allegedly independent research projects

They claim the **European Union (EU)** and some the world's greatest scientific minds have traditionally supported the precautionary principle. They say that it is ridiculous to aggravate our European allies on this questionable issue.

Group 1 has requested that the Administration alter their position. They were told to present their arguments to the Office of Strategic Initiatives, which develops presidential positions after reviewing historical data, consulting experts, and monitoring public opinion.

Group 2 represents officials of the **Food and Drug Administration (FDA)** and the **U.S. Department of Agriculture (USDA)**. The USDA group includes officials from the **Animal and Plant Health Inspection Service (APHIS)**, the **Food Safety and Inspection Service (FSIS)**, and the **Foreign Agricultural Service (FAS)**. These agencies have negotiated mutually acceptable import-export requirements with the EU and its member countries. They have joined together to support the position of the Uruguay Round of the GATT. The GATT consensus, despite EU objections, was that trade measures must have a scientific basis. Without science-based requirements they say the world will return to the pre-GATT situation of uncontrolled protective quotas, tariffs, and **technical barriers to trade (TBT)**. These barriers squelch productivity, encourage inefficiency, cause economic chaos based on non-competitiveness and protectionist sanitary measures, and contribute to global starvation. They say use of precautionary principles permits total politicization of trade policies.

Members of Group 2 admit that the United States invoked precautionary measures by banning feeding of ruminant offal to livestock and by prohibiting U.S. citizens from donating blood if they spent over six months in the United Kingdom. They say these measures were based on established risk-assessment procedures and were necessary to protect from BSE and its side effects in the face of extraordinary uncertainty. They say this was an unusual situation and not an endorsement for general application of the flawed precautionary principle.

The Office of Strategic Initiatives has scheduled a meeting with supporters of the precautionary principle (Group 1) and USDA and FDA officials (Group 2). They will allow spokespersons from each group thirty minutes to present their case.

Each group should choose a spokesperson and advisor to present their arguments and meet to prepare their case. The discussion leader will then appoint two newspaper reporters who will attend all sessions and prepare, without mutual consultation, 200-word news articles to be distributed the following day. Attendees should elect two official spokespersons who will witness all proceedings and prepare fifteen-minute invited speeches summarizing the presentations. Both speeches must be presented to all at the next meeting.

After a break, the spokespersons will meet with the Director and Assistant Director of the Office of Strategic Initiatives (selected by attendees) and present their arguments with everyone observing. The Director and Assistant Director of the Office of Strategic Initiatives will have thirty minutes to prepare a decision for presentation. Then the selected speakers will summarize the proceedings.

Following the two talks there will be a twenty-minute question and answer session for all participants. Time should be allowed for critiques and closing questions.

Discussion Topic 7: Mexican Cattle and Tuberculosis (TB) Control

The Issue

In 1993, the USDA published a proposed regulation aimed at expediting cattle trade between Mexico and the United States as part of the **North American Free Trade Agreement (NAFTA).** The proposal tightened TB requirements on live cattle moving from Mexico to the United States. It recommended that Arizona, California, New Mexico, and Texas provide increased border security, more inspections, increased control of movement of Mexican cattle, and increased control over quarantined feedlots within their borders.

The border states objected. They presented a counter proposal saying Mexican officials should take additional responsibility for controlling TB in their country. They also proposed that Mexico be permitted to export cattle into the United States only from TB-free areas. The Joint Mexican-U.S. TB Working Group was created to provide leadership for Mexican control efforts.

The U.S. government pressured Mexico to take positive action and they did. Nonetheless, TB-infected cattle of Mexican origin continued to appear in U.S. slaughterhouses. USDA officials, eager to finalize the TB-eradication program continued pressuring Mexico to take firmer local control efforts or stop exporting live cattle to the United States. More than a decade later the situation resurfaced.

Discussion Strategy

The attendees should be divided into four groups as follows:

Group 1 represents trade officials who have been charged to increase trade with Canada and Mexico to advance the goals of the NAFTA. As they attempt to sell U.S. manufactured goods and high-tech items in Mexico, U.S. trade officials are continually told that trade is a two-way street. The Mexican officials assert that cattle moving to U.S. feedlots and stocker operations are placed under excessive restrictions because Mexico has TB. They are told this is a guise to impose protectionist measures.

U.S. trade officials are under pressure from the administration to resolve this controversy. They have tried unsuccessfully to persuade the **Animal and Plant Health Inspection Service (APHIS)** to reduce restrictions on Mexican cattle so the United States can increase market access for other products south of the border.

Group 2 represents APHIS officials who have been frustrated in efforts to eradicate TB. Each year around 200 cases of TB are identified in slaughterhouses throughout the United States. Many of these are known to originate in Mexico. Others are suspected of being of Mexican origin but lack positive identification. Group 2 feels interstate movement of Mexican cattle is a large part of the problem. They are considering new regulations requiring more inspections, restricting Mexican-origin cattle from moving within states, and increased control over feedlots within the states.

Group 3 represents a consortium of agricultural officials from Texas, Arizona, New Mexico, and California. Officials from seven other feedlot states have joined them. Group 3 feels the USDA should do more to exclude Mexican cattle and is shirking its responsibility by expecting states to do the job. They say Mexican cattle pass through their territory and end up in over twenty states where they could spread TB.

Group 4 represents livestock dealers and feedlot operators. They are resisting the efforts of Groups 2 and 3. They say U.S. cattle are too expensive, in short supply, and unavailable when needed. They insist that border-state officials are in cahoots with U.S. livestock organizations to raise prices by excluding Mexican competition.

Group 4 says TB is really not a problem because no cows die from it, and people don't get it by eating meat from infected cattle.

The media has picked up the issue. The Secretary of Agriculture has been told to straighten it out and has scheduled a public hearing. He has invited representatives of the four concerned groups to present their cases and propose measures to address the matter.

Each group should meet to prepare a case and choose a spokesperson and advisor to present the arguments. Attendees should elect two newspaper reporters who will attend the public hearing and prepare, without mutual consultation and on deadline, 200-word news articles to be distributed to attendees the following day. Attendees can also elect speakers to summarize the public hearing for the annual meeting of the National Association of State Veterinarians and for the joint House-Senate Committee on Agriculture. Both speeches must be presented to all attendees at the next session.

All participants will attend the public meeting. The spokespersons will present their cases and answer questions from the audience.

Discussion Topic 8: Compulsory or Voluntary Disease Reporting

The Issue

Disease reporting is a major component of livestock health infrastructures. **Monitoring, surveillance and reporting (MS&R) systems** are essential for healthy livestock and to prioritize animal health research and regulatory programs. **National animal health reporting systems (NAHRS)** can credibly reflect a country's livestock health status and assure the safety of its animal products for international trade.

In most countries, disease reporting is a cooperative effort involving national, state, or provincial authorities; livestock producers and processors; and the veterinary, diagnostic, academic, and regulatory communities. Despite several attempts, the United States has never established a viable, fully participatory NAHRS.

In October 2001, an Animal Health Safeguarding Review recommended that the **United States Department of Agriculture (USDA)** clearly define its NAHRS as a cooperative, not voluntary, program for all industries and states that request USDA certification of animal products for export.

To date, the USDA has stopped short of proposing regulations requiring states to report livestock diseases. The U.S. reports to the **Office International des Epizooties (OIE)**, while reasonably accurate, are developed in an inconsistent and piecemeal fashion.

Livestock diseases have moved to center stage in international trade. The health status of exporting countries has become a key issue in measures imposed on imported livestock products. The need for an NAHRS repeatedly surfaces in trade negotiations.

Some states have resisted reporting livestock diseases based on principle. Others lack the legal authority. Some states are suspicious of the federal government's use of the information and regard public reporting as a violation of the proprietary confidentiality of producers and processors. Many state veterinarians and industry leaders resist compulsory NAHRS because they feel other countries don't accurately report and the information can be used against them. For these reasons, USDA efforts to establish an NAHRS have stalled.

On the global scene, the quality of animal disease reporting by national governments is regarded as an indicator of national credibility, a measure of each country's animal health infrastructure, and the soundness of their export certifications. Several countries are initiating compulsory NAHRS that will provide competitive advantages in the quest for market access.

A group of concerned USDA employees, state veterinarians, and diagnostic laboratory personnel has decided to act. They don't want the competitive position and international credibility of the United States to suffer.

Discussion Strategy

The attendees should be divided into four groups as follows:

Group 1 represents the concerned USDA employees, state veterinarians, and diagnostic laboratory personnel who want to do something about a U.S. NAHRS. They are preparing a presentation for the upcoming annual meeting of the **U.S. Animal Health Association (USAHA)**. They believe the country's international image is tarnished by lack of support for a credible NAHRS. When pressed by their foreign counterparts they are ashamed to admit that only about half of the states regularly submit an annual livestock health report and that the U.S. submissions to the OIE are based on lack of information rather than positive data.

Group 2 represents a consortium of veterinarians, agricultural organizations, livestock producers, and meat processors that oppose compulsory livestock disease reporting because it infringes on states' rights and proprietary confidentiality of private enterprises. They have gathered support from colleagues who fear a compulsory reporting system will have more negative than positive effects on trade. They are preparing a response to the Group 1 presentation.

Group 3 represents the USDA's NAHRS Steering Committee. The USAHA has decided to hold a symposium on the subject and has invited Group 3 to open the session with a historical update and clarification of the current status of livestock disease reporting in the United States. The NAHRS Steering Committee (Group 3) is comprised of USDA officials, academicians, laboratory diagnosticians, and industry groups. They have agreed to report, but have indicated that NAHRS is pretty much on hold because many states are unable or unwilling to participate. The steering committee had recommended that the NAHRS report the presence or absence of OIE List A and List B diseases without naming their location unless emergencies exist or regionalization efforts are needed.

Group 4 is the USAHA Board of Directors. They will attend the symposium, meet later, and determine if they should take action on the issue.

Each group should choose a spokesperson and advisor to present their case at the symposium. They should meet to prepare fifteen-minute presentations for the symposium witnessed by all attendees.

After the groups have chosen their representatives, attendees should select two newspaper reporters who will attend the symposium and prepare 200-word news articles to be distributed the following day. They should also select two spokespersons to prepare fifteen-minute invited speeches. Speaker #1's talk is for the National Association of Livestock Health Officials. Speaker #2's speech is for the National Cattlemen's Association and the National Poultry Producers Federation.

At the symposium, discussion leader(s) will moderate and time each group's presentation and allow twenty minutes for audience questions.

At the next session the board of directors will present their decision, the newspaper articles will be distributed, and the assigned speeches will be presented.

Then there will be a twenty-minute question and answer session and twenty minutes for critiques, closing questions, and summaries. Attendees who didn't participate throughout the process may be asked to present spontaneous summaries to close the exercise.

Discussion Topic 9: Pressures from Producer Organizations

The Issue

Livestock producer and processor organizations strive to represent the best interests of their members. They prepare educational materials, monitor proposed laws or regulations affecting their industries, and lobby legislators to support beneficial proposals.

Livestock health policy (LHP)-makers often receive requests for proposed policy changes that will benefit producers. They must weigh conflicting requests against the best interests of the livestock industries and the public at large.

For the **United States Department of Agriculture (USDA)** this often forces choices between protecting consumers and serving the livestock industry. Sometimes this dual mission is addressed by calling state agricultural agencies' departments of agriculture and consumer services.

In the mid 1990s, the **Animal and Plant Health Inspection Service (APHIS)** clarified its mission of protecting U.S. agriculture and added enhancement of foreign markets to its goals. This left consumer protection to the **Food Safety and Inspection Service (FSIS)**, although APHIS always considered prevention of zoonoses a major objective.

Recently, farmers have pressured USDA and APHIS to protect livestock producers from environmentalists and animal welfare advocates whose activities appear overly restrictive, irrational, destructive to small farmers, and inflationary for food prices.

Spurred on by members from agricultural states, the U.S. Senate has commissioned the National Academy of Sciences to establish a panel of experts to study effects of lobbying by industry and other interests on quality, price, and availability of livestock products.

Discussion Strategy

The attendees should be divided into five groups. Each group has been asked to testify on the issue before a National Institute of Health (NIH) panel that consists largely of academicians. The groups should be as follows:

Group 1 represents a coalition of poultry producers and processors. They recommend a complete overhaul of agricultural and food-safety regulations because they feel the federal bureaucracy is infringing on their freedom by establishing excessive, ineffective, unnecessary, and burdensome inspection and disease-control mandates.

Group 2 represents USDA officials. They present a mixed message. This is partly due to vagaries of the reorganization that moves parts of APHIS into the Department of Homeland Security to help protect against bioterrorism. It also results from the sometimes-conflicting functions of protecting both the livestock industries and consumers while enhancing trade. Some USDA officials say reorganization is essential, and others say the multiple missions are closely related and could both be successfully accomplished with adequate budgets.

Group 3 represents the cattle and swine industries. They say they are capable of meeting public expectations for safe and wholesome low-priced foods if the government would get the environmentalists and animal welfare advocates off their backs.

Group 4 represents selected environmental and animal welfare representatives. They say the livestock industries are profit driven, without public consciences, and out of control. They insist on stricter control to protect the environment and the rights of animals.

Group 5 is the NIH panel. They are attempting to prepare an agenda for their first meeting and are holding a hearing to gain insight into the items needed for the report. They have invited Groups 1–4 to participate in the hearing.

Each group will meet to prepare for the hearing, which will be attended by all. The groups have been asked for twenty-minute presentations that suggest legislative initiatives they deem necessary to benefit the public at large. Each group should choose a spokesperson and advisor to present their case and the points they considered in developing it. Then each group should meet to prepare their case and present it to Group 5, the NIH panel, while all attendees listen.

The discussion leader(s) will time each group's presentation and allow twenty minutes for audience questions after the four groups have reported.

At the next session Group 5 will present a list of issues and positions it will include in its report. Then time will be allowed for critiques and closing questions.

Discussion Topic 10: **Foot-and-Mouth Disease (FMD)** Eradication Policies

The Issue

Media coverage of the 1999-2001 British FMD outbreak alerted the world to the financial impact of and controversies surrounding its control or eradication.

Within the United States, which has been FMD-free for over sixty years, public concern has generated debate about how the country should respond when FMD appears. The issue is being aired constantly in printed media and on radio and television talk shows.

Information about FMD's potential for global spread due to increasing travel and international commerce has convinced everyone that its introduction into the United States is inevitable. Most veterinarians and USDA officials agree.

When pressed as to the best method to handle an FMD outbreak, the animal health community appears to lack a unified position. They try to avoid taking sides by explaining the complexity of the issue in incomprehensible and vague language. They appear divided and confused.

The public is becoming emotional and vocal as finger pointing increases. It seems that the less they know, the more opinionated people become. They are demanding statements from public officials, politicians facing election, and livestock health authorities in support of widely divergent viewpoints.

Individuals in a position to intelligently address FMD agree that the best bet is to prevent its introduction. They seek increased funding for border security; baggage, mail, and cargo inspections; immigration controls; disease monitoring and surveillance; animal identification; diagnostic laboratories; and research.

Experts say FMD will have long-term economic impact, cause a significant rise in food prices, and reduce the competitiveness of the United States in the global marketplace. They contend FMD is extremely contagious and difficult to diagnose because it resembles many other conditions. They add that it can spread before infected animals show characteristic symptoms and that it attacks cattle, swine, sheep, goats, and free-roaming wild species. The many different types of FMD virus complicate its control. FMD viruses are resistant to many disinfectants and environmental influences and require different, only partially effective, vaccines with short duration of immunity and limited shelf lives.

Informed, uninformed, and misinformed spokespersons seem to fall into four general categories. All are extremely vocal. The groups supporting each position represent mixed interests that differ on other issues. The groups are environmentalists, animal rights and animal welfare advocates, veterinarians, livestock producers and processors, and state and national livestock health officials.

Discussion Strategy

The participants will represent an expert panel selected to recommend policy to the **United States Department of Agriculture (USDA)** and should be divided into four groups as follows:

Group 1 says the United States should invoke the **stamping out method** and slaughter all infected and exposed animals until the disease is eradicated. They consider vaccinations a desperate action to be used as a last resort when all else fails.

Group 2 insists the disease should be ignored and permitted to run its course without intervention until all susceptible animals are either dead or immune. In their view, animals permanently disabled and suffering should be killed humanely for meat. They say this approach is humane, environmentally sound, and recognizes that FMD is part of nature's plan.

Group 3 says all cattle, swine, sheep, and goats in the country should be immediately vaccinated, at government expense, against all known FMD viruses and continually revaccinated. They say this will prevent the disease and resolve the issue.

Group 4 indicates that each outbreak should be addressed individually depending on the virus type, the species involved, and the extent of spread through the nation. Their suggested strategy requires initial test and slaughter, massive use of immuno-stimulating preparations, and vaccination only if the stamping out method appears unsuccessful. Group 4 suggests a high-level scientific decision-making body called the U.S. FMD Authority be established immediately. They say the FMD Authority should establish decision-making criteria for dealing with FMD outbreaks and should be empowered to authorize stockpiling of equipment, vaccines, test reagents, and other essential biologicals and pharmaceuticals.

Each group should meet, choose a spokesperson and an advisor to present their arguments, outline their case, and prepare a fifteen-minute presentation for a meeting of all groups.

The spokespersons and advisors from the four groups will assemble for the meeting before an audience comprised of the remaining attendees. Before the meeting begins, a reporter from both the *Washington Post* and the *St. Louis Post-Dispatch* should be designated. They must meet a six-hour deadline for a written 200–300 word story on the meeting to be presented as the final item on the session agenda.

The discussion leaders will moderate the group meetings and insist on timely closure. They will also force timely conclusion of each presentation at the joint meeting. After the groups have made their presentations, the discussion leaders will allow twenty minutes for audience questions. Then all attendees will complete a secret multiple choice ballot to select the arguments that

- Are most clearly and convincingly presented
- Are most scientifically sound
- Are in the best national interest
- Should be chosen by the USDA

During a break, the discussion leaders will tabulate the results and report to all participants. The two reporters will then read their stories, and discussion will follow.

Glossary

Accredited veterinarian—A veterinarian approved by the **United States Department of Agriculture (USDA)** to perform official functions in State-Federal Cooperative Programs under conditions outlined in 9 CFR 161.

Active immunity—A degree of acquired specific protection against a pathogenic organism, cancer cell, toxin, or other foreign substance in bodily tissues or fluids. Active immunity results from exposure or vaccination and a resultant specific recognition, processing, production, and mobilization of protective antibodies or cells programmed to carry out specific protective responses.

Adjuvant—A substance that enhances the activity of pharmaceuticals or vaccines by increasing their effectiveness or prolonging their presence in the body.

African horse sickness—A highly fatal mosquito-borne viral OIE List A disease of horses present in parts of Africa and the Middle East that attacks the respiratory or cardiovascular system. It is regarded as exotic in the Western Hemisphere.

African swine fever—A highly contagious and often fatal viral infection of swine that exists as hidden infections in wild warthogs and certain tick species in parts of Africa and occasionally spreads to Europe and the Caribbean. It is an OIE List A disease regarded as exotic in North America.

Akabane—An insect-borne viral infection of cattle; present in parts of Africa, Southeast Asia, and the Middle East and considered exotic to North America and Europe. It causes mild, usually unobserved, infections in adult cattle but, more seriously, it infects the fetus causing abortion or birth of calves with multiple congenital defects.

American Association of Veterinary Laboratory Diagnosticians (AAVLD)—An organization dedicated to the dissemination of information on the diagnosis of animal diseases and to the coordination of the diagnostic activities of regulatory, research, and service laboratories. www.aavld.org

American Veterinary Medical Association (AVMA)—The national veterinary association of the United States. Its goal is the advancing of veterinary medicine in public health, biological sciences, and agriculture. It is the authorized voice of the U.S. veterinary profession. www.avma.org

Analytes—Substances measured or detected in diagnostic tests.

Animal Agriculture Coalition—An organization of U.S. animal-industry groups working together to advise the **United States Department of Agriculture (USDA)** and encourage industry-sensitive policies, procedures, and regulations.

Animal and Plant Health Inspection Service (APHIS)—The **United States Department of Agriculture (USDA)** agency responsible for the health of animals and plants. APHIS has regulatory authority over livestock health, food safety, exotic-disease exclusion, animal welfare, and expansion of foreign markets for livestock products. www.aphis.usda.gov

Animal Health Infrastructure—The basis, permanent foundation, and cohesive guiding force for livestock health, food-safety, and international marketing programs. Infrastructures include regulatory authorities, diagnostic and inspection services, exotic-disease exclusion activities, and emergency response programs.

Anthelmintics—Compounds used to destroy parasitic worms in the intestinal tracts of animals.

Anthrax—An often fatal OIE List B zoonotic disease of livestock caused by the spore-forming toxin-producing bacterium *Bacillus anthracis*. Anthrax occurs in livestock in areas of alkaline limestone soils throughout the world. Infected animals die. The bacteria are disseminated through the body and form resistant spores when exposed to air. The spores survive for years in the environment and provide a source of infection. Human infection occurs when spores gain bodily access through broken skin, inhalation, or rarely from eating meat of animals dead of anthrax. Early treatment with antibiotics is sometimes successful.

Antibiotics—Substances produced by living organisms, or synthesized, that are harmless to mammalian cells but can kill or inhibit the growth of sensitive bacteria.

Antibodies—Specifically active immunoglobulins produced by immunocompetent cells in response to foreign substances (**antigens**) that enter the body. Antibodies circulate in the body fluids, recognize and incapacitate organisms carrying the stimulating antigen, provide a significant component of immunity, and can be measured for diagnostic purposes.

Antigen—Any molecule capable of stimulating a specific immune response. Antigens are present on viruses, bacteria, toxins, and protozoa. They are the active portions of vaccines.

Antimicrobial resistance—The property of some bacteria to be unaffected by specific antibiotics. This resistance can be natural or acquired. It is sometimes attributed to the misuse of over-the-counter or prescription antimicrobials or to the use of antibiotics in livestock.

Antimicrobials—Chemical or biological compounds, including antibiotics, produced naturally or synthesized, that exert negative effects on microbial agents such as bacteria, viruses, and fungi.

Area Veterinarian in Charge (AVIC)—A veterinary official from the **Animal and Plant Health Inspection Service (APHIS)** responsible for agency activities in a state or group of states.

Association of Official Analytic Chemists (AOAC)—A not-for-profit international organization dedicated to building worldwide confidence in analytic results by providing fit-for-purpose methods for assuring quality measurements. Also known as AOAC International. www.aoac.org

Avian encephalomyelitis—A globally distributed viral infection of the nervous system of chickens, turkeys, and many other avian species. It is usually evident only in young birds, which exhibit tremors, paralysis, and sometimes death.

Avian influenza—A highly infectious, globally distributed viral infection of commercial poultry, migratory waterfowl, and pssiticine birds. Multiple viral strains, distinguishable by serologic typing, exist in nature and tend to mutate causing changes in virulence. **Highly pathogenic avian influenza (HPAI)**, also called fowl plague, is an OIE List A disease that is exotic in the United States and many other countries.

Bacterins—Killed bacterial vaccines.

Biologicals—Products originating from living organisms, such as animals, animal cells, or animal pathogens, also called biologics. In this book, usually substances or products, such as vaccines, serums, and diagnostic reagents, used in the prevention, treatment, or diagnosis of animal disease.

Biosecurity—Combined actions undertaken to prevent transmission of biological agents, including pathogenic organisms or biological toxins, to human or animal populations by natural routes of transmission or by the intentional activity of bioterrorists.

Bluetongue—An insect-transmitted, non-contagious, sometimes fatal OIE List A disease of sheep characterized by fever, reddening and swelling of extremities, ulcerations of the mucous membranes of the mouth, and swelling and sometimes blue discoloration of the tongue. Sheep, cattle, and other ruminants are readily infected in vector-infested ecosystems within thirty-five to forty degrees of the equator, or during insect seasons elsewhere, where midges of the genus *Culiciodes* are present. Infection is unobserved in most species except sheep.

Botulism—An intoxication caused by ingestion of preformed toxins produced by the spore-forming bacterium *Clostridium botulinum* in the absence of oxygen. The potent botulism toxin causes life-threatening muscle paralysis in animals and humans.

Bovine herpes mammallitis—A herpes virus infection of cattle manifested by ulcers on the teats; can resemble lesions caused by foot-and-mouth disease.

Bovine shipping fever—A transmissible respiratory disease complex of cattle stressed by shipping, commingling, and exposure to multiple viral and bacterial infections. Affected cattle develop fever, rapid respiration, nasal discharge, and often a terminal pneumonia associated with bacteria of the genus *Pasteurella* or *Manheimia*.

Bovine spongiform encephalopathy (BSE)—An inevitably fatal OIE List B disease, also known as "mad cow disease," characterized by progressive neurological dysfunction. BSE is caused by a newly discovered class of pathogenic agents called **prions**, which are subviral in size, detectable by molecular techniques, resistant to most disinfectants and sterilization procedures, and transmitted by the ingestion of meat or certain by-products of infected cattle.

Bovine tuberculosis (TB)—A chronic infection caused by the bacterium *Mycobacterium bovis*, which principally affects cattle but occasionally infects humans. Affected individuals experience chronic respiratory disease and gradual debility. For over 50 years the **United States Department of Agriculture (USDA)** has worked to eradicate bovine TB by border controls, testing, herd quarantines, carcass inspections, and the tracing of infected animals to their origin. While formerly extensive, it is now rare in United States.

Bovine viral diarrhea—A globally ubiquitous, contagious, viral infection of cattle characterized by erosions of the gastrointestinal mucosa, sometimes called mucosal disease. Cows infected during pregnancy can abort, produce calves with congenital anomalies, or give birth to persistently infected offspring that serve as permanent sources of infection.

Brucellosis—An infection with bacteria of the genus *Brucella*. Bovine brucellosis in cows, caused by *Brucella abortus*, and porcine brucellosis, caused by *Brucella suis*, can both infect humans causing undulant fever, a chronic debilitation, muscle and joint pain, and intermittent fever. *Brucella abortus* is transmitted by the placenta and discharges of aborting cows or by the consumption of unpasteurized milk from infected cows.

Camplobacteria—A genus of bacteria, once called vibrios, that dwell in contaminated food and water and in the intestinal tract of animals, birds, and people. They are excreted in the feces and are a cause of human food-borne gastroenteritis, diarrhea, and occasionally abortion and fatal meningitis.

Cattle tick fever—An OIE List B parasitic disease that causes the rupture of red blood cells and is characterized by fever, weight loss, anemia, and jaundice. Its reservoir is in healthy carrier animals in Mexico and Central America. Transmission is by ticks. It has been eradicated from the United States, which remains free due to requirements that cattle moving northward across the southern border be dipped in tick repellents and inspected for tick infestation. Also known as bovine babesiosis, tick fever, or Texas fever (formerly called bovine piroplasmosis).

Center for Epidemiology and Animal Health (CEAH)—A **United States Department of Agriculture (USDA)** program located at Fort Collins, Colorado, that conducts epidemiological studies, interprets animal-disease monitoring and surveillance data, evaluates and plans disease-control programs, and conducts quantitative risk assessments. www.usda.aphis/vs/ceah

Center for Veterinary Biologics (CVB)—The division of the **Animal and Plant Health Inspection Service (APHIS)** charged with the evaluation, licensing, inspection, and regulation of veterinary biologicals to assure purity, potency, safety, and efficacy of vaccines and diagnostic reagents in the United States. www.aphis.usda.gov/vs/cvb

Cervids—Deer, elk, moose and other members of the family *Cervidae*.

Chief veterinary officer (CVO)—Usually a nation's highest ranking animal health official.

Chronic wasting disease (CWD)—A slow-acting transmissible spongiform encephalopathy of deer, elk, and other cervids characterized by brain lesions, excess salivation and urination, gradual weight loss, and eventually death. CWD is found among free-ranging and captive animals in Western United States and Canada.

Classical swine fever (hog cholera)—A sometimes-fatal OIE List A viral disease of swine characterized by fever and hemorrhages of the skin and internal organs. It is present in many parts of the world and is exotic to the United States since its eradication in 1978. It is similar in appearance to African swine fever, but the two are caused by different viruses.

Cloning—The production of genetically engineered identical replicas of animals.

Clostridia—A globally distributed genus of spore-forming and toxin-producing bacteria that inhabit the soil and the intestinal tracts of most animals and cause gastroenteritis in humans.

Coalition for Animal Agriculture—A loosely organized group of U.S. livestock producer and processor organizations that meets to develop positions on agricultural policy and advise the **United States Department of Agriculture (USDA).**

Code of Federal Regulations (CFR)—www.access.gpo.gov/nara

Codex Alimentarius Commission (CODEX)—A subsidiary of the **Food and Agriculture Organization (FAO)** of the United Nations. CODEX is the international body designated by the World Trade Organization to set standards for foods, food residues and contaminants, and pharmaceuticals.

Confinement livestock operations—Farming operations in which cattle, swine, or poultry are reared in close confinement as opposed to grazing freely in pastures.

Contagious bovine pleuropneumonia (CBP)—A frequently fatal OIE List A bacterial pneumonia of cattle present in parts of Africa, Asia, and the Middle East and regarded as exotic elsewhere.

Council for Agricultural Science and Technology (CAST)—An organization composed of scientific societies, corporations, and individual members that disseminates information and issues analyses to the public, the scientific community, and the media.

Creutzfeldt-Jacob disease (CJD)—A chronic, fatal, degenerative disorder of the human nervous system that occurs sporadically worldwide in approximately one out of a million people. Until 1993, when **Variant Creutzfeldt-Jacob disease (VCJD)** was recognized in England, CVD was regarded as a genetic or metabolic defect. It is now regarded as a **prion**-induced spongiform encephalopathy.

Deoxyribonucleic acid (DNA)—Sometimes called desoxyribonucleic acid, this highly stable molecule present in living cells transmits genetic information by providing templates for production or replication of new DNA or ribonucleic acid (RNA) molecules. Both DNA and RNA direct the production of proteins and form the basis of genes and chromosomes that direct hereditary processes. Laboratory procedures, called recombinant DNA technology, which involve severance of DNA strands and the insertion of new bits of DNA into the nuclei of cells, can alter the properties of organisms. Techniques for detecting the DNA of specific microorganisms are used in the diagnosis of animal diseases.

Diphtheria—An acute, contagious, sometimes fatal, human disease caused by the toxin of the bacterium *Corynebacterium diphtheriae,* which enters the bloodstream and damages the kidneys, heart, and nervous system and produces a characteristic membrane in the lining of the throat that impedes eating and breathing. Vaccination of infants has virtually eliminated diphtheria in most developed countries. Diphtheria can be transmitted by unpasteurized milk.

E. coli—A ubiquitous bacterial species of the genus *Escherichia,* with multiple subspecies, a few of which are pathogenic. *E. coli* inhabits the intestinal tract of most animals and humans and whose presence in the environment or in foods indicates fecal contamination. Some *E. coli* are extremely pathogenic for young or immunologically compromised individuals, but most are avirulent for mature healthy individuals.

E. coli **O157/H7**—A specific, highly pathogenic bacterium of the genus *Escherichia* that causes food-borne gastroenteritis, colitis, and sometimes hemolytic uremic syndrome in humans.

Embryo transfer (ET)—The implantation into donor females of fertilized ova that result from planned matings and are harvested by various methods.

Emergency Disease Guidelines—Disease-specific instructions for the recognition, diagnosis, response, control, and eradication of exotic diseases of livestock produced by the **Animal and Plant Health Inspection Service (APHIS)**; sometimes called "the red books."

Emerging diseases—Diseases that have been recently recognized or seem to be increasing in prominence, seriousness, or importance.

Endemic diseases—Diseases present and firmly established in a country or region.

Environmental Protection Agency (EPA)—www.epa.gov

Enzootic bovine leukosis (EBL)—A widely distributed OIE List B disease that is a persistent, usually inapparent, viral infection of cattle. It is caused by the bovine leukemia virus and in some high-incidence herds the cattle exhibit tumor masses that result in condemnations at slaughter. Some countries have EBL-control programs and restrict importations from infected herds or countries.

Enzootic diseases—Diseases permanently ensconced in animal populations.

Ephemeral fever—An insect-transmitted viral infection of cattle and water buffalo that causes epidemics of fever, debility, and sometimes paralysis. It occurs in parts of Australia, Africa, Asia, and the Middle East and is apparently exotic elsewhere.

Epidemiology—The study of the distribution and transmission of diseases in populations.

Epizootiology—The now defunct term for veterinary or animal epidemiology.

Equal national treatment—The principle in the **World Trade Organization (WTO) Sanitary and Phytosanitary (SPS) Agreement** that espouses nondiscrimination in application of import measures between countries where similar health conditions prevail.

Equivalency—The component of the WTO SPS Agreement indicating that signatory countries agree to acknowledge that similar levels of risk mitigation can be achieved by different methods. Examples of equivalency are the use of different disinfectants and washing techniques to achieve similar levels of sanitation, or the use of different tests to diagnose the same disease.

Etiology—The medical term for the cause of a disease; the study of causes of disease.

European Commission (EC)—The governing body of the **European Union (EU)**.

Exotic diseases—Diseases absent from a country or region; also called foreign animal diseases (FADs).

Fast track authority—The power granted to the administration to negotiate treaties and trade agreements that can be approved or disapproved, but not amended, by Congress. It gives credibility to national representatives. Also known as trade promotion authority.

Federal Register—A journal published on each regular business day by the U.S. government containing notice of decisions and rulings by government agencies; discussions of organizational matters including changing responsibilities and authorities; notices of petitions and applications filed with government agencies; and notices of investigations, meetings, and public hearings relevant to LHPs and other issues. It contains drafts, called dockets, which outline proposed rules, regulations, or international standards. This provides opportunity for public viewing and comment. www.access.gpo.gov/nara

Food and Agriculture Organization (FAO)—A branch of the United Nations that provides food and agricultural assistance to needy nations.

Food and Drug Administration (FDA)—Part of the Department of Health and Human Services. www.fda.gov

Food Animal Residue Avoidance Databank (FARAD)—A USDA-supported online decision support system and data bank that offers livestock producers, veterinarians, and other interested parties information on the availability, legal uses, dosages, and withdrawal times for drugs used on livestock. www.farad.org

Food Safety and Inspection Service (FSIS)—Part of the USDA. www.fsis.usda.gov

Foot-and-mouth disease (FMD)—An OIE List A, highly contagious, rapidly spreading, viral disease of ruminants and swine characterized by vesicle formation on the mouth and feet, lameness, and debilitation with long term economic impact on infected countries. Its control is complicated by the many different virus types, which survive many environmental influences.

Footrot—A globally ubiquitous bacterial infection of ruminants that causes swelling and necrotic interdigital ulcerations, pain, and severe lameness. It is frequently associated with *Fusobacterium necrorphorum,* but multiple bacteria are usually present.

Foreign Agricultural Service (FAS)—www.fas.usda.gov

Foreign Animal Disease Diagnostic Laboratory (FADDL)—at Plum Island, NY. www.arserrc.gov/naa/home/piadc.htm

Foreign Animal Disease Diagnosticians (FADD)—Designated, qualified veterinarians who conduct foreign animal disease (exotic disease) investigations. www.farad.org

Free Trade Area of the Americas (FTAA)—The proposed trading bloc that may expand the North American Free Trade Agreement (NAFTA) to include all countries of North and South America and the Caribbean.

General Agreement on Tariffs and Trade (GATT)—An organization that originated following World War II to reduce tariffs, quotas, and other barriers to trade. The GATT has over 100 member countries and multiple commodity agreements. Its agricultural provisions were assigned to the **World Trade Organization (WTO)** and became the WTO **Sanitary and Phytosanitary (SPS) Agreement**.

Genetically modified organisms (GMO)—Organisms produced by the transfer of nuclear material between individuals or species: includes clones, transgenic animals, plants, and microbes with genetically altered characteristics.

Glanders—An OIE List B, zoonotic bacterial disease of horses that causes fever, rapid respiration, thick nasal discharge and ulcerating nodules in the skin, respiratory passages, and internal organs and is frequently fatal. Glanders is present in parts of Asia and the Middle East. It is considered exotic elsewhere.

Globalization—The rapidly growing international movement toward integration and interdependence of economic, monetary, and governmental activities of nations that is expanding the domain of political and trade relationships and providing challenges for governments, individuals, and cultures.

Harmonization—Governmental and industry efforts to cooperatively strive for international standardization of diagnostic tests, surveillance systems, import requirements, quarantine procedures, animal identification policies, vaccine standards, and risk assessment/risk management systems as recommend by the WTO SPS Agreement.

Hazard Analysis and Critical Control Point (HACCP)—The basis of a food-safety program that focuses inspections on points in the food chain that have the highest risk of acquiring, supporting, or propagating agents responsible for food-borne illness.

Helminths—Parasitic worms including tapeworms, flukes, and nematodes.

Highly pathogenic avian influenza (HPAI) (fowl plague)—A virulent form of avian influenza, a viral disease of poultry categorized as an OIE List A disease. Most avian influenzas are milder and not classified as HPAI.

Human immunodeficiency virus (HIV)—The virus, probably of wild primate origin, that is globally endemic in human populations and causes acquired immunodeficiency syndrome (AIDS).

Identification (ID)—In animal health contexts, usually referring to animal identification systems that enable trace-back of carcasses to farm of origin.

Indemnity—Payments to compensate for losses incurred as a result of regulatory actions.

Infectious bovine rhinotracheitis (IBR)—A globally ubiquitous viral respiratory infection of cattle characterized by fever, rapid respiration, and nasal discharge. Cattle infected during pregnancy often abort. Many infected animals intermittently shed virus for prolonged periods.

Infectious laryngotracheitis (ILT)—Also called avian infectious laryngotracheitis, an OIE List B disease that is a highly contagious, acute viral respiratory disease of chickens and pheasants.

Infrastructure—The basis, permanent foundation, and cohesive guiding force for the domestic animal health programs and international agricultural activities of a country, including disease control, surveillance, border security, and diagnostic capacity.

Insectoacaricides—Chemicals that kill insects, ticks, and mites and may produce harmful residues in treated animals or the products they produce.

Inspector in Charge (IIC)—Title of the chief inspector, usually a veterinarian, in a USDA inspected meat or poultry packing plant.

Integrated production systems—Livestock production systems in which livestock and poultry are reared, fed, harvested, and marketed under the same ownership; sometimes called intensive management practices.

International Animal Health Code—A volume published by the OIE that lays out international standards for the movement of livestock and livestock products, disease reporting, and maintaining healthy animal populations.

International Organization for Standardization (ISO)—A non-governmental international organization, also called the International Standards Organization, established in 1947 to establish general and specific standards for global trade in all articles of commerce and to encourage cooperation in intellectual, scientific, technological, and economic activities including laboratory management, test methodology, and animal ID procedures. www.iso.org

International Plant Protection Commission (IPPC)—The World Trade Organization (WTO)-designated standard-setting organization for plant health; the plant-health counterpart of the OIE.

Johne's disease—A contagious, globally ubiquitous, bacterial infection of cattle, small ruminants, and cervids characterized by a long incubation period followed by chronic diarrhea that causes loss of weight, productivity, and condition. Death eventually ensues. Also called bovine paratuberculosis.

Land Grant System—The cooperative state-federal program that encourages and supports teaching, research, and information dissemination in colleges of agriculture, home economics, and veterinary medicine in the United States.

Leptospirosis—An acute or chronic infection with any of a variety of spiral-shaped bacteria of the genus *Leptospira* that persist in the kidneys of most mammals, including humans. *Leptospira* are excreted in the urine, which serves as a source of infection. Acute leptospirosis is manifested as fever, jaundice, liver and kidney malfunction, bloody urine, and sometimes death.

Lesion—Any tissue abnormality, either visible grossly or microscopically, with or without impairment of body function. Most lesions are caused by disease or trauma.

Listeria—A ubiquitous genus of bacteria with reservoirs in the soil and the gastrointestinal tract of livestock, fish, and birds. In mammals it can produce abortions and sometimes fatal encephalitis. In sheep it is sometimes called circling disease. The most important *Listeria* species, *L. monocytogenes*, occasionally infects humans causing fever, malaise, abortion, and sometimes death. Serious outcomes are most common in immuno-compromised and newborn individuals.

Livestock—Animals and poultry reared in captivity for commercial production of meat, milk, eggs, and by-products. Livestock includes poultry, swine, cattle, sheep, and goats. Wild species, such as deer, elk, bison, llamas, alpacas, ostriches, and emu, when reared in captivity, may be considered livestock and subject to LHPs.

Livestock health infrastructure—The collective activities and programs that serve as a basis, permanent foundation, and cohesive guiding force for a country's domestic livestock health programs and the sanitary (health) aspects of international marketing of livestock and livestock products.

Livestock health policies (LHPs)—The traditions, practices, laws, regulations, administrative procedures, and standards that guide, manage, govern, and police the production, transportation, processing, and marketing of livestock products throughout the world.

Lumpy skin disease—An occasionally fatal, OIE List A disease of cattle present in parts of Africa and the Middle East but regarded as exotic elsewhere. It is caused by a poxvirus and is suspected of being transmitted by direct contact and insects.

Malignant catarrhal fever (MCF)—An invariably fatal, contagious viral infection of cattle manifested by fever, inflammation of the nose and eyes, lesions of the gastrointestinal mucosa, and encephalitis. Sheep-associated MCF, present in the United States, and African MCF are caused by different viruses.

Modified live virus (MLV)—A virus weakened in the laboratory so it induces immunity but not disease when used as a vaccine.

Monitoring, surveillance, and reporting (MS&R) system—The complete package of disease-specific testing, general oversight, documentation, and communication of the health status of a country's livestock population. It comprises a key component of the national livestock health infrastructure.

Multi-jurisdictional Authority—Regulatory oversight of animal health and food safety vested in several government agencies, often accompanied by limits placed on national governments regarding their preemptive authority over subnational units and territories.

Mycotoxins—Poisonous substances produced by fungi.

National animal health reporting system (NAHRS)—The name for the systems responsible for the gathering, collating, summarizing, and transparently reporting of the health and disease status of the livestock populations of a country.

National Association of State Departments of Agriculture (NASDA)—www.nasda.org

National Cattlemen's Beef Association (NCBA)—www.beef.org

National Center for Disease Control and Prevention (CDC)—An Agency of the U.S. Public Health Service with headquarters and laboratories in Atlanta, GA. The CDC conducts educational activities and laboratory and field investigations of human disease problems to fulfill its mission of disease prevention and health promotion. www.cdc.gov

National Institute for Animal Agriculture (NIAA)—A national LHP forum in which livestock producers, scientists, veterinarians, regulators, and business leaders meet to address domestic and global issues facing animal agriculture. www.animalagriculture.org

National Poultry Improvement Program—A cooperative state-federal program to improve the health of U.S. poultry by certifying states, flocks, and hatcheries as free of certain infectious diseases. Certification involves the application of standardized sanitation, testing, record-keeping, and surveillance procedures. The poultry diseases involved include several *Salmonella* and mycoplasma infections of economic significance to poultry production. Addition of avian influenza to the list is under consideration. www.aphis.usda.gov/vs/npip

Negligible risk—A mutually agreed upon measure of risk so low that parties agree to accept risks at or below this level. Also known as tolerable risk, no significant risk, *de minimus* risk.

Neosporum caninum—An intracellular protozoan parasite that causes paralysis, skin disease, and pneumonia in dogs. It also infects cats, goats, sheep, and cattle and is a cause of bovine abortion.

Newcastle disease—An OIE List A virus infection of chickens and wild birds having global distribution. Some viral strains attack the nervous and respiratory systems. The more widely distributed, more virulent, and highly fatal strains attack the gastrointestinal and respiratory tracts. This form, called exotic Newcastle disease or viscerotrophic velogenic Newcastle disease, is an exotic disease in the United States and is subject to eradication by test and slaughter.

Nipah virus—A newly recognized, highly contagious, often fatal viral infection of swine and humans characterized by fever, difficult breathing, occasional neurological signs, and sudden death. Currently confined to Southeast Asia, swine and people in contact with pigs are believed to have contracted the virus from wildlife.

North American Plant Protection Organization (NAPPO)—The regional component of the **International Plant Protection Commission (IPPC)**, the **World Trade Organization (WTO)**-designated standard-setting organization that generates guidelines for the safe international movement of plants and plant products.

Office International des Epizooties (OIE)—The world's oldest international veterinary organization, with goals to develop and maintain a worldwide animal-disease reporting network and to facilitate world trade by minimizing the risk of spreading livestock diseases. The OIE is the **World Trade Organization (WTO)**-designated international standard-setting organization for livestock health. It prepares criteria for disease-free status of countries and recommends sanitary measures such as testing, quarantine, and health certification procedures for the safe international trade in livestock. The OIE publishes the *International Animal Health Code*. The Code describes livestock diseases and recommended testing, vaccination, health certification, and quarantine measures for international movement of livestock, poultry, germ plasm, and related commodities. It also publishes the *OIE Manual of Standards for Diagnostic Tests and Vaccines*. www.oie.int

OIE List A diseases—Fifteen livestock diseases determined by the OIE to require urgent reporting because of their capacity to cause serious economic losses, rapid international spread, or human illness.

OIE List B diseases—Approximately 70 livestock diseases determined by the OIE to be less urgently reported than List A diseases but nonetheless reportable because of their potential to cause economic losses, international spread, or human illness.

Papular stomatitis—A globally distributed benign poxvirus infection of cattle that produces mouth lesions that can be confused with vesicular diseases and other diseases producing ulcerations of the oral mucosa.

Paramyxovirus infections—Infections caused by members of a large family of viruses, Paramyxoviridae, which infect most animal species and include human mumps and bovine rinderpest. Newcastle disease virus and about ten other paramyxoviruses infect the respiratory tracts of multiple avian species throughout the world. Most cause mild disease.

Passive immunity—A degree of short-lived disease protection against an infectious agent or toxin conferred by antibodies produced in one animal transferring to another individual via blood transfusion, injection of immune serum or globulin concentrates, or by drinking the colostrum (first milk) of an immune mother.

Pathogen—An organism capable of causing disease.

Persistent infections—Infections that remain in the body, usually undetected, permitting infected persons or animals to serve as sources of infection for prolonged, occasionally intermittent, periods.

Peste des petits ruminants—An OIE List A viral disease of sheep and goats characterized by fever, erosions of the mouth and gastrointestinal tract, diarrhea, and death. It is present in parts of Africa and the Middle East and regarded as exotic elsewhere.

Polymerase chain reaction (PCR)—A procedure for amplifying minute portions of nucleic acids to achieve quantities detectable with various molecular technologies, thus permitting identification of disease-producing agents that would otherwise be unrecognizable.

Porcine reproductive and respiratory syndrome (PRRS)—A contagious viral infection of swine manifested by abortion, stillbirths, mummified fetuses, and pneumonia among surviving litter mates.

Precautionary principle—The often-debated contention that suspicions of risk should be acted upon until positively disproved. This runs contrary to the belief that regulatory measures should be based on sound science, and the invoking of this principle is often regarded as a device to protect noncompetitive industries from importations of products for which no valid risks can be established.

Prions—Subviral, proteinaceous particles resistant to disinfectants and many sterilization techniques. Prions are believed to induce **bovine spongiform encephalopathy (BSE)**, chronic wasting disease of deer and elk, and other **transmissible spongiform encephalopathies (TSEs)**.

Protozoa—Non-bacterial single-celled microorganisms, most of which are free living. Some cause diseases like malaria, trichinosis, and trichomoniasis.

Pseudorabies—A viral infection of swine, also known as mad itch or Aujeszky's disease, that is highly fatal for piglets and causes respiratory disease or neurologic disorders resembling rabies in older pigs. It can be transmitted to cattle, sheep, goats, and numerous wild species.

Psittacosis—A globally distributed zoonotic infection caused by *Chlamydia psittaci*, a bacterium found mostly in psittacine birds such as parrots and parakeets. Also called parrot fever, avian chlamydiosis, and ornithosis, it is common in wild birds, including pigeons, but occurs occasionally in domestic turkeys and rarely chickens. Humans acquire the infection by inhalation of dust from feathers or bird droppings and develop fever, depressed appetite, and a debilitating cough with the expression of green mucous in advanced stages. The infection is treatable with tetracycline.

Q-fever—An acute enzootic, usually inapparent, globally distributed, infection of cattle, sheep, goats, and other animals caused by *Coxellia burnetti,* a member of the Family Rickettiaceae that shares properties of both viruses and bacteria. The infection can cause infertility or abortion in ruminants and an occasionally fatal influenza-like disease in humans who can acquire it via tick bites, inhalation, or by drinking unpasteurized milk from infected animals.

Qualititative risk assessment—A procedure that characterizes risk in nonnumerical terms such as negligible, minimal, moderate, or maximum likelihood of occurrence of events or diseases.

Quality assurance programs—Disease-control and food-safety procedures, often voluntary, that improve productivity and product quality by adhering to standard management practices in livestock production or processing operations.

Quantitative risk assessment—A procedure that characterizes risk numerically, usually in terms of probabilities of occurrence of events or diseases.

Quarantine—A period during which an animal or person is kept in isolation to prevent the possible spread of disease. The conditions and time of quarantine are usually based on the mode of transmission and the period of communicability of the disease.

Rabies—An often-fatal saliva-transmitted OIE List B disease of warm-blooded mammals characterized by a highly variable, and frequently long, incubation period, fever, malaise, various unusual behaviors, and sometime indiscriminate biting attacks on animals or people.

Regionalism—Political and economic unity and loyalties within adjourning geographic areas with common ecosystems, populations, and social and cultural characteristics; often resulting in common trade policies.

Regionalization—Division, for trade purposes, of areas into regions including countries, parts of countries, groups of countries, or groups of parts of countries.

Rift Valley fever—An often fatal, mosquito-borne, viral OIE List A disease of ruminants and humans. It is present in Africa but exotic elsewhere.

Rinderpest—A highly contagious, often-fatal viral OIE List A disease of cattle and wild cloven-hoofed animals that causes ulceration of the gastrointestinal tract. Rinderpest is endemic in parts of Africa and regarded as exotic elsewhere.

Risk—In animal health, the term is often used to indicate the likelihood of disease introduction or the seriousness and possible consequences of a disease.

Risk analysis—The collective notions of risk assessment, risk communication, and risk management.

Risk assessment—The process of identifying a hazard and evaluating its risk. In animal health, risk assessment usually signifies the process of identifying and estimating, either qualitatively or quantitatively, the seriousness and possible consequences of specific diseases.

Risk communication—Exchange of information about risk, leading to risk management decisions and risk mitigating measures.

Ruminants—Four-stomached, cud-chewing, hoofed mammals (Ruminantia) such as cattle, sheep, and goats.

Salmonella—A globally ubiquitous and sometimes pathogenic genus of bacteria with multiple species that inhabit the intestinal tracts of animals and humans and are excreted in the feces. Many *Salmonella* contaminate foods and cause disease if acquired in adequate doses by susceptible individuals. Salmonellosis is probably the most common zoonotic disease.

Sanitary and Phytosanitary (SPS) Principles—The principles of the **World Trade Organization (WTO) Sanitary and Phytosanitary (SPS) Agreement**. They require that SPS measures be scientifically sound, equitably applied (**equal national treatment**), harmonized with international standards, transparent, undertaken with consideration of equivalence, risk-assessment based, and applicable on a regional basis.

Sanitary measures—Actions designed to promote the health of humans or animals. Phytosanitary measures deal with plant health.

Scrapie—A **transmissable spongiform encephalopathy (TSE)** of sheep, and rarely goats, characterized by a prolonged incubation period, locomotor incoordination, and behavioral changes including rubbing against objects, staggering, tremors, walking in circles, progressive weight loss, and ultimately death.

Screwworms—The flesh-eating larvae of certain subtropical and tropical flies, principally *Cochliomyia hominivorax* in the Americas and other species elsewhere, which deposit eggs in fresh wounds on animals and occasionally humans. Upon hatching, their eggs produce larvae that penetrate flesh and unless treated can produce death. Screwworm flies have been eradicated from the United States, most of Mexico, and much of Latin America by a joint Mexico-United States Screwworm Eradication Program based on insecticide applications, surveillance, and the release of sterile males that mate with females and foil successful reproduction.

Serology—The study of serum, the clear liquid remaining after blood has clotted. Serological tests are used to diagnose diseases and identify infectious agents.

Serotype—A variation or subdivision of an infectious agent distinguishable by serology.

Serum—The clear cell-free portion of the blood remaining after clotting or centrifugation. Serum contains measurable antibodies useful in disease diagnosis.

Sheep pox and goat pox—Sometimes fatal diseases of sheep and goats characterized by widespread eruptions of the skin due to closely related poxvirus infections. Both diseases are on OIE List A and present in parts of Eastern Europe, Africa, and Asia. They are regarded as exotic to the Western Hemisphere.

Sheep scabies—Persistent, contagious skin inflammation, often called mange or sheep scab, caused by one of several skin burrowing mites, some of which are exotic to the United States.

Shigellosis—A sometimes food-borne, occasionally fatal, acute infection of the human gastrointestinal tract causing fever, diarrhea, and vomiting. Humans are the major reservoir and the usual source of infection. Transmission may result from ingestion of contaminated water, milk, or food.

Sore mouth—A globally ubiquitous, contact-transmitted, zoonotic, poxvirus infection of sheep and goats, also known as contagious ecthyma, contagious pustular dermatitis, or orf, that produces papules, pustules, and scabs on the mouth and lips.

Stakeholder—An individual with a vested, usually financial, interest in an area. Major stakeholders in livestock health are producers, processors, and marketers of animal products.

Stamping out method—The traditional disease-eradication procedure applied to exotic diseases. The method involves the identification, quarantine, testing, and slaughter of infected herds or flocks, followed by the cleaning and disinfecting of contact premises and controlled repopulation.

Staphylococci—A genus of bacteria with multiple species, some of which produce powerful toxins causing food poisoning, pneumonia, or hospital-acquired infections in humans and a variety of acute and chronic infections in livestock. Antimicrobial resistance sometimes makes treatment difficult.

Stem cell technology—Procedures for manipulating and cultivating stem cells, which are primitive, non-specialized cells capable of differentiating into almost any component of the body. Stem cells are found in the bone marrow and other blood-forming organs. This technology offers hope of replacement of defective or diseased body components and organs.

Surveillance (active)—Disease-specific, proactive regular observation, testing, and control activities.

Surveillance (passive)—Observation and investigation of suspicious health events.

Swine vesicular disease—A relatively mild viral disease of swine that produces lesions identical to FMD, vesicular exanthema of swine, and vesicular stomatitis and complicates their diagnoses. It is exotic to the United States and much of the world but has appeared in parts of Europe and Asia.

Technical barrier to trade (TBT)—Non-tariff obstacles imposed on importations based on specialized scientific concepts or market considerations; these barriers are frequently regarded as being placed to protect domestic industries.

Tetanus—An acute, often fatal, neurological syndrome exhibiting stiffness and muscle spasms caused by neurotoxins produced by the bacterium *Clostridium tetani* when it multiples in tissues under anaerobic conditions, such as in puncture wounds. Also called lockjaw, tetanus can occur in humans and most livestock.

Titer—A measure of concentration of a substance in solution. Determined by testing serial dilutions until they no longer react to standard reagents. In animal health, titers usually express the level of disease-specific antibodies in serum and are one indication of an animal's immune status.

Total quality management (TQM)—A program encouraged by breed associations and livestock health organizations to address all aspects of animal health and food safety by the conscientious application of sanitation, disease-preventive measures, residue-avoidance procedures, and other assurances that products have optimum quality and wholesomeness. Specific procedures vary with the production-management system and geographic area.

Toxoids—Inactivated toxins used for immunization.

Trade promotion authority (TPA)—A level of authority, also known as fast track authority, sought by national governments, that permits officials to negotiate international trade agreements without the approval of representative legislative bodies such as the U.S. Congress. It bestows credibility upon national representatives and reduces endless haggling.

Transmissable mink encephalopathy (TME)—A rare, frequently fatal, neurodegenerative **transmissible spongiform encephalopathy (TSE)** of mink with an apparent incubation period of eight to twelve months. The clinical signs include incoordination and irrational behavior. It produces spongiform lesions similar to other TSEs. It was speculated that TME may result from feeding mink with meat from downer (non-ambulatory) cows. This conjecture was never confirmed but has been used by the European Union (EU) as evidence that **bovine spongiform encephalopathy (BSE)** is present in the United States.

Transmissable spongiform encephalopathies (TSEs)—A group of chronic neurodegenerative animal and human diseases caused by highly resistant proteinaceous particles called **prions**. They are characterized by prolonged incubation periods, extended neurological manifestations, and death.

Transparency—The obligation and expectation that importing countries clearly articulate the underlying scientific bases of sanitary measures imposed upon commodities entering their territory.

Trichinosis—Infestation with the larvae of the protozoan parasite *Trichenella spiralis,* causing a condition that is usually asymptomatic in swine but can cause serious disease and sometimes death in people. Prevention requires thorough cooking of pork and the meat of carnivores and bears.

Trichomoniasis—A venereal protozoan infection caused by *Trichomonas fetus* that causes bovine infertility.

Tuberculosis (TB)—A chronic respiratory infection with bacteria of the genus *Mycobacterium* transmitted by respiratory discharges disseminated by coughing and sneezing. Initial infection is often unnoticed but it can progress, or be reactivated, and be fatal. Human TB is caused by *M. tuberculosis,* and bovine TB is caused by *M. bovis,* which occasionally infects people. The principal lesions are rounded lumpy growths called tubercles.

Typhoid fever—A generalized, sometimes fatal disease of humans caused by one of multiple types of the bacterium *Salmonella typhi.* It is usually transmitted by consuming contaminated food or water. Humans are the reservoir and the usual source of infection.

U.S. Animal Health Association (USAHA)—An organization that serves as a forum for communication and coordination among state and federal governments, universities, industry, and other groups on laws, regulations, policies, and programs concerning animal health and disease control, animal welfare, food safety, and public health. www.usaha.org

U.S. Code of Federal Regulations—Annually revised volumes summarizing permanent regulations developed by government agencies under authority of laws passed by Congress and signed by the President. Prior to publication in the annual updates, new regulations and effective dates are published in the Federal Register. www.access.gpo.gov/nara

U.S. Fish and Wildlife Service—An agency of the Department of Interior charged with conserving wildlife and habitats, migratory birds, and endangered species through conservation and education programs. They have authority over the import and export of plants, wildlife, or caged birds protected by domestic statute or international treaty. www.fws.gov

U.S. Trade Representative (USTR)—The lead individual on U.S. international trade issues. The Office of the USTR operates out of the Office of the President.

United States Department of Agriculture (USDA)—www.usda.org

User Fees—Fees imposed for government-conducted services to make benefiting parties partially offset the costs of those services.

Variant Creutzfeldt-Jacob disease (VCJD)—Also know as new variant CJD, this disease differs from classic CJD by having earlier ages of onset and slightly different clinical signs and microscopic lesions. The agents of CJD and VCJD are biologically indistinguishable. VCJD probably is acquired by eating **bovine spongiform encephalopathy (BSE)**-contaminated meat. Its recognition caused criticisms of British handling of BSE, allegations that agricultural interests neglected consumer safety, and the transfer of animal health responsibilities from agricultural to consumer oriented agencies in the **European Union (EU)**.

Vector-borne diseases—Diseases transmitted by intermediate hosts. The intermediate hosts are usually insects, but sometimes mammals (as with rabies) or birds (as with psittacosis).

Vegan—A strict vegetarian who consumes no animal products and sometimes refuses to wear items of animal origin like wool or leather.

Venezuelan equine encephalomyelitis (VEE)—An acute OIE List B, mosquito-transmitted, often-fatal viral infection of horses that can be prevented by vaccination. VEE is endemic in Central America and northern South America. It entered the United States from Mexico in 1971 and was eradicated. It is now considered exotic.

Vesicles—Blisters produced by infections rather than friction.

Vesicular diseases—Diseases characterized by vesicle formation.

Vesicular exanthema of swine—A viral disease of swine, sometimes called San Miguel sea lion disease, that produces vesicular lesions causing lameness and lack of appetite. These symptoms are identical to FMD, swine vesicular disease, and vesicular stomatitis, thus complicating their diagnoses. It is now considered exotic to the United States and most of the world.

Vesicular stomatitis—An OIE List A viral disease, presumably transmitted by insects and present in northern South America, Central America, and periodically in the southwestern United States. It is considered exotic elsewhere. The disease affects horses, cattle, and small ruminants. It produces vesicles in the mouth and on the feet and teats of cattle that are indistinguishable from those caused by FMD.

Veterinary Medical Officer (VMO)—A veterinarian employed by a regulatory agency to perform official duties.

Veterinary Services (VS)—The national veterinary agency of a country who has authority over animal disease-control, animal welfare, and livestock regulatory activities.

Vibriosis—An old name for camplobacteriosis, a venereal bacterial disease that causes infertility and abortion in cattle. Bacteria of the genus *Camplobacteria* are spiral or comma-shaped and are present in the gastrointestinal tracts of animals and humans and sometime cause gastroenteritis.

Virulent—Able to produce disease.

Virus-Serum-Toxin Act—A law passed by Congress in 1913 and amended in 1985. It charged the **United States Department of Agriculture (USDA)** to assure that animal vaccines, serums, and diagnostic reagents produced or imported into the United States are pure, potent, safe, and effective. The law is implemented by the **Center for Veterinary Biologics (CVB),** which issues product licenses and import permits.

Viscerotrophic velogenic Newcastle disease—A highly virulent and rapidly transmissible form of Newcastle disease of chickens; also called exotic Newcastle disease in the United States.

West Nile fever—A mosquito-borne viral infection that can be fatal to birds, horses, and humans. Previously considered exotic to the United States, it was introduced in 1999 and has spread over much of the country.

Withdrawal time—The time period after the administration of pharmaceutical or biological products that animals or their products must be withheld from markets to avoid human consumption of potentially harmful residues.

World Trade Organization (WTO)—An organization created by the **General Agreement on Tariffs and Trade (GATT)** to implement and adjudicate, with force of international law, a series of 28 agreements governing international trade.

World Trade Organization (WTO) Sanitary and Phytosanitary (SPS) Agreement—One of 28 WTO agreements, this one deals with human, animal, and plant health issues in international trade.

Zoonotic—Capable of transmission from animals to humans. Zoonotic diseases are called zoonoses.

Index

G

L

M

Made in the USA
Las Vegas, NV
19 September 2026

e66506ad-4d61-441d-a7bd-88a9584f5b0eR01